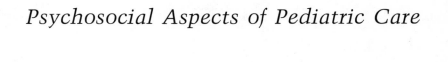

Psychosocial Aspects of Pediatric Care

PSYCHOSOCIAL ASPECTS OF PEDIATRIC CARE

Edited by

ELIZABETH GELLERT, Ed.D.

Associate Professor
Department of Psychology
Hunter College
of the City University of New York
New York, New York

Grune & Stratton
A Subsidiary of Harcourt Brace Jovanovich, Publishers
New York   San Francisco   London

Library of Congress Cataloging in Publication Data
Main entry under title:

Psychosocial aspects of pediatric care.

  Includes bibliographies and index.
    1. Sick children—Psychology. 2. Children—Diseases—
Social aspects. I. Gellert, Elizabeth [DNLM:
1. Child psychology. 2. Pediatrics. WS105.3 P974]
RJ47.5.P785   618.9'2'001   78-16682
ISBN 0-8089-1091-4

Grune & Stratton, Inc.
111 Fifth Avenue
New York, New York 10003

Distributed in the United Kingdom by
Academic Press, Inc. (London) Ltd.
24/28 Oval Road, London NW 1

Library of Congress Catalog Number 78-16682
International Standard Book Number 0-8089-1091-4

Printed in the United States of America

Contents

Preface

This handbook is designed to fill a gap in the literature about child behavior written specifically for pediatricians and other pediatric staff. It concerns aspects of child (and adolescent) psychology that have particular relevance for the medical practitioner whose patients are children and youth. Although there are now at least two periodicals published in the United States which focus on pediatric psychology, there are few up-to-date textbooks in this field.

This volume spans a wide array of topics. It comprises contributions of pediatricians, child psychiatrists and psychologists, and a Child Life Worker. Although most aspects of child development are relevant to pediatric practice, there are some special topics, usually missing in child psychology texts, that are of special concern to pediatric staff. Such topics constitute the subject matter of this book. The topics have been selected with the editor's experience as a pediatric psychologist as a guide. Among them are chapters dealing with the child's interpretation of illness, children's reactions to hospitalization, the psychological management of terminal illness in pediatrics, the uses of hypnosis in pediatric settings, psychological testing of children, various types of psychopathology as they are encountered in pediatric practice, and numerous additional subjects.

Many medical schools now include child psychiatry or child psychology in their curriculum; this book may serve as a text or starting point for use in such inservice programs. It may also serve as a reference for pediatricians in private practice as well as for others whose work brings them into contact with pediatric patients.

The editor wishes to thank the contributing authors for the chapters—all of which are original—that they have written for this book. Their industriousness and flexibility, as well as their knowledge, have made this volume possible.

ELIZABETH GELLERT

Contributors

Ellis I. Barowsky, Ph.D.
Assistant Professor
Department of Curriculum and Teaching
Special Education Program
Hunter College of the City University of
  New York
New York, New York

Jules Bemporad, M.D.
Director of Children's Services
Associate Professor of Psychiatry
Massachusetts Mental Health Center
Harvard Medical School
Boston, Massachusetts

James D. Block, Ph.D.
Chief Psychologist
  and Director of Clinical Studies
Maimonides Developmental Center
Brooklyn, New York

Gaston E. Blom, M.D.
Professor of Psychiatry and Elementary
  and Special Education
Department of Psychiatry
Michigan State University
East Lansing, Michigan

Peter Blos, Jr., M.D.
Psychiatric Consultant
Associate Director
Child Development Project
Department of Psychiatry
School of Medicine

University of Michigan
Ann Arbor, Michigan

Betty C. Buchsbaum, Ph.D.
Clinical Assistant Professor
New York Hospital
Westchester Division
Cornell Medical Center
Department of Psychiatry
White Plains, New York

Elizabeth Crocker, M.Ed.
Director
Child Life Department
Izaak Walton Killam Hospital for
  Children
Halifax, Nova Scotia, Canada

Lloyd O. Eckhardt, M.D.
Assistant Professor
Department of Psychiatry and Pediatrics
University of Colorado Medical Center
Denver, Colorado

Stanford B. Friedman, M.D.
Professor of Psychiatry and Human
  Development
Professor of Pediatrics
Director, Division of Child and
  Adolescent Psychiatry
Head, Behavioral Pediatrics
University of Maryland School of
  Medicine
Departments of Psychiatry and Pediatrics
Baltimore, Maryland

Eleanor Galenson, M.D.
Clinical Professor
Department of Psychiatry
Albert Einstein College of Medicine
New York, New York

G. Gail Gardner, Ph.D.
Associate Professor of Clinical Psychology
Assistant Professor of Pediatrics
University of Colorado Medical School
Denver, Colorado

Elizabeth Gellert, Ed.D.
Associate Professor
Department of Psychology
Hunter College of the City University of
  New York
New York, New York

Edward Goldson, M.D.
Director
Family Care Center
The Children's Hospital
Assistant Professor of Pediatrics
University of Colorado
Denver, Colorado

Margaret C. Heagarty, M.D.
Associate Professor of Pediatrics
Cornell Medical College
New York Hospital
New York, New York

Robert Miller, M.D.
Assistant Clinical Professor
Department of Psychiatry
Albert Einstein College of Medicine
New York, New York

Anita R. Olds, Ph.D.
Consultant
Environmental Facilities for Children and
  Child Development
Cambridge, Massachusetts
Lecturer
Eliot-Pearson Department of Child Study
Tufts University
Medford, Massachusetts

Richard M. Sarles, M.D.
Associate Professor of Child Psychiatry
  and Pediatrics
Director, Child Psychiatry—Pediatric
  Liaison Service
Departments of Psychiatry and Pediatrics
University of Maryland, School of
  Medicine
Baltimore, Maryland

Edward Sperling, M.D.
Associate Clinical Professor
Department of Psychiatry
Albert Einstein College of Medicine
New York, New York

Dane G. Prugh, M.D.
Professor
Departments of Psychiatry and Pediatrics
University of Colorado Medical Center
Denver, Colorado

Charles Wuhl, M.D.
Clinical Instructor
New York Medical College
New York, New York

Psychosocial Aspects of Pediatric Care

CHILDREN THINK ABOUT ILLNESS: THEIR CONCEPTS AND BELIEFS

Peter Blos, Jr., M.D.

INTRODUCTION

Basically, children are researchers. This ranging curiosity includes their own bodies, how they function, and why things go wrong, as they invariably do. For every question there must be an answer which the child obtains by a mixture of observation, thought, fantasy, previous experience, and prior explanation. But the effectiveness of this research is limited by intruded affect, and the child's current level of cognitive function, need for defense, and opportunities for observation.

This chapter reviews some of the studies by adults that have explored children's ideas, concepts, and understanding of matters pertaining to their body's health, illness, treatment, and death. It then discusses the applicability of this material to clinical work with children.

Firm distinctions between cognition and knowledge on the one hand and fantasy and belief on the other are problematic at best; for heuristic purposes I will separate them. *Knowledge* will be defined as those cognitive elements which represent reality. These elements must be representative of the highest level of reasoning and reality recognition of which a certain age child is capable and they serve an explanatory function for the child. Children's *fantasy* will be defined as representative of that group of thoughts which reflect affective distortion of reality and a less than age-appropriate use of logic.

As Piaget[27] has stated, children function with a dual system of looking at the world—reality and fantasy—and they consider that both approaches yield verities. A hierarchical arrangement of these views does not occur until adolescence. Since the 1940's many studies and reports have commented on the emotional effect of hospitalization, surgery, and chronic illness on children.[34] (See chapters 3, 6, 4.) Correctly, much emphasis is given to the importance of preparing children for such events, conveying to children in age-appropriate language the experiential realities in store for them, and providing appropriate emotional protection. There is an awareness in these studies of the child's conceptual ability, the disrupting effect of anxiety, and the child's use of fantasy to fill in the gaps of knowledge.

Such research, however, has told us little about the actual cognitive content of children's knowledge of their bodies and illness, and research that explores children's knowledge directly is sparse and hard to find. The few studies available explicitly or implicitly rely upon Piagetian concepts of cognitive development. For example, that particular and characteristic aspect of prelogical thinking are egocentricity, concreteness, consistency of objects, and moral causality; while the more mature aspects of thinking are characterized by reversibility of mental operations, capacity for transformations, synthetic operations, and a capacity for abstraction.

In the specialized inquiry to follow we will see what happens when these modalities of cognition are turned on a unique object for the child: his own body. Much is mystery here because the body is enclosed by skin; often the only evidence of things going on are proprioceptive, kinesthetic, and tactile. Furthermore, since the touched and the toucher are one, this evidence is unique and reality testing is difficult in the absence of another's validation. An inner mental representation develops of one's own body in space—the body image—but at the same time there also resides within, a sense of self. Clearly, the cognitive capacity for observation and thinking will often be contaminated by the emotions aroused by what is happening to the self, *my* self, *my* body. The feelings and thoughts of others about bodily functioning will also be influential, and will affect body image and sense of self.

To assist children in the cognitive-affective process of learning about their bodies, health, illnesses and vulnerabilities, and treatment procedures, it is valuable to know how children think about these issues, how best to elicit information about such thinking, and how best to correct any wrong conclusions. Cognitive mastery and emotional mastery inevitably complement one another. Health professionals must learn not only to understand what a child is saying but also to communicate effectively in both domains of a child's thinking.

Concepts of Illness and Disease

Children's ideas and theories about illness and disease have most often been investigated by presenting a child with a stimulus picture illustrating some scene of illness. In these studies the examiner's discussions may vary in directness, but all are designed to cover certain specific questions regarding the origins of illness. Some investigators have utilized a direct interview method, sometimes providing the child with the opportunity for projective play with dolls. These techniques have been used primarily when speaking with the child about his own specific current illness. (The effect of the differing methodology on the data has not been a subject for discussion in the literature.)

Subjects for the studies to be reviewed here have been both well and sick children. Sick children have been studied who are acutely ill, chronically ill, or ambulatorily convalescing. Few authors have made specific comparative studies of the well and sick[11,35,36] although Lynn, Glaser, and Harrison[18] compared children with severe illness (rheumatic fever) and transitory common illness. No studies have been found that compared conceptualizations of illness as perceived by different severe illness groups even though there are indications that overt and occult illness, e.g., cardiac disease[6] and orthopedic problems,[30] are perceived and handled differently by children.[3,5]

WELL CHILDREN'S IDEAS OF ILLNESS CAUSALITY

Nagy[22] in 1948 was the first to report specific observations on well children's theories about becoming ill. Her work is mostly descriptive and does not focus on the developmental cognitive aspects. She does note, however,[23] that few children between 8 and 12 years of age take into consideration multiplicity of causation in regard to the origin of disease. (An age breakdown is not given in the study, so a developmental look at the data within the age range is not possible.) In her studies of 5–11 year old children's ideas about germs she states that "the majority of children kept until the end of childhood the idea that if any germ reaches the body, one necessarily falls ill without regard to the status of the germ or the condition of the body."[24]

In 1956, I studied the healthy child's understanding of the causes of disease.[4] Forty-two healthy children (21 girls and 21 boys, 5–10 years of age) were interviewed using nine stimulus pictures. These pictures were designed to be illustrative of a variety of disease situations, e.g., stomach ache, getting a cold, transmission of germs, parental illness. To focus the problem, each picture was presented with a few introductory sentences; the child was then invited to tell the examiner what was going to happen next. The examiner freely followed or probed the child's explanatory thinking: Why will the person in the illustration become ill? How did this happen?

The first response for all ages was frequently a cliché, probably culturally determined. "He'll catch cold because he got cold," or "She'll have a cold because she got wet." Gellert[11] also found this to be true. Only further discussion with the child would reveal his or her own ideas. With some of the younger children, questioning the cliché only produced a restatement or a voice tone-change while repeating the statement. Both responses are representative of syncretistic thinking, i.e., the statement is the reason.

Material obtained from one picture will serve to illustrate the results obtained. This picture shows two boys. One is in the act of taking a chair away from the other. The latter has a handkerchief in one hand but is clearly shown to be coughing a fine spray directly at the first boy. The examiner's introductory statement was, "These two boys are having a fight about the chair. As you can see one of them has a cold and he is sneezing on the other one's face. Will that boy (E. points) get sick?" All children answered in the affirmative; however, the typical explanatory cliché mentioned above was not heard, probably because the examiner stated it in the introduction: One boy sneezes in the face of the other. Further discussion revealed different perceptions as to how he became sick.

Three stages in the development of a capacity for logical thinking about respiratory illness transmission were discernible.

Stage 1: Descriptive. Explanation of causality is made by enumerating conditions, situations, or actions contiguous with the onset of illness and offering this as explanatory of cause. An example:

(Male, 5:1) (Why do you think he gets sick?) 'Cause that boy is coughing near him. (Well, but why does he get sick?) See, a boy is near and he coughs at you or sneezes and that means you get a cold.

Note that the embellished explanation is essentially a restatement, an example of syncretistic thinking. For him "features bound together within the raw material of observation seem . . . to be related . . . by causal connection."[27] Precausal thinking, in which motive and cause are confused, is also inferable here; but in response to other pictures it is even more convincing.

State 2: <u>Exploratory</u>. Here a specific reality factor is perceived as being associated with the onset of illness, but the thought process is still basically syncretistic. An example:

> (Male, 7:1) Uh, oh (Why?) Why? Because he sprayed his breath all over him, all over his face. (Would that make him sick?) Yes. 'Cause his germs come in his breath, you can see that on the paper. (What do the germs do?) They make him sick. (How?) Because it's somebody else's germs and not his.

Further development in the thought process can be seen. The child has begun to lose some of his egocentrism and subjectivity and is beginning to perceive some association between cause and effect. An agent (the germ) exists and serves an explanatory function even though it is still utilized in the descriptive mode of the previous stage.

Stage 3: <u>Causative</u>. A mechanism is postulated involving several steps, which may or may not be physiologically correct but which are used to relate a given effect to its cause. An example:

> (Female, 9:11) Well, maybe; I'm not sure but I think he would because the germs would spread). (How do they spread?) Well, when you cough, everyone has germs, and when you cough you can't see the germs come out but they spray and give other people what you have. (?) Well, the germs, I guess they'd spread out to the other person, they'd go in his mouth and nose and then if he was a healthy child, well, it wouldn't be so bad.

Here is evidence of relatively mature modes of causal thinking. Implied are intermediary steps which lead from cause to effect. In addition, we begin to see examples of multiple causality and a shift from the absolutism seen earlier. Specifically, health and vulnerability are implied concepts that appear for the first time. They contribute to the child's cautious and relativistic statement concerning the certainty with which illness will occur. The child is now aware that one can get a cold or a stomach ache in more than one way, and that even if exposed one may not become ill.

In looking at the response to the other pictures utilized in my study, these same three categories of causal thinking are sustained. A significant leap in conceptual capacity for these healthy children was demonstrated between the oldest group (9–10 years of age) and the two younger groups (5–6 years of age, $p = <.01$; 7–8 years of age, $p = <.05$). This finding was confirmed by Gellert's observations[12] in her study of children's knowledge about their bodies.

TRANSGRESSION AS CAUSALITY

Over the last thirty years the majority of clinical studies on the emotional impact of illness report evidence that children think of illness as punishment for bad or prohibited behavior. Gellert[11] found that two-thirds of her 102 subjects (4–16 years of age; 72 hospitalized, 30 well) stated or implied that the illness of the child in the picture used was partially or wholly a result of breaking rules or neglecting recommended actions. More than one-quarter of the group blamed the story child's illness entirely on consciously perpetrated transgressions. (Unfortunately, an age breakdown is not given in the study so we do not know if this reaction changes with age.) However, Gellert did show that there was a difference in this regard between ill and well children.

> Well children showed a greater tendency to explain illness in terms of human action or default. It is interesting that this difference was largely due to the fact that

the well children made a significantly greater proportion of statements blaming persons in the protagonist's environment for his disorder. . . . The tendency to blame the story child himself for getting sick was almost equal in the two groups.[11]

Evidently, thinking about causality of illness changes when a child becomes ill. Dubo,[8] studying children with tuberculosis; Brazelton, Holder, and Talbot,[6] studying children with rheumatic fever; and Schechter,[30] reporting on children with orthopedic problems, report a high incidence of children who believed that their own affliction was a punishment for misbehavior. Lynn et al,[18] in studying children with rheumatic fever in contrast to those with transient common illnesses, found that they held strongly to the concept of self-causality as an explanation. Bergmann,[3] in her study of hospitalized children, presents clinical evidence of ill children's confused thinking on causality. Moreover, she demonstrates that the private worries and guilts which normal children often suffer about such things as family secrets, masturbation, and menstruation, can invade the thought processes of ill children and, by association with the illness, be perceived as causative.

Elizabeth (10:6) who has rheumatic fever, has a deep secret. It may be reconstructed as: my dead father was an Indian. He was bad (died of alcoholism). She is afraid that the doctors will find this out through their frequent blood tests. Poignantly she tells Bergmann, "If a father has bad blood would the children have it too? . . . I don't want anyone to know that I had a bad father. Could they find out from my blood?"

Ernest (8:0), who has rheumatic fever with signs of chorea, is discussing with Bergmann how upset he was about other boys on the ward who exhibited sexual play. He discloses that his name for his sexual organ was *weiner.* When told in the course of the conversation that grownups use the word *penis* he becomes upset and says " 'Penis?' You said it was 'penis'? But then does one get sick from touching it, because Gary touched it and he got sick and they gave him penic-illin!"

Peters[26] made a specific attempt to study conceptual thinking in twenty-four ill children, (8–11 years of age) who were hospitalized, but ambulatory, when interviewed. Her assessment instrument was a modified Thematic Apperception Test followed by a direct interview.

In three-fifths of the fifty-five illness stories for which causal agents were specified, the ill character caused his own illness; in nearly one-third of the stories other people were cited: and in one-tenth of the stories the environment was held responsible. Girls in the sample designated the action of the ill character as causing illness more frequently than did boys. Boys showed a tendency to specify other persons and environmental agents as causal agents more frequently than girls. There was a tendency for the assignment of self-causality of illness to decrease with increasing age.[26]

Peters goes on to elaborate that the texts themselves reveal a "pervasive implication that the illness resulted from disobedient or imprudent behavior."[26] The only study of hospitalized children to offer contradictory conclusions is that by Gofman, Buckman, and Schade.[15] These investigators studied 100 children by asking, in a single interview, four questions clearly directed to each child's own hospital experience. However, Brazelton et al[6] had earlier commented on the need to gain the child's confidence since ideas of self-causality, wrongdoing, and punishment tend not to come up for many sessions; and Lynn et al[18] later showed that children can discourse much more freely when the illness is projected upon other children or upon a doll. One must suspect that the method chosen by Gofman et al predetermined their conclusions.

CONCEPTUALIZATION UNDER STRESS

Barnes[2] focused on levels of consciousness as exhibited by children's response in the Intensive Care Unit (ICU) following cardiac surgery, and the children's later recall of their stay in the ICU. There were 13 subjects from 6 to 13 years of age, with the majority from 7 to 11 years of age. Observations, drawings, and interviews provided the data. It was concluded that:

> the children were very alert to ICU phenomena, especially treatments and procedures. The children's responses also clearly demonstrated a high frequency of distortion of the phenomena, especially in events which occurred in a room. Children who had had deaths of relatives and other experiences leaving memory traces, recalled those deaths and emotional experiences while recovering in the ICU.[2]

Unfortunately the research design did not include later meetings with the children to study the transformations of thinking which might occur over time. For instance: Would distortion, fantasy, and dream life take over after the stress situation, with its attendant alertness and reality organization, had receded into the past?

Concepts of Health

As has been stated, children's health beliefs and their development have rarely been investigated. Although Nagy[22] studied children's theories concerning various aspects of human biology, her focus was primarily on concepts of becoming ill rather than on being well, i.e., healthy.

In 1965, Rashkis[28] studied the development of children's understanding of health by using a play interview technique with fifty-four well children, 4–9 years of age. She was primarily interested in inquiring about "the meaning of health, personal and social responsibility, the attitude of others toward health and health prevalence." When these children were asked, "What is it like to be well?" the most common response was in the "not sick" category, e.g., "You are not sick"; "When you were sick and got all better"; "We have to be over our cold." However, within the sample significantly more of the older children described the presence of health as an experience of a pleasurable state, e.g., "You feel sunshiny"; "Feel good"; "You are happy and peppy and could dance around in circles."

Rashkis goes on to state that:

> Irrespective of age the children recognize the limitations of their ability to keep themselves well and are aware of human vulnerability to illness. Eating is regarded as the most important self care activity in fostering health and together with the protective image of the adult, appears to figure significantly in the children's ways of coping ideationally with the potential threat of illness. An increasing trust in the physician is observed.[28]

but it does not become significant until the 8–9 year-old level.

Five years later, Gochman and his colleagues[13,14] tried to approach this subject by an investigation of children's perceptions of their vulnerability to health problems and accidents. His normal subjects (7–17 years of age), were asked a series of questions such as, "How likely are you to catch a cold (have an accident, cut your finger, and the like) in the next year?" Nothing was known of the subjects' health history or family health experience. Analysis of the data demonstrated that at some indeterminate time before the age of 7 years, children apparently acquire a consistent hierarchical pattern of health problem expectancies which remain stable over time.[14] It was inferred that children's expectancies regarding dental problems attain consistency at an earlier age than non-dental problems.[14] (Is this related to the universal experience of losing teeth, or to the high attention given to teeth-brushing at an early age?) The study showed that girls had a higher level of expectancy of health problems than boys, older children had a higher expectancy than younger children, and non-inner-city children had a higher expectancy than those from the inner city.[13] It was clearly demonstrated that, at 10 years of age, expecting to be healthy concurrently means to a child that he will not expect to get sick. Since such ideas were not expressed by younger children, this was interpreted as evidence of learning or education. It must be pointed out, however, that this idea may not be an issue of knowledge per se, but may reflect the development of a complex mental operation—reversibility—which Piaget[27] says becomes possible at about 10 years of age.

The paucity of data on health is relieved by a different and interesting study done by the Connecticut State Board of Education.[7] Five thousand children (grades K-12) were surveyed to ascertain their interests, questions, and (implicitly) their ideas about matters pertaining to general health. Much rich anecdotal material here reflects an age-appropriate style and content.

In grades K-2, the primary health concern is "not to be sick"; this corroborates Rashkis's findings.[28] The range of interest in this age group of children is wide, "here and now"—oriented, and much governed by their own experiences. The question, "What do you want to know about the body?" elicits some of the following: "What makes blood?"; "When I eat fast, I choke. I don't like spinach"; "When I'm cold, I shiver."

Third-graders respond to the question, "What is a healthy person?" with a variety of ideas having to do with behavior and appearance: "Doesn't play with matches"; "Lifts weights"; "Isn't too fat or too skinny"; "Combs her hair"; "Smells clean." Fourth-graders respond to the same question differently and with greater depth: "Is physically fit"; "Does a certain amount of walking and running and does exercises"; "Eats everything he should, the right vegetables, not too much fattening food or candy, eats a well-balanced diet"; "Keeps clean, washes hands and face before meals, takes a bath every night or so, brushes his teeth, doesn't live in dirty surroundings." The authors conclude that for these two grades there is a high degree of interest in the parts, function, and appearance of the body; the causes, effects, and cures of diseases; and the origin, development, and care of babies.

The authors also point out that the fourth-graders' questions accurately reflect Gesell's findings about children of this age: namely, they are introverted, and prone to examine themselves and their bodies. I would also underscore that the form of their concepts illustrates the general concern shown at this age for the rules, be it a game or the care and feeding of the body. It is not surprising that when a child of this age becomes ill, he sees it as a consequence of not having followed the rules to the letter which likely he has not. Another resolution of the dilemma of causation is to call the illness "not fair." This will immediately be recognized as a characteristic response of this age group to the injustices of the playground, school, and home.

Where do children get their ideas about health? Few investigators have addressed this question. Mechanic reports that maternal influences on children's health attitudes are substantially less than anticipated.[20] However, the study is not a convincing one, and by itself, this information is hard to assess. Lewis and Lewis,[17] studying television as a common source of children's health concepts, demonstrated that commercials have a considerable impact. Children from 10 to 13 years of age, viewing commercials pertaining to health, thought 70% of them to be true, while nearly half of the children believed all messages viewed. The acceptance of commercial health messages was higher in the lower socioeconomic group.

It is interesting to note that no study examining the ill child's concepts of health was found. It may be presumed that health professionals, parents, and ill children believe health to be so obvious in the face of disease and illness that it does not deserve study. Yet it would be of interest to see if concepts of health and the terms in which they are defined would vary with the severity of illness, chronicity, or residual defect experienced. Would we see a conceptual regression, an idealization, or some other kind of distortion? This information would seem to be of use in understanding children with long-term illness or permanent handicap, since by helping such children correct distortions, some disappointment and disillusionment might be prevented.

Concepts of Death and Dying

In recent years there has been considerable interest in the area of death and dying. (Since this is specifically taken up in chapter 5, I will restrict myself to reviewing a few studies which explore the physically well child's concept of death.) Schilder and Wechsler in 1934[31] were the first to explore ideas about death with children directly. The population was seventy-six children (5–15 years of age), on the psychiatric ward of Bellevue Hospital. They concluded that, for these children their own death was not within probability and they did not think about it. But they were quite capable of believing in the death of others and could discuss it freely. "Death does not appear as a natural end of life; it is the result of the hostility of others; it is a punishment meted out for wrong doing (by extension, the punishing agent may be God)."

In 1940, Anthony[1] extensively studied 117 normal English school children and their ideas about death. Her findings revealed they all knew of death, readily thought of it, and could speak of death without difficulty. They associated it with ideas of retaliation and reparation.

Nagy[21] using a classroom setting in Hungary, sought the views of 4–10 year-old children about death. Her findings corroborated those of the previous researchers, including the fact that children throughout this age range are interested in the subject. In addition, she found that for many children death is personified, and that before the age of 8 or 9 years the child cannot comprehend the process of dying.

Rochlin[29], in individual play sessions, studied 3–5 year-old children who had led relatively trauma-free lives. These children had thought about death and had heard about it; their ideas were clearly the result of their own thinking and observing, not that of teaching. Death was recognized by these children as an arrest of vital functions that comes about "not due to natural causes but as a result of strife, defiance of authority and retaliation, (and) hostility." "In sum, death is the outcome of certain relations between people."[29]

In a healthy, Catholic, Canadian population, Gartley and Bernasconi[10] confirmed the finding that children can speak of death and related matters in quite a matter-of-fact way. In contrast to previous findings, however, this group of children could speak of their own death with some credibility although it was placed in the vague and distant future. Death was considered to be final and irreversible. Although death was not personified as Nagy had found, it would appear from the study that these children felt

God, His angels, and heaven to be quite real, concrete, and personified. Fast and Cain, studying a healthy child population in bereavement found that "all the misconceptions about death which we were able to detect implied that the deceased still lived."[9] Perhaps the conceptual issue is not whether death is permanent or reversible, but rather which concept fulfills the emotional need of the child to "experience a continued relationship to the person who has died".[9]

In general, normal children from about 3 years of age are capable of conveying to us their thoughts about death. From 3 to 5 years of age, death is seen as violent and comes as a retaliation for being bad, but may not be permanent. The dead are often animate, so they have needs, they can think, feel and move; in fact, death is like another life.

Many opportunities exist in the well young child's thinking to confuse going away, or going to sleep (separation) with death as he understands it. Four-old-old John, who knows that his grandfather died recently, asks soberly, "When is grandpa coming for dinner?" His tone conveys that John misses him, but also contains the implication that grandpa is depriving him by not coming, thereby making him feel sad.

Between the ages of 6 and 10, death becomes more real, final, universal, and inevitable; but it is not until the latter part of this period that one's own fragility can be acknowledged. Early on, death may be personified and therefore one's wits, skill, and speed permit one to escape. During this period the objective facts of death become more interesting, and conceptual differentiation is made between the living and the nonliving, the animate and the inanimate. By the end of this period, death can be placed among other general processes and principles which govern the world.

In adolescence, the intellectual and cognitive tools of the adult are present but their use is threatened by the pubertal upsurge of intense bodily change accompanied by changes in emotional lability. Death may be viewed as a philosophical problem of life, or it may be challenged and denied by risk-taking. For some adolescents the childhood idea that death is not permanent still lingers. Suicide for the adolescent is frequently conceived of as retaliation, but also as reversible: "I can watch and enjoy the sorrow of my parents. They will be sorry at the way they treated me." Recall Tom Sawyer and Huck under the church pews attending their own funeral and becoming teary-eyed at their eulogy! In fact, most observers believe that for all of us it is not truly possible to conceive of our own death and that throughout our adult lives the childhood concepts linger on.

Views of Mental Illness

Two investigations have explored children's understanding of their peers' mental illness.[16,19,25] In the first study, five brief descriptions of children were prepared. One reflected a normal child's behavior in an upsetting situation, and four reflected behavior characteristic of common psychopathological entities ranging from mild to severe. The subjects were normal fourth to sixth grade children. The second study used the same methodology. Both teams of investigators found that the subjects clearly discriminated disturbed from normal behavior. Neither group found any sex differences. Novak[25] reports that his subjects did not discriminate between the clinical severity of the descriptions (which may reflect the social relations approach in his experimental design). In contrast, Marsden and Kalter found that their subjects did "make distinctions among degrees of disturbed behavior roughly in accord with those made by clinicians. Moreover their perceptions of emotional disturbance are for the most part independent of their fondness for or dislike of the disturbed peer and are not related to intelligence scores."[19]

Kalter and Marsden went on to explore children's concepts of etiological factors in the causation of mental illness, using the same methodology but now stressing the question: "How did this boy get to be the way he is in the story?" They report that "fourth- and sixth-graders seem to hold specific views of the etiology of childhood emotional disorders."[16] However, for each portrayed mentally ill child the subjects showed little consensus about the etiology. From the data obtained five categories of etiological theory were constructed: (a) inappropriate parenting, (b) modeling, (c) peer scapegoating and rejection, (d) problems internal to the central figure, and (e) other, i.e., infrequent or idiosyncratic ideas. Sixth-graders showed more clearly articulated views about etiology and tended more often to cite the category called inappropriate parenting as causative, than did the fourth-graders. The clarity of etiological explanation was not related to the degree of psychopathology.

The primary persons referred to by the sample as being etiologically culpable were self, parents, and peers. Evidently, in both physical and mental illness, the healthy ten- to twelve-year-old child sees primary causality lying with the most important people: self and parents. As Kalter and Marsden do not give any information about the content of poor parenting or self-causality, we do not know if, in the etiology of mental illness, such factors as transgression, blame, and wrongdoing are seen as causal. From the literature and clinical practice, however, there is no doubt that mentally ill children are convinced that their symptoms and suffering are the result of wrongdoing or thinking. This is true even for those who defensively externalize the problem.

Children's Concepts of Treatment

Data about well children's ideas and beliefs concerning treatment do not appear to be available; there also seem to be no studies examining well children's concepts about health personnel and the mechanisms of treatment.

Peters[26] examined the treatment concepts of ambulatory hospitalized children. In the projective stories told, the story character was the agent of treatment in less than one-tenth of the treatment references. On direct questioning, 15 of the 24 children could think of no way in which they could contribute to their own recovery. The other 9 children could see only very passive contributory roles for themselves, such as staying in bed. In 66% of the children's references to treatment, the intent was considered to be helpful. But for one-third of these references the context and wording suggested strong overtones of punishment or hostility, and direct hostile intent of treatment was evidenced in about 10% of the references. In general, the younger the child the more likely he was to designate the motivation of treatment as hostile to him.

In the stories, 54% of the references to the mode of treatment were to penetration. Almost half referred to a surgical penetration even though none of the children were hospitalized for surgery. It is interesting to note that treatment by ingestion and limitation of activity, the most commonly experienced mode of treatment for any child, registered infrequently (7% and 11%, respectively).

Lynn et al[18] noted that both rheumatics and nonrheumatics revealed a high incidence of anxiety in the structured doll play about such treatment and diagnostic elements as injections and blood sampling, medication, surgery (although none of these child patients had been admitted for surgery), pain, physical restriction, and hospitalization. The children's ideas about the mechanism of action which would make the treatment modality lead to recovery was not explored.

The picture changes when we look at children who have been hospitalized for a long time. Brazelton et al[6] and Schechter[30] each give numerous anecdotal examples in which children see treatment modalities as evidence of staff malevolence and of a desire to hurt the child patient. Since none of these studies are systematically reported, comparisons are not possible, but it does seem that the perception of good intent of treatment (as shown in Peters's study,) wanes during hospitalization. Brazelton et al observed that among the rheumatic fever patients, the "passive children seemed to interpret their restrictions as punishment rather than as measures necessary for their welfare. The more active children rebelled against their restrictions but in so doing appeared anxious.'[6]

Barnes'[2] study reflects another aspect of the child's attitude toward the helping person. In recalling the ICU period, the children most often talked about the nurses, who were perceived as helpful. The doctors, next most frequently mentioned, evoked fear; the children wished for the nurse to be present whenever the doctor examined them. Parents were also talked about, but not nearly so much, in the immediate stress situation and in the later discussion about the ICU experience. The professional identity of the author, in this case a nurse, was not discussed in relation to these findings. It should be noted that no study has included the professional role of the investigator among the variables to be considered.

Children's View of Research Hospitalization

Schwartz,[33] prompted by the ethical and legal considerations of informed consent with children, studied the hospitalized child's knowledge and ideas concerning participation in a research project. Fifty hospitalizations of a purely research nature of 36 children (4–18 years of age) were examined. Of the 36 children, 26 were being studied for short stature. Each child, and his or her parents, were prepared over an extended period of time prior to hospitalization.

The results are startling. For children younger than 11 years of age, no evidence appeared in two psychiatric interviews, child-to-staff or child-to-child ward communication, or psychological testing that any child was cognizant of what research meant— this despite the facts that research had been openly discussed in the prehospital period, and that the unit was clearly identified as a research ward. Past the age of 11, only 6 of the 19 children mentioned anything which could be interpreted as a reference to research, e.g., guinea pig, specimen, experiment. Of those six, five had symptoms of overwhelming anxiety. Four of the six viewed the hospitalization as a mixture of treatment and research. The two remaining subjects viewed the hospitalization as being purely for research purposes and signed themselves out.

It is hard to know what conclusions should be drawn from this report. Since the concept of research is intellectually manageable by those less than 11 years of age, one can only conclude that fears of being the object of research were so intense that the whole idea had to be banished from awareness. Apparently the preparation offered had not in any way met the emotional needs of these children and their parents.

DISCUSSION

As we have seen in this review, children's concepts of illness, health, and treatment are dependent upon their level of cognitive development. This should be no surprise to anyone who spends time with well children in the family, school, or wherever they congregate. Usually adults are amused, surprised, or nonplussed at concrete or syn-cretistic thinking, but tend not to engage the child in further elaboration. In subject matter which is painful or depressing, or in talking with a child who is suffering, this tendency is even stronger. Our impulse is not to follow the cues which the child offers us that indicate his awareness of his reality. In what follows, I would like to discuss the implications of the reviewed material for clinical work with sick children.

Below the age of 3 years, thinking on issues of causality, especially about one's own pain or vulnerability, is focused on the relationship with the parents. It is the parents' presence or absence that is important; they are the powerful, all-knowing, and protec-tive ones. Thinking at this age is highly egocentric, and practical explanations or reasons provide little support against the onslaught of fear, pain, and separation. The child's research methodology is to obtain data via all the senses. The data obtained from parental mood, affect, and emotional stance to which the young child is so particularly sensitive must be stressed. All the data procured by the child are put together via concrete cognitive operations in a linear, non-Aristotelian, primary process manner so that strange conclusions often result.

Statements of fact, or warnings such as "This will hurt" or "I am going to leave you now" will be understood by the child younger than 3 years of age. But the reasons for them will not be perceived as explicatory. Although reasons given to the child of this age are more for the adult's own emotional needs, they will reflect the trust and honesty of the adult-child relationship. That explanations will not be understood as such, and cannot be expected to facilitate cooperation, must not lead adults to feel that they should not be stated. On the contrary: Simple explanations are valuable. Their tone is important at the time and the very act of offering them establishes a model and baseline of truthfulness. Moreover, it leaves the way open for further explication and elaboration when the child is not under stress or is simply older. In contrast to this, the natural protective impulse to try to shield the child from parental affect may result in emo-tional isolation that may be frightening.

In the 3–7 year-old age range, thinking about causality is prelogical and egocentric, but the child's vocabulary is increasing enormously. Syncretistic thought, juxtaposition of events, confusing the different meanings of the same word, e.g., "cold" for both temperature and respiratory illness, and the use of the word as thing or cause will make any logical explanation subject to distortion or mimicry. However, unless we listen carefully, we may fail to realize that this has taken place. We need to keep in mind that children in the process of cognitive learning often fool adults into believing that they understand the explanation and that it answers their questions about causality. Believ-ing in the magic of our own explanation, we adults fail too often to detect the confusion.

Does this mean we should not explain to children about health and illness, germs and medicine? No. It means we must give as simple and true an explanation as possible while staying attuned to the reverberations of the inevitable distortions. We must remember that children need new facts, new words, and new examples if their knowl-edge base and cognitive ability are to grow. That fact and fancy, at this age, will exist very comfortably side by side must not be forgotten.

At about the age of eight to nine years, there is a quantum leap in conceptual ability in the realm of causality. More complex mental functions are now possible; a major landmark is being reached and the child's formal mental processes now facilitate understanding. In Piagetian terms this is the era of sophisticated concrete operations which will move into the formal mental operations of adolescence. The third- and fourth-graders of the Connecticut Board of Education study[7] who were so curious about their bodies and how they work reflect these changes. New, practical, pragmatic, realistic reasoning ability makes the middle school years a time when all kinds of facts are learned. For these children explanations, drawings, and explications are very useful in gaining cooperation and, indeed, in allaying anxiety. Reality is a very powerful force and one that a youngster at this age can utilize more and more effectively in coping with explicit difficulty. No longer is a person exposed to measles or a cold doomed to come down with the illness. Intermediary steps between cause and effect are known and understood, complexity is acknowledged, and rationality is valued. Now the logic of Sherlock Holmes begins to be enjoyed. Research into the why's and wherefore's of disease, illness, and treatment as well as many other mysteries of life can be entered into with pleasure because the mental capacity is there.

In those studies which examine the effect of short-term hospitalization and illness or surgery, reality seems to be the common ground on which both adults and children can meet stress. Barnes[2] noted how reality-oriented her cases were during their stay in the Intensive Care Unit and in their recall of these events several days later. Vernon et al point out in their review that in a variety of studies done on successful preparation of children for hospitalization, the single common element was the provision of "factual information concerning the things the child will experience during hospitalization."[34] Peters's[26] study of treatment showed a high incidence of perception of benevolent intent regarding the helpful and healing intention of doctors and nurses, although the younger children were more suspicious.

Long-term hospitalization and illness as well as severe threats to life itself can be expected to erode the beneficial effects of reality-based knowledge, and I believe that the studies of Brazelton et al,[6] Dubo,[8] Schwartz,[33] and Schecter[30] all illustrate this. Yet the effects of serious illness, prolonged convalescence, or lifelong disability upon cognitive abilities has not (to my knowledge) been explicitly studied in children. It is well known that, in general, high anxiety level interferes wih good thinking and reality testing. From the data reviewed it would appear that the duration and intensity of stress for children differentially affects the amount of cognitive distortion. In addition, the younger child will distort reality more readily, whereas the older child will have greater tolerance (all other things being equal).

The stress-induced change in thought content reflects a waning of confidence and a loss of reality focus indicative of an emotional regression, as all the authors state. I think that a cognitive regression is implied as well. By "cognitive regression" I mean a loss of age-appropriate, specific cognitive abilities under the duress of stress and affective pressure. In the use of this term I mean also to suggest that there is an invasion of affect that distorts the perception of pragmatic realities and cognitive abilities, and as a result, fantasies become real. I do not mean that this regression would necessarily be reflected in all areas of thought; rather, it would occur in specifically sensitive spheres. The concept of cognitive regression alerts us to the idea that there is an optimum cognitive-affective balance that allows good learning to take place. When this balance is upset by an overload of affect, learning, along with the utilization of knowledge already obtained, will be impaired.

If these hypotheses are true they might generate a rule of thumb for helping children understand their illnesses as well as the needs for hospitalization, procedures, doctors, nurses, and medicine. In preparation for hospitalization, surgical procedures, and other brief encounters with medical issues, reality knowledge is most helpful. To know what is going to happen and how it will be experienced increases the feeling of mastery. But if stress is prolonged (for whatever reason), information will not be utilized well because of a cognitive regression. At such times an opportunity for emotional expression is imperative.

A good example of the importance of a cognitive-affective balance, the ability to evaluate it, and the courage to respond to it is shown by Schowalter et al.[32] They report on a sixteen-year-old girl with chronic kidney disease, a failed kidney transplant, and considerable suffering under dialysis. Following a shunt revision which clotted, she refused further help and wished only to be allowed to die. Her parents concurred. Although the situation was very difficult for the staff, it was determined that the girl and her parents had assessed the situation as accurately as anyone could on both the cognitive and affective levels, and their decision was respected. It was reported that she died an unusually peaceful uremic death with her parents by her side.

The report by Schwartz[33], mentioned earlier, suggests an alternative picture wherein the concept of cognitive regression might have been helpful. The chronically ill children under study were of such an age and ability that they could have been expected to understand the concept of research, and to understand that their hospitalization was solely for such a purpose. Yet under the circumstances reported, wherein those under 11 years of age could not even acknowledge research and those older did so only with great anxiety, we must suppose that something like a cognitive regression had occurred. One could suggest that sufficient affective support had not been provided and therefore the information concerning research hospitalization could not be assimilated at age-appropriate levels. At this point, additional realistic and cognitive information could not be assimilated; neither would it undo the repression of previously acquired factual material. This state of affairs will only be remedied when the attendant fantasies and fears are elicited and are allowed some expression and resolution. As this process occurs, there can be a resumption of ongoing and positive cognitive processes, including the recall of factual material and the acquisition of new and relevant knowledge.

The characteristics of cognitive regression as I see them are (a) a seeming lack of age-appropriate cognitive ability in a specific area; (b) denial of any knowledge about the area, as though to say, "I am incapable of knowing this kind of information"; and (c) no evidence of impaired mental processes in emotionally neutral areas. These three points would occur in the presence of stress, especially stress of prolonged duration. The function of the regression would be a defensive one since awareness of certain knowledge in consciousness would cause intolerable anxiety. It is for this reason that providing further information in an attempt to "reach" the child would be to no avail. The anxiety must have been reduced first.

When a child who is ill or hospitalized says "I don't know" in response to questions such as "What is the matter?" or "Why are you here?", there are two possibilities: Either he really does not know, and some reality information may be very helpful; or what he knows (or thinks he knows) is so scary that he can't remember, and then some affective support and opportunity for ventilation may be in order. When reality is not grasped by a child with the intellectual capacity to do so, then affect has interfered and must be dealt with first.

How can one get a child to reveal these affective distortions of reality? The reviewed research shows that thoughts, concepts, feelings, and ideas can be more easily expressed via displacement than directly. Children expressing thoughts and feelings about themselves in displacement appear to some to be so disingenuous that it is hard to believe that they could not say the same things directly. Yet we accept displacement easily, albeit with a smile, if an adult requests some information "for a friend." The same is true for the child. Putting some distance between self and topic by using dolls, puppets, or drawing can be very helpful. Even framing the discussion in terms of "a boy or girl I know" rather than in the directly demanding "you" can facilitate the exchange of information.

Finally, knowing what children think about disease and why they think that they, in particular, got sick helps us to catch the cues they send us in their words and manner. It does little good to tell children routinely that they are not the cause of their illness, and that they should not feel responsible for their illness because it could happen to anyone. Any child is more likely to feel that such a statement is "out of the blue," intrusive, uninteresting, or simply totally unrelated to his own thinking. Only when the child has indicated that the thought or feeling we express is just below the surface of his own awareness can we assist in delivering his feelings up to the light of reason. Because confidence is a prerequisite, this will require both attention to and time spent with the child.

CONCLUSION

The literature on children's understanding and knowledge about their bodies, health, illness, treatment, and death has been reviewed with focus on the cognitive aspects. In general, researchers reported a distinct change in children's thinking on these matters at about 8–9 years of age, a change that reflects the child's improved ability to think in a reality-oriented, causal manner. The majority of researchers found that in many children, well and ill alike, causality in illness was related to wrongdoing, and illness was perceived as punishment. These convictions were most notable in the younger child, and they decreased with age. Healthy children's views of death and dying were briefly reviewed. In reviewing children's concepts of mental illness, research hospitalization, health, and treatment, it was noted that research is very sparse. Comparative studies of the well and ill child's conceptualizations are rare. No studies were found on ill children's concepts of health, how treatment works, the comparative conceptualizations of children with different illnesses, and the impact of stress on children's conceptual abilities and ideas about illness.

In the discussion, an attempt was made to show how information about children's knowledge and their cognitive processes could prove useful in the handling of sick children, in providing for their treatment, and in improving communication between them and health care personnel. The concepts of cognitive regression and cognitive-affective balance were put forth in an attempt to draw attention to both the cognitive and affective aspects of learning and knowledge.

There is much to be learned in this area. In addition, we must integrate our awareness of children's cognitive knowledge with our knowledge of their emotional and fantasy response to illness and its impact on the body. Sensitive clinicians know a great deal by intuition and insight, but such knowledge needs articulation. Armed with more knowledge, we may be better able to assist children in their mastery of the trauma of long- and short-term hospitalization, chronic illness, and physical handicap.

REFERENCES

1. Anthony, S. *The child's discovery of death: A study of child psychology.* New York: Harcourt, Brace, 1940.
2. Barnes, C. M. Levels of consciousness indicated by responses of children to phenomena in the intensive care unit. *Maternal Child Nursing Journal,* 1975, *4,* 215–290 (Monograph No. 4).
3. Bergmann, T. *Children in the hospital.* New York: International Universities Press, 1965.
4. Blos Jr., P. An investigation of the healthy child's understanding of the causes of disease. Unpublished dissertation, Yale University, 1956.
5. Blos Jr., P., & Finch, S. M. Sexuality and the handicapped adolescent. In J. A. Downey & N. L. Low (eds.), *The child with disabling illness: Principles of rehabilitation.* Philadelphia: W. B. Saunders, 1974, pp. 521–540.

6. Brazelton, T. B., Holder, R., & Talbot, B. Emotional aspects of rheumatic fever in children. *Journal of Pediatrics*, 1953, *43*, 339–358.

7. Byler, R., Lewis, G. & Totman, R. *Teach Us What We Want to Know*. New York: Mental Health Materials Center, Inc., 1969.

8. Dubo, S. Psychiatric study of children with pulmonary tuberculosis. *American Journal of Orthopsychiatry*, 1950, *20*, 520.

9. Fast, I., & Cain, A. C. Fears of death in bereaved children. Paper presented at the Annual Meeting of the American Orthopsychiatric Association, Chicago, 1964.

10. Gartley, W., & Bernasconi, M. The concept of death in children. *Journal of Genetic Psychology*, 1967, *110*, 71–85.

11. Gellert, E. Children's beliefs about bodily illness. Paper presented at the meeting of the American Psychological Association, New York, 1961.

12. Gellert, E. Children's conceptions of the content and functions of the human body. *Genetic Psychology Monographs*, 1962, *65*, 293–405.

13. Gochman, D. S. Children's perceptions of vulnerability to illness and accident: A replication, extension and refinement. *HSMHA Health Reports*, 1971, *86*, 247–252.

14. Gochman, D. S., Bagramian, R. A., & Sheiham, A. Consistency in children's perceptions of vulnerability to health problems. *Health Service Reports*, 1972, *87*, 282–288.

15. Gofman, H., Buckman, W., & Schade, G. H. The child's emotional response to hospitalization. *American Journal of Diseases of Children*, 1957, *93*, 157–164.

16. Kalter, N., & Marsden, G. Children's understanding of their emotionally disturbed peers: II. Etiological Factors. *Psychiatry*, 1977, *40*, 48–54.

17. Lewis, C. E., & Lewis, M. A. The impact of television commercials on health-related beliefs and behaviors of children. *Pediatrics*, 1974, *53*, 431–435.

18. Lynn, D. B., Glaser, H. H., & Harrison, G. S. Comprehensive medical care for Handicapped Children: III. Concepts of Illness in Children with Rheumatic Fever. *American Journal of Diseases of Children*, 1962, *103*, 42–50.

19. Marsden, G., & Kalter, N. Children's understanding of their emotionally disturbed peers: I. The Concept of Emotional Disturbance. *Psychiatry*, 1976, *39*, 227–238.

20. Mechanic, D. The influence of mothers on their children's health attitudes and behavior. *Pediatrics*, 1964, *39*, 444–453.

21. Nagy, M. H. The child's theories concerning death. *Journal of Genetic Psychology*, 73, 1948, 3–27.

22. Nagy, M. H. Children theories concerning the origin of diseases. Proceedings and papers of the 12th International Congress of Psychology, Edinburgh, 1948. London: Oliver and Boyd, 1950, p. 96.

23. Nagy, M. H. Children's ideas on the origin of illness. *Health Education Journal 9*, 1951, 6–12.

24. Nagy, M. H. The representation of germs by children. *Journal of Genetic Psychology*, 83, 1953, 227–240.

25. Novak, D. W. Children's reactions to emotional disturbance in imaginary peers. *Journal of Consulting and Clinical Psychology*, 42(3), 1974, 462.

26. Peters, B. M. Concepts of hospitalized children about causality of illness and intent of treatment. Unpublished Ph.D. dissertation, University of Pittsburgh, 1975.

27. Piaget, J. *Judgment and reasoning in the child*. New York: Humanities Press, 1928.

28. Rashkis, S. R. Child's understanding of health. *A.M.A. Archives of General Psychiatry*, 12, Jan. 1965, 10–17.

29. Rochlin, G. *Griefs and discontents: The forces of change*. Boston: Little, Brown and Co., 1965, pp. 63–120.

30. Schechter, M. D. The orthopedically handicapped child. *A.M.A. Archives of General Psychiatry*, 4, March 1961, 247–253.

31. Schilder, P. & Wechsler, D. The attitudes of children toward death (1934). In L. Bender (ed.),

Contributions to developmental neuropsychiatry. New York: International Universities Press, 1964, pp. 132–160.

32. Schowalter, J. E., Ferholt, J. B., and Mann, N. M. The adolescent patient's decision to die. *Pediatrics, 51*(1), 1973, 97–103.

33. Schwartz, A. H. Children's concepts of research hospitalization. *New England Journal of Medicine, 287*(12), 1972, 589–592.

34. Vernon, D. T. A., Foley, J. M., Spiowicz, R. R., & Schulman, J. L. *The psychological responses of children to hospitalization and illness: A review of the literature*. Springfield, Ill.: Charles C Thomas, 1965.

35. Waechter, E. H. The responses of children to fatal illness. In M. Duffey (ed.), *Current concepts in clinical nursing*. Vol. III. St. Louis: Mosby, 1971, pp. 115–127.

36. Waechter, E. H. Children's awareness of fatal illness. *American Journal of Nursing, 71*, June 1971, 1168–1172.

WHAT DO I HAVE INSIDE ME?
HOW CHILDREN VIEW
THEIR BODIES

Elizabeth Gellert, Ed.D.

INTRODUCTION AND METHODS

Children's conceptions of illness and of medical procedures obviously must be influenced by their ideas about the contents and functioning of the human body. Although the literature is replete with references to children's emotional reactions to illness, hospitalization, and so forth, very few systematic investigations have concentrated upon pediatric patients'—or healthy children's—conceptions of the working of their bodies. This chapter reports the findings of one such pilot effort and refers to the few related studies published thus far. Although the data were gathered more than a decade ago, recent informal replications did not differ notably from the findings to be presented. *

The subjects of the study were 96 boys and girls,† all but four of whom were hospitalized for a variety of somatic disorders or symptoms. Their age ranged from 4 years, 9 months to 16 years, 11 months. The majority of the children came from lower- to middle-class homes; 95% were white. According to their own statements, they had received little or no formal instruction about human anatomy and physiology.

The subjects were interviewed individually, using a standard questionnaire and outlines of front and back views of child figures (see Figures 1 and 2). The children filled in the outlines with a pencil, as requested. The examiner recorded the children's verbal responses during the interview. Since the length of the questionnaire was restricted by the limited attention span of most children, it was decided to focus upon body parts that are common loci of illness. The final questionnaire follows here.

---

* For a more detailed account of this study, see Gellert.[3]

† $N = {<}96$ for some questionnaire items included after data collection began.

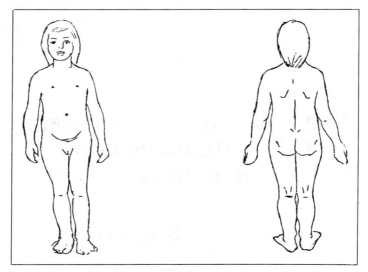

Fig. 1.   *Female outline to be filled in. (Reduced from original size.)*

1. What do you have inside you? Tell me as many things as you can think of that are inside you.
2. a. Show me the head.
        What is in the head? Tell me all the things that are in the head.
    b. Make a circle on the pictures where, and about how big the heart is. What does the heart do? What is it for? What would happen if we didn't have a heart?
    c. Show me some places where you have bones. (Try for a minimum of five locations.) What do we have bones for? What would happen if we didn't have any bones?

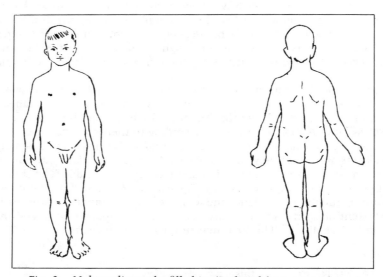

Fig. 2.   *Male outline to be filled in. (Reduced from original size.)*

    d.   Make a circle about where, and about how big the stomach is. What does the stomach do? Show me where the food goes after you swallow it. (Sketch in diagram.) And then? And then? (If excretion is not mentioned spontaneously, ask, "Does it ever come out anywhere?" If answer is affirmative, say, "Show me where it comes out.")

    e.   Make a circle about where, and about how big the ribs are. Why do we have ribs? What for? What would happen if we didn't have ribs?

    f.   Make a circle about where, and about how big the liver is. What does the liver do? What would happen if we didn't have a liver?

    g.   What do you think we have a skin for? What would happen if we didn't have a skin?

    h.   Make a circle where, and about how big the lungs are. How many lungs are there? What do we have lungs for? What would happen if we didn't have lungs?

    i.   Do you have nerves? Any nerves? (If no, ask "Does anybody else? Who?") What are the nerves for? What else? What would happen if we didn't have any nerves?

    j.   Make a circle where, and about how big the bladder is. What do we have a bladder for? What would happen if we didn't have a bladder?

    k.   How come we have bowel movements? What for? Where do bowel movements come from? (Probe for derivation from food, stomach, intestines.) Show me (on the diagram). What would happen if we didn't have bowel movements? About how often, how many times, should people have bowel movements? About how often do you have bowel movements?

3.   a.   What do you think is the most important part of you? If you picked one part of you as the most important, which one would you pick? Why? What makes it the most important?

    b.   Are there any parts of you that you could live, or get along without? Which ones?

Every effort was made to obtain maximum information form each question by using repeated probes such as, "What else . . . and what else."

RESULTS

In answer to the first question, which asked about bodily contents, three unexpected factors complicated the analysis of the data.

1.   Subjects varied in their interpretation of what constitutes the inside of the body. Some considered only the trunk, others included the skin, etc.

2.   Some subjects' responses reflected the notion that bodily contents are not stable; e.g., people might have nerves sometimes and not at others.

3.   Some responses seemed to imply that individuals differ from one another with regard to the parts their bodies contain.

The mean number of bodily ingredients listed rose rather steadily from means of 3.3 (4-6 years of age) to 13 (15–16 years of age) with a sharp rise occurring at 9 years of age. The number listed per subject ranged from zero to 34 ingredients. Parts mentioned by at least half the sample were bones, blood vessels, heart (and parts thereof), and blood. In the present study as well as in Tait et al.,[6] reproductive organs were included rarely (4%) and not before preadolescence. Since the subjects were pediatric patients, it is not surprising that their lists often included items associated with illness, e.g., appendix, tonsils, gall stones, pus. The youngsters in Tait's study, most of whom were not ill, manifested the same tendency. Very few children mentioned nonmaterial ingredients such as "a soul," "Jesus," "health," or "a spirit." However, some seemed to think that "the pulse," "reflexes," and a "windbag" were inside them.

The youngest children typically thought they contained what they had ingested and egested, e.g., food, liquids, bowel movements, and blood, although none at any age mentioned sputum or perspiration. By contrast, from 11 years of age forward, materials related to ingestion and egestion were no longer listed. With this group, the most prevalent items were permanent body parts related to the musculoskeletal and the circulatory systems. Contrary to the reports of Fraiberg[1] and Schilder and Wechsler,[5] the majority of subjects below 8 to 9 years of age also mentioned bones, brain, and eyes. Even below 7 years of age, 24 different bodily ingredients were known to some of the 20 children sampled.

When quizzed about the head's ingredients per se, 78 out of 92 children mentioned the brain; 55, the eyes; 45, the ears; and 24 the teeth. Neck, nerves, and chin were included rarely. Similarly, teeth, tongue, and mouth were listed surprisingly infrequently. Only one mentioned muscles as such, but some reflected awareness of "movers": "The part where you swallow"; "When you chew it moves"; and "joints between the eyes." As reported by Nagy,[4] children 5–11 years of age stated that the brain is made of bone (probably confusing it with the skull), blood, skin, flesh, cells, and other miscellaneous contents. Cells and nerves were mentioned rarely, and then only by her oldest subjects. Nagy's subjects most frequently thought that the brain is for thinking and other intellectual activities. In her study, answers such as, "for working," or "moving," declined with increasing age.

The importance attributed to a particular body part may affect psychological reactions to its impairment. Moreover, one could hypothesize that such valuations shift intraindividually as a result of problems encountered with a particular body part. The present investigation did not test the latter hypothesis, but it did inquire into views regarding the relative importance and dispensability of various organs. Tables 1 and 2 present the results.

By far, the body part most frequently judged to be the most important was the heart. Next in frequency, beginning with children 9–10 years of age, was the brain. Seven subjects—all but one less than 11 years of age—cited the eyes. Parts possibly associated with breathing, e.g., lungs, nose, throat, mouth were rated most important by 11 of the 72 children who were asked about this. The particular body part's role in ordering vital processes or its indispensability for living were the reasons given by the majority of children for judging their choice most important. However, some very young children apparently judged the importance of a body part according to the amount of time it takes to take care of it, e.g., "The feet; you have to take good care of them . . ."; "You have to scrub them between your toes, which is real hard." Surprisingly, no subject cited bones or muscles as being most important. Neither did anyone list vitalisms such as "soul" or "spirit" in this connection.

With regard to dispensable body parts (see Table 2) a great variety was mentioned: sometimes realistically, sometimes unrealistically (the latter probably because of ignorance). With increasing age the absolute number of dispensable parts mentioned per subject, rose from a mean of 2.1 to a mean of 4.9, dropping off slightly (4.7) in the oldest group. At least one 5-year-old child expressed a conviction that may be quite prevalent during the preschool period, namely, that he needed *all* his parts to live. Such a view might contribute substantially to emotional reactions to the loss of any body part. Eleven children considered hair to be indispensable, a finding that may account for some youngsters' extreme resistance to having it cut. There was a general trend to

Table 1[3]   The Most Important Part of the Body

Part	Age in years and months						Total group N = 71
	4–6.11 N = 18	7–8.11 N = 13	9–10.11 N = 21	11–12.11 N = 7	13–14.11 N = 8	15–16.11 N = 7	
Heart	3	4	9	4	5	1	26
Brain	—	—	1	2	3	2	8
Eyes	2	1	3	—	—	1	7
Head	1	—	2	1	1	—	5
Lungs	—	1	2	1	—	1	5
Stomach	3	—	1	—	—	—	4
Nose	2	1	—	1	—	—	4
Whole body	1	—	1	1	—	—	3
Legs	2	—	—	—	—	—	2
Hair	1	—	—	—	—	—	1
Feet	1	—	—	—	—	—	1
Liver	—	1	—	—	—	—	1
Throat	—	1	—	—	—	—	1
Bladder	—	—	1	—	—	—	1
Mouth	—	—	1	—	—	—	1
Teeth	—	—	—	—	—	1	1
Nervous system	—	—	—	—	—	1	1
Five senses	—	—	1	—	—	—	1
"French fries"	1	—	—	—	—	—	1
Don't know	1	4	—	1	—	—	6
Total responses	18	13	22	11	9	7	80

Note: Some children listed more than one part as being their most important. Hence the total number of responses is greater than the total number of children.

consider parts dispensable if they were considered capable of regeneration or artificial substitution, if they were associated with surgery, or if they were one of a pair (lung) or of many (finger).

Among the organs specifically referred to in the questionnaire, the size and location of the heart were more generally known than those of any other parts, except the bones. Even 60% of the 4 to 6-year-old children placed it relatively correctly in the body outline they were given. By 7 years of age, most of the children knew that the heart is an important part of them. Around this age, they usually explained its function by describing the heart beat, e.g., "The heart ticks," "beeps," "makes a noise," "goes in and out," "shakes"; or by asserting that "we need it to live." Occasionally, they ascribed religious or psychological functions to the heart. For example: One youngster said, "The heart is where God lives"; another claimed, "The heart makes you dream." One five-year-old child described the function of the heart as follows:" . . . 'Cause God made it that we could live; the heart makes you do all the things you're supposed to do. It shakes. It sort of makes you get a little bit of energy; without a heart you'd sort of die; you'd be sort of buried—have to get buried, you know."

During midchildhood, an increasing proportion (43% of children 9–10 years of age) associated heart function with being able to breathe. At least some of these children believed that heart beats and respiration either are identical or coincident. After the age of 11 years, the association of heart function with breathing became deemphasized. By the age of 13 years, most subjects explained what the heart does

Table 2[3]   List of Body Parts Reported to be Dispensable

Body part	Age group in years and months						Total group N = 71
	4–6.11 N = 15	7–8.11 N = 13	9–10.11 N = 21	11–12.11 N = 7	13–14.11 N = 8	15–16.11 N = 7	
Appendix	—	—	2	3	6	2	13
Arms							
(plural)	1	2	3	3	4	2	15
Arm (one)	—	—	2	1	1	1	5
Belly button	1	—	—	—	—	—	1
Blood (some)	—	—	—	1	—	—	1
Bones	—	—	—	—	—	1*	1
Bosoms							
(nipples)	1	—	—	—	—	—	1
Bowels							
(part of)	—	—	—	—	—	1	1
Brain	1	—	—	—	—	—	1
Cheeks	1	—	—	—	—	—	1
Chest							
(left side)	1	—	—	—	—	—	1
Chin	1	—	—	—	—	—	1
Ears (plural)	1	—	2	1	1	1	6
One ear	—	—	2	1	—	—	3
Eardrum	—	—	1	—	—	—	1
Outside							
(ear)	—	—	1	—	—	—	1
"Hearing"	—	—	1	—	—	—	1
Eyes (pl.)	1	1	3	3	1	2	11
One eye	—	—	1	—	1	—	2
Eyeballs	—	—	1	—	—	—	1
Fat (some							
excess)	—	—	—	1	—	—	1
Feet (pl.)	—	—	3	—	1	1	5
One foot	—	1	—	—	—	—	1
Fingers (pl.)	—	2	2	—	—	2	6
One finger	—	1	3	—	1	1	6
Gallbladder	—	—	—	—	—	1	1
"Generative							
organs"	—	—	—	—	—	1	1
Hair	3	1	5	1	—	1	11
Eyebrows	3	—	—	—	—	—	3
Eyelashes	1	—	—	—	—	—	1
Sideburns	—	1	—	—	—	—	1

by referring in some manner to its role in supplying blood to all parts of the body: "The heart beats blood out to the blood vessels."

Although the term *circulation* was frequently used to describe blood flow, there was no evidence that subjects, even by adolescence, understood that blood returns to the heart from the various regions of the body. However, with increasing age, a growing proportion of children mentioned the interaction of the heart with other organs and body parts." [4]

In comparison with the heart, knowledge about the lungs was sparse and vague. They were rarely listed (8%) below 9 years of age and were omitted by the majority even

Table 2³(Continued)

| Body part | Age group in years and months | | | | | | Total group |
	4–6.11 N = 15	7–8.11 N = 13	9–10.11 N = 21	11–12.11 N = 7	13–14.11 N = 8	15–16.11 N = 7	N = 71
Hands (pl.)	—	—	3	1	1	—	5
One hand	—	—	—	—	—	1	1
Head	1	1	—	—	—	—	2
Heart	—	—	—	—	—	1*	1
Heel	1	—	—	—	—	—	1
"Insides" (some)	—	—	—	—	1	—	1
Kidneys (pl.)	—	—	—	—	1	1*	2
One kidney	—	—	1	1	2	2	6
Legs (pl.)	1	1	3	3	4	2	14
One leg	1	1	2	1	1	1	7
Liver	—	—	2*	—	—	—	2
Lungs (pl.)	—	—	1	—	—	—	1
One lung	—	—	—	—	1	1	2
Mouth	1	—	1	—	—	—	2
Muscles	—	1	—	—	—	—	1
(in one leg)	—	—	—	—	—	1	1
Nails	2	—	1	—	—	—	3
Nose	1	—	1	—	—	—	2
Pituitary gland	—	—	—	—	1	—	1
Ribs	1	—	—	—	—	1	2
One rib	—	—	—	—	1	1	2
Shoulders	1	—	—	—	—	—	1
"Something on the side"	1	—	—	—	—	—	1
Spleen	—	—	—	—	1	—	1
Stomach	—	1	—	—	—	—	1
Part of stomach	—	—	—	—	1	—	1
Teeth	—	—	1	2	1	—	4
Testes	—	—	—	—	1	—	1
Thyroid gland	—	—	—	—	1	—	1
Toes	—	1	2	—	—	1	4
One toe	—	—	2	—	1	1	4
Tongue	—	—	—	1	1	1	3
Tonsils	—	—	1	2	2	1	6
Ulcers	—	—	—	—	1	—	1

beyond that age. (Could such indifference account for the increase in smoking among adults despite its alleged harmfulness to the lungs?) Like Nagy's[4] findings, ideas about the location of the lungs, particularly among younger subjects, were often wrong. Between 7–11 years of age, almost 50% thought that the lungs are in the neck, throat, or head. Other placements circled were on the back, arms, knees, shoulders, or abdomen. Beyond 10 years of age fairly correct placement occurred in the majority of cases. However, even when the lungs were placed in the right location, their size tended to be grossly underestimated by most children at all ages, and more so by the younger ones. The lungs were sometimes sketched in like windpipes or like ribs. Five out of 57 subjects thought they had only one lung, while other estimates of their number went as high as 100! The correct number was given by 72% of the subjects. (Confusions regarding the number of many body parts were quite commonly found.) Below the age of 7 years, most children would not theorize about the purpose of having lungs. However, some of the older children expressed ideas such as these: The lungs are for chewing, for hair, to make the mouth water, for walking, singing, connecting the arms to the trunk, and to contain the body's blood. Nagy[4] reported that her subjects often thought of air primarily circulating in the head. In the present study, it was not until 9 to 10 years of age that the majority mentioned the lungs' relation to breathing.

Among the ideas of 49 children about the functions of the skin, personal appearance tended to be emphasized by the younger subjects (4–8 years of age), e.g., "To not make see the blood and bones." Also, children of this age often expressed the idea that the skin keeps the body "together"; "So blood won't fall out"; "it helps keep everything in." After 9 years of age, protection from noxious aspects of the environment was mentioned by the majority as the function of the skin. This idea did not appear in subjects less than 8 years of age. (It is not surprising that many youngsters are upset by injections and other perforations of the integument since they tend to consider its intactness as almost vital to their bodily integrity). Most children seemed to think of the skin as being moistureproof, and only one (10 years of age) mentioned the skin's role in respiration. Unfortunately, explanations of perspiration were not sought in the study.

The most frequently listed ingredients of the body were the bones (74%). Their most predominantly mentioned locations were in the extremities and in the head. The function of bones to maintain bodily shape, uprightness, and to effect motility was generally recognized by the age of 11 to 12 years. Even the majority of nine- to ten-year-old children said that the bones give shape, form, structure, hardness and/or strength. From 9–10 years of age forward, all subjects could cite one or more reasons for having bones. Strangely, only three of the 93 subjects associated the function of bones with growing. Five thought that bones provide needed material such as blood, calcium, and iron. Despite the high degree of awareness and comprehension about bones which prevailed, none of the subjects considered them their most important part. Counteraction to "shrinking," to "folding in," or to "contracting into a ball" or into "shapelessness" was the only function that was mentioned with rather stable frequency at all ages. Although correct responses increased with age, only four young subjects could mention no function of the bones and wrong responses were almost totally absent in their answers. Had it been feasible to extend this investigation to even younger children, it is likely that the ubiquitousness of bones within the body would not have been known to at least some children. (The investigator recalls the astonishment of one 4-year-old child when he was told that he had bones inside him.)

Although general information about bones was common, accurate knowledge about the ribs was not. Only 13 out of 96 subjects spontaneously listed the ribs as a bodily ingredient. Before the ages of 9 to 10 years, less than 25% located them in the thoracic region. Two small circles above the pelvis, along the sides of the body, reflected 25% of the 7– to 10-year-old children's concept of the ribs' location. In a small subsample ($N = 12$), the modal concept of the number of ribs in the body was two! The most prevalent ideas expressed about rib function were (a) related to protection of other body parts, and (b) related to maintenance of shape, structure, or form of the trunk. Of the 88 subjects asked, 34 would offer no ideas about functions of the ribs and only three related them to breathing. Thirteen children thought that the ribs helped them bend, move the arms or legs or both, lie down, sit up, or stretch. Apparently many people learn about ribs at a late age—if at all!

In the total sample, only 8% listed nerves among their ingredients. For the most part, the younger children in the sample either knew little or nothing about the nerves or expressed wrong conceptions. When questioned, eight children, all below 9 years of age, denied that they had nerves. Some subjects thought that only adults have nerves and others expressed the notion that it is possible to have nerves at some times and not on other occasions. A substantial proportion (25%–44%) in all but the oldest group connected nerves with negative emotions such as nervousness, anger, fear, or worry. Nerves also occasionally were considered to counteract negative states: (You have nerves) "So you won't keep on being too nervous. . ." "If you get too nervous you won't stay alive"; or, to "absorb shock—like at the base of your teeth." One interesting opinion asserted that nerves cause allergy. The variety of diverse functions ascribed to nerves was among the largest for any body part included in the questionnaire. "With increasing age there was a steady rise in the following explanations (of nerve function): conducting messages between the brain and parts of the body, the control and stabilization of mental activities. . . (and) sensory perception."[3]

Sensory perception was the most frequently mentioned purpose of nerves beyond the age of 9 years. From that age on, 32% also "mentioned the role of the nerves in maintaining bodily integrity by serving as a warning system against possible harm from the external environment."[3] By 15–16 years of age, only occasional mistakes were found in the children's explanations of what the nerves do.

It will be remembered that several questions concerned with the digestive system were included in the questionnaire. For reporting purposes, the digestive system will be considered to include any body part which is actually (or allegedly by a subject to be) associated with the vicissitudes of food and liquids from ingestion to egestion. (In analyzing the data, it became apparent that responses might have been even more diverse and informative than they were, if subjects had been asked to trace the course of food and to trace the course of liquid, air, and the like.)

Below the age of 9 years, no subject spontaneously listed the stomach as being one of his ingredients, although almost all of the children proved to have some ideas about it when questioned specifically. Since the stomach is the locus of frequent and vivid sensations, this finding is surprising. It may have been due to a semantic confusion, since the colloquial use of the word *stomach* often refers to the entire interior and exterior abdomen. Some of the younger children may have interpreted the term in this fashion, and therefore did not list it as being inside themselves. For males, the fact that the visible genitalia may be considered to be external to the body, may have accounted for the sparse listings.

Although all children had conceptions regarding the location of the stomach, the majority (particularly among the younger children) drew it below its true location. Nagy[4] found the same tendency. As mentioned, the prevalence of this response may have been due to the colloquial use of the word *stomach* to refer to the belly. Another factor which may have contributed to the low positioning of the stomach is that many sensations related to eating, e.g., feelings of fullness, nausea, gurgling, and the like, often emanate from parts below the stomach. Since the children usually associated the stomach with eating, and since most subjects showed little or no knowledge about the intestines, they might have inferred that the stomach is located where those sensations were experienced. Until the age of 13 years, the majority overestimated the size of the stomach, often drastically so. Answers regarding the function of the stomach are summarized in Table 3. Its role in digestion was mentioned either without definition or described in rather rudimentary terms. It would have been interesting to ask specifically about the meaning and process of digestion. However, some conceptions voiced were that food enters blood; that it is ground or chewed to make it smaller; that it dissolves into liquid; that it comes to rest, or that it becomes stored. Five youngsters explained that food is transformed into energy.

When asked where food goes after it is swallowed, even the youngest children

27

Table 3³   Children's Ideas About the Function of the Stomach

	Percent per group						
	Age group in years and months						
Explanatory category	4.9–6.11 N = 20	7–8.11 N = 19	9–10.11 N = 23	11–12.11 N = 9	13–14.11 N = 13	15–16.11 N = 11	Total group N = 95
1. *Don't know*	30	—	—	—	—	—	6
3. *Function related to breathing*	15	21	13	—	—	—	11
4. *Function related to blood*	10	16	13	—	—	—	8
7. *Stomach runs everything else; most important organ*	—	—	4	—	8	—	2
10. *Function related to containing internal organs—i.e., to hold our insides; (the term, "stomach," probably used to refer to the entire trunk).*	—	11	—	—	8	—	3
8. *Stomach is essential to life*	15	16	13	—	15	9	13
5. *Function related to having strength or energy*	11	5	4	—	15	9	6
6. *Function related to growth in height or volume*	5	11	—	—	—	9	4
11. *Stomach is a "relay" station—i.e., spontaneous mention that food goes elsewhere from the stomach.*	—	5	39	22	15	27	16
9. *Function related to any aspect of digestion —i.e., food softens, grinds, turns food around; dissolves, makes food smaller; digests food; transforms food into person, bones, fat, blood*	—	21	30	67	77	73	37
2. *Function related to food and/or eating —i.e., food is stored, kept, held, rests in stomach; food goes from stomach elsewhere; to eat; for food.*	70	95	96	100	92	100	91

traced it to the abdominal region, though not always to the stomach. "A few thought that food goes through the lungs or heart as it passes through the chest on the way to the stomach."[3] From the abdominal region, food was either channelled to other body parts or considered to be discharged. It was not until the ages of 12 to 16 years that the majority (67%) said that some food stays in the body and some is eliminated. Among the very young, some thought that food just stays in the abdomen and goes no further. Below the age of 7 years, a frequently encountered notion was that food keeps going downwards until it reaches the feet, sometimes traveling after that to other parts (neck, head, arms) or being eliminated altogether. Children younger than 8 years of age (40%) did not think that food ever "comes out anywhere" and 13% thought that it can only come out the way it entered, i.e., orally, by throwing up or being turned upside down. The existence of the esophagus (or any counterpart thereof) was usually unknown below the age of 10 years. Reference to the intestines was not made by the majority before the age of 14 years and even then they were sometimes located above the stomach; sometimes the sequence of the small and large intestines was reversed. There was evidence of confusion regarding the number of the body's intestines, although they were always referred to plurally.

Some expressed conceptions of the vicissitudes of food after it is swallowed are diagramed below:

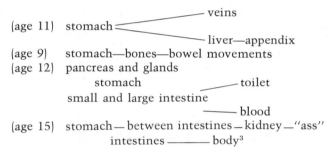

Among the least known digestive organs in the inquiry was the liver. (The spleen was even less known; none of the subjects in the trial phase of this research knew what it was, and so it was deleted from the questions adopted.) No children below the age of 9 years, and only 19% of the total sample, spontaneously listed the liver as one of their ingredients. Alleged location(s) of the liver(s) (some subjects thought they were paired) attested to prevailing misconceptions: legs, head, chest, total body, and various areas of the abdomen. The liver's size almost always was considerably underestimated. Most subjects did not come up with ideas regarding the function of the liver, and some did not think they had one unless they had eaten one. (Again one is tempted to make a hypothetical connection between the low significance attributed to the liver by most children in the sample, and the apparent indifference to the dangers of liver disease among adult alcoholics. It would be important to take the intervening step of sampling adult ideas about the liver to explore this potential relationship further. In addition to partial but correct responses about liver function that began to appear from the age of 9 years forward, alleged theories about its role included: It "helps us think"; "helps us bend our knees"; "is for the skin"; "protects the heart from being scratched"; "makes you look fat."

The questions about bowel movements, per se, were added when data-gathering already was underway. Thus, only 75 subjects had the opportunity to answer them; of these children, 69 offered explanations of their derivation and function. Table 4 summarizes these responses.

Table 4³   The Derivation and Function of Bowel Movements

	Age in years and months						Total group N = 75
	4.9–6.11 N = 15	7–8.11 N = 14	9–10.11 N = 21	11–12.11 N = 7	13–14.11 N = 9	15–16.11 N = 9	Percent per group
1. Don't know; no answer	7	21	10	—	—	—	8
2. So that we can go to the toilet	47	21	19	43	11	—	24
3. So we won't go in our pants	20	—	—	—	—	—	6
4a. Any reference to food or eating in association with bowel movements	47	27	67	57	78	56	55
4b. To make room for more food; to allow us to eat more	13	14	10	14	11	22	13
4c. Bowel movements are derived from food —i.e., they come from what we eat; food turns into b.m.'s	40	21	52	29	—	44	35
5. Bowel movements come from the kidneys (and other visceral organs)	—	—	—	14	—	22	4
6. We have b.m.'s to keep from getting too full, fat, stuffed, clogged; to avoid bursting or exploding	13	36	67	43	67	44	41
7. To maintain health and/or life; to avoid discomfort, illness, pain, medical intervention; to stay alive—(bursting and exploding excluded)	47	43	67	43	56	67	51
8. To dispose of waste, excess and/or unneeded material—("bad" things excluded)	—	—	24	14	56	67	23
9. To dispose of noxious material—i.e., poison, bad things	—	14	—	—	11	—	4

Strangely, although many children considered constipation (not having bowel movements) a serious, even terminal condition, none mentioned enemas or laxatives in this connection although presumably most subjects had experienced such treatment. (However, they were not specifically asked, "What could be done about it if you didn't have bowel movements?")

In view of some prevalent attitudes in most North American societies, surprisingly few children referred to bowel movements as being noxious, dirty, or dangerous, although they were often associated with health. With increasing age of subjects, there was a change from viewing the productions of bowel movements as social requirements

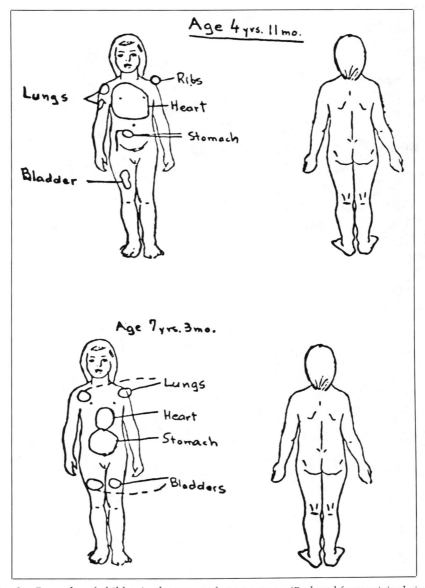

Fig. 3. *Examples of children's placement of some organs. (Reduced from original size.)*

("you go toilet 'cause Mommie tells you to") to seeing them as mechanical necessities (to make room for more food). Some connection of feces with food was made by the majority from the age of 9 years forward. Of 44 subjects who were asked how often they should defecate (care was taken to couch this question in words the child understood), 19 said three to seven times a day, and 12 said twice a day! The generality of and the explanation for this finding need to be pursued further, but it is tempting to hypothesize that children (and adults) feel obligated to defecate more than once daily, particularly since more than half the subjects queried felt that they did not defecate as

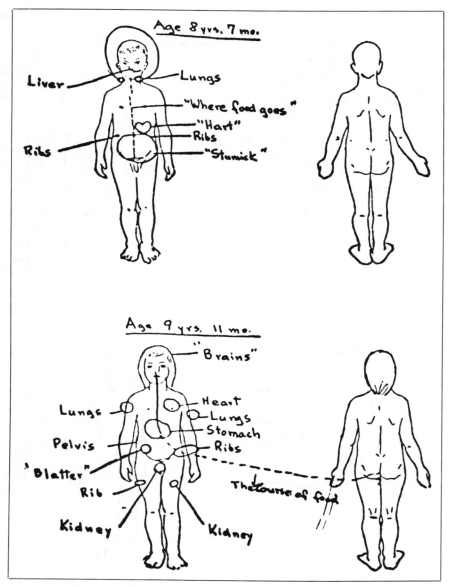

Fig. 4.   *Additional examples of children's placement of organs. (Reduced from original size.)*

often as they should. This finding may well reflect Western emphasis upon "regularity."

Another excretory function, urination, was explored indirectly by asking about the bladder's location and function. The degrees of ignorance and confusion expressed about this organ were astonishing. Some of it may have been caused by a lack of distinction between the gall bladder and the urinary bladder. However, until the age of 13 to 14 years, a minority associated the bladder with urination. (Unfortunately, the investigator did not ask specifically about ideas regarding the origin of urine.) In this connection, some children confused the alimentary and urinary tracts. In the Tait et al. study,[6] wherein subjects were required to draw the body interior, only 6% of 300 adults

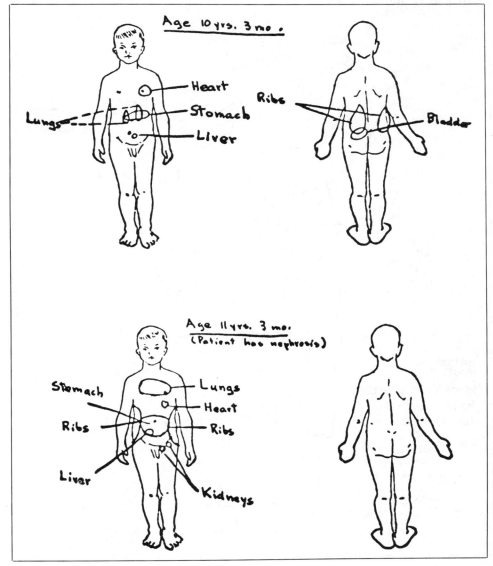

Fig. 4. (Continued.)

included the urinary bladder, and none of 22 sixth-graders sketched it in. In view of the very palpable sensations often emanating from the bladder, this apparently prevalent finding warrants further exploration.

CONCLUSION

The foregoing material is only a small sample of the information and notions some children acquire about the contents and functioning of the human body. Although much of this material may seem astonishing to an adult, it often is quite reasonable to a

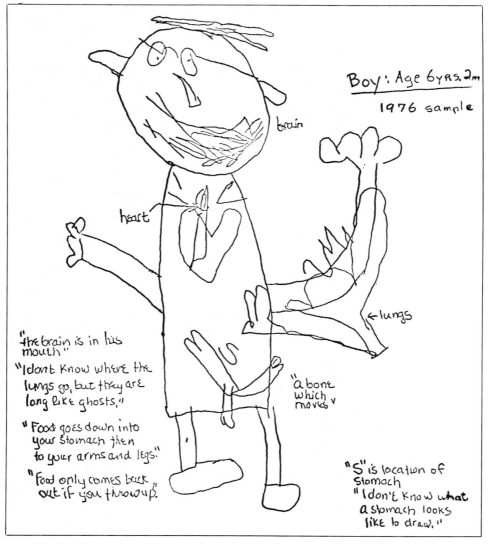

Fig. 5. *Spontaneous drawing of self with contents. (Reduced from original size.)*

child, given the sensations, observations, and verbally transmitted lore available to children at different ages and at their various cognitive stages of development. Obviously, as sometimes indicated in the questionnaire, many more questions related to the current topic would have elicited illuminating replies from the current subjects, as well as from other healthy or hospitalized children. Figures 3, 4, and 5 illustrate some representative graphic and verbal responses from a pediatric and a well sample of the child population.

The writer has found that many children know more about their bodies than has been supposed by some experts (see Fraiberg[1]). Nevertheless, the children's ideas (and probably those of many adults as well) about bodily construction and functioning are often vague, false, or nonexistent.

In the interests of health care and of explanation of specific illnesses, it might be advantageous to teach children early and accurately about their bodies. It should be noted, however, that there is no current evidence that such understanding prevents or even reduces the emotional trauma often associated with illness.

Numerous instructional materials for learning about the human body are available: Books such as *What's Inside of Me?* (Herbert S. Zim, New York: Morrow & Co., 1952); replicas of adult human bodies that, organ by organ, can be taken apart or assembled, for example, The Visible Man and The Visible Woman (Renwall Products, P.O. Box 428, Arlington, New Jersey, 08016), might be useful for such teaching. Unfortunately, many of these educational aids omit the genitalia.

It seems likely that children who have been exposed to specific and correct information about their bodies would be better informed about the body than those who have not. This hypothesis cannot be taken for granted, however, since little is known as yet about the development of the capacity to understand complex processes such as blood circulation, respiration, digestion, and the many others involved in human physiology. It is also yet unclear just how explanations should be couched to be appropriate to different age or intelligence levels.

In summary, the writer, who has worked as a psychologist in pediatric settings, is reminded of an incident reflecting this problem. A 7-year-old girl who was about to undergo surgery was "prepared" for the forthcoming event by a half-hour explanation given by an experienced child psychiatrist. When subsequently asked about what the doctor had told her, the young patient's inscrutable reply was, "Search me!"

REFERENCES

1. Fraiberg, S. *The magic years.* New York: Scribners, 1959.

2. Gellert, E. A developmental study of children's ideas about the content and function of the human body. Paper presented at the meeting of the Eastern Psychological Association, New York, April, 1960.

3. Gellert, E. Children's conceptions of the content and functions of the human body. *Genetic Psychology Monographs,* 1962, *65,* 293–405.

4. Nagy, M. H. Children's concepts of some bodily functions. *Journal of Genetic Psychology,* 1953, *83,* 199–216.

5. Schilder, P., Wechsler, D. What do children know about the interior of the body? *International Journal of Psychoanalysis,* 1935, *16,* 345–350.

6. Tait, C. D. & Archer, R. C. Inside-of-the-body-test. *Psychosomatic Medicine,* 1955, *17,* 139–148

YOUNG CHILDREN'S PERCEPTIONS
AND REACTIONS
═══════════TO HOSPITALIZATION═══════════

Ellis I. Barowsky, Ph.D

Adjustment to the exigencies of life is a developmental process, with the individual's abilities to cope predicated upon the previous establishment of healthy experiences and relationships. Hospitalization, which requires separation as well as adjustment to potentially threatening events, is one of these exigencies. Preparation, support, and protection from physical and psychological pain, while meeting the developing individual's daily needs, are indeed important; however, they cannot forestall or thwart anxieties which occur naturally. Recognition of those factors which contribute to maladjustment is essential in that their minimization will better help the child to cope with new and often frightening experiences.

One must be cautioned, however, against following a recipe approach in the prevention of any anxieties or stresses resulting from a new situation; such a conclusion would be extremely naive. Our only hopes are to recognize sources of stress, and accordingly to prepare the individual better on developmentally appropriate affective and cognitive levels. Thus the individual can anticipate and cope with such sources before they become overwhelming and threaten healthy functioning. In writing within the structure of a developmental model, there is no more appropriate manner in which to begin than to refer to the primary precipitant of infantile anxiety: separation.

Separation Anxiety

"We must remember that a child who lives in a world of vanishing objects perceives his human world on the same basis. It is not only glasses and key cases and teddy bears that have no existence when he cannot perceive them; mothers and fathers, loved persons, are subjected to the same primitive reasoning. They appear and disappear in a ghostly fashion, like dream people. And, unlike the furniture of the object world, these human love objects are necessary for the child's existence and his inner harmony."[17]

The message conveyed by this passage from *The Magic Years* as well as the information provided by the works of Spitz,[27,28] Bowlby,[7,8] and others has provided a firm base upon which the anxiety and psychopathy of prolonged estrangement of the mother-child unit and temporary separation from the love object have been seen as causing dire psychosocial consequences to the developing young child.

For a long time the issue of separation anxiety has played almost a noncontested role in explanations of the child's reaction to separation and to the disengagement precipitated by hospitalization, almost to the exclusion of other significant and contributing factors. More recently, however, staunch support of the mother-child relationship as an exclusive factor in child development has waned, and the more comprehensive interrelationships of psychosocial deprivation have received more emphasis.[10]

Nevertheless, the manifestations of separation anxiety are clinically valuable. They can be seen in those behaviors that become evident in the disruption of the proximity between two individuals after an affectional tie has been formed.[12] More specifically, the child's crying, sucking, for example, although approaching teleological explanation, nevertheless appear to be attempts to reestablish close physical contacts with a mother or mother surrogate after contact has been suspended. "The intensity of this attachment behavior may be heightened or diminished by situational conditions,[1] a factor to be noted in any attempt to gain understanding of a child's reaction to a strange physically and psychologically threatening environment. Underlying these fears is a lack of experience and of emotional maturity, for penultimate in the signs of maturity is the capacity of the individual to be alone.[30]

In certain cases of psychosocial deprivation, such as those of the institutionalized child and of children forming attachment late in infancy, object relations are affected[13] and emotional homeostasis may be undermined or compromised.

While the factor of separation anxiety cannot be underscored sufficiently for children at certain developmental stages, additional critical factors (some of which act as a catalyst to the manifest anxiety) are indeed influential in determining the course and reaction to hospitalization for most children.

Moreover, Fraiberg's[17] "vanishing of objects," may further be applied to the changes, temporary alterations, or disappearance of routines to which the child has been accustomed. Separation (hospitalization) disrupts parent-child, sibling, peer, and child-object relations and must be viewed in this perspective. The removal of the child from his accustomed routines often includes disruptions of school attendance, alterations in achievement of developmental milestones, and distortions of certain at least relative consistencies in the child's daily experience upon which he relies for security. The child's routines are displaced by the routines of the hospital, new restrictions, new people, as well as by the limitation in movement dictated by the nature of the illness requiring hospitalization.[12,19,21]

In essence, the child's potential reactions to this new situation and the demands placed upon him are dependent upon a matrix of interacting factors: age at hospitalization, the dynamics of the family's interaction, duration of hospitalization, number of prior hospitalizations, the nature of the illness, preparation for hospitalization, visitation arrangements for parents, therapeutic procedures to be performed, methods available to the child to reduce his distress reaction, postoperative reactions of parents, and postoperative medical treatment. These factors, as well as ideation normative for respective developmental stages, influence the child's reactions to and perceptions of hospitalization.

Age at Hospitalization

For the infant from birth to about 6 months of age, the separation of hospitalization, although it disrupts the parent-child relationship, is not accompanied by the prolonged rebelliousness, distress, and overt anxiety often manifested in the toddler. We do know, however, that even at this early age maternal and stimulus deprivation is not without its peril and influence on the child's physical and emotional development. The effect of separation from the home environment appears to be secondary to the effect of separation from the figure who represents the security of satisfying both bodily and emotional needs. Further, the detrimental effect of multiple providers of emotional and therapeutic care adds to the number of strangers in the infant's life and detracts from his integrated functioning. This combination of the mother's absence and the presence of strangers will generally elicit overt distress behavior and will further interfere with the child's exploration and learning from the environment. Realization of the presence and interaction of such factors has prompted more unified attempts to administer service, particularly to the disabled infant whose deficit remediation rests upon the skills of numerous specialists.[5]

Since the child of about 6 or 7 months has already formed somewhat of an attachment to its mother, it is not difficult to surmise the confusion which may ensue after separation. The child cannot yet understand that objects can exist when they are out of sight, and thus the "internal harmony" suggested by Fraiberg is now in jeopardy. The child from 2 to 4 years has not yet developed the concept of time, and although he may be aware that his parents will return to visit him, he can not judge when this will happen. He may therefore maintain a high level of anxiety in such anticipation, at the same time remaining unresponsive to establishing new relationships in his new setting. The infant's reactions to threats to his emotional integrity are not short-lived. Studies have shown that resulting disturbances are not confined to the period of hospitalization, but also may persist from preschool age to later adolescence. Using the population of children admitted to hospitals in Great Britain during the first week of March 1946, and following subsequent posthospitalization adjustment, Douglas[15] reported that 22% of the children upon returning home exhibited deterioration in their behavior. Problems most frequently reported included increased nervousness, difficulty in control, and problems relating to sleep. Less frequent areas of disturbance included loss of bladder control, temper tantrums, eating problems, and speech defects. These disturbances were found to be related to the age at which the child was hospitalized as well as to the duration of hospital stay.

A follow-up of these children in adolescence indicated sustained deficits in academic skills areas, attitudes toward work, behavior problems, and delinquency. The prevalence of these problems appeared to be a function of the frequency and duration of the hospitalization before the age of 5.[11,15]

Psychosocial Risk

Nonmedical conditions surrounding the period of hospitalization appear to play a significant role in the child's reaction and subsequent adjustment. Quinton and Rutter[25] found a significant relationship between psychosocial disadvantage of the child's family, multiple hospitalizations, and subsequent posthospitalization conduct and behavioral disturbances in children. In a sample of 10-year-old children, behavioral and psychiatric problems were increased after hospitalizations when two or more of the following factors existed:

1. The child was currently living in a broken home.
2. The mother showed psychiatric disturbance.
3. The father had police connection.
4. The child had been in the care of the local authority.
5. The home was seriously overcrowded (more than 1.5 persons per room) or there were four or more siblings.
6. The father had an unskilled or semiskilled occupation.

These factors would tend to place the patient under greater stress prior to the hospital admission, and the distress experienced by separation may have an interacting effect upon the resulting behavior.

Two cases illuminate the operation of certain of these risk factors.

M. was a 3½-year-old female child with spina bifida who was admitted to a major New York City hospital for a surgical procedure which involved the relocation of a dislocated hip. On a previous occasion she had been hospitalized for similar procedures. During the month prior to her admission, her parents separated and the father left the state to seek employment. The mother was receiving assistance for psychological problems which related to the break-up of the marriage a well as to the child's management. The hospital admission was initially uneventful. However, upon returning home M. became withdrawn, difficult to manage, and showed regression in certain behaviors such as the loss of previously attained bladder control. Further, she refused intervention as a physical therapy outpatient (with which she had been cooperative prior to hospitalization) and refused to interact with other children in a therapeutic nursery that she had been attending.

While separation at M.'s age may have been traumatic in itself, the added factor of the family's discord, possible perceived abandonment of the father, once the mother's need for psychological assistance may have served indirectly as a catalyst to the posthospitalization disturbances.

G. was a 4 ½-year-old male child referred as an outpatient for a neuromuscular evaluation. When brought to the medical facility for the procedure which involved psychological, physical, and occupational therapy diagnostic evaluation, he demonstrated phobic behavior toward the facility as well as severe avoidance of the respective therapists: he carried his mother's set of keys which he refused to give up even momentarily, and he further refused to use the center's bathroom facilities when it proved necessary. An interview with G's mother and observation of the mother-child interaction indicated a pathological symbiotic relationship in which the mother, who was mildly agoraphobic, unconsciously was maintaining the child's behavior. Even after being "weaned" from his mother over the course of numerous sessions, he continued to carry the keys as a transitional object, a behavior which was encouraged by G.'s mother.

In the cases of M. and G., whose ages placed them at risk, poor family relations and parent psychopathology may have exacerbated their anxieties surrounding separation and hospitalization.

The expenses of hospitalization in conjunction with a depressed socioeconomic level add further pressures and stresses to the family, and may result in the concomitant deprivation of the needs of other family members. This is particularly true of the family of the chronically ill or physically disabled child, where the costs of prosthetic and orthotic devices, medically related therapies, and medication, add further strain and contribute to the psychosocial risk. Although this deprivation may be borne as a martyrdom, or as repentance for guilt feelings surrounding the birth of a delayed or disabled child, it may also be manifested as resentment and rejection of the child. The resulting lack of attachment between parent and child may place additional stress upon the child patient and render him vulnerable to the anxieties surrounding hospitalization.

PREPARATION FOR HOSPITALIZATION

In an attempt to understand the importance of proper preparation, let us recall the conditions which prevail at the times when hospitalization becomes necessary. First, the child's medical need is provided by a virtual stranger. Second, the routines which provide the child with order to his life are disrupted and new routines take their place. Third, individuals who provide the emotional security necessary to maintain the child's "inner harmony" and integrity are separated from him. Fourth, it is quite possible that a painful procedure is to be employed, or as Haller[19] refers to it, a "premeditated injury" is inflicted. Moreover, this procedure is performed when the child is psychologically vulnerable due to the disordering of his environment and estrangement of love objects. Under such conditions of stress, the child may seek to assume a prior stage in his development when he was more secure, thus regressing to infantile behavior. He may further assume psychological postures inconsistent with his present stage of development.

To prevent the undermining of the emotional support which is provided by the parent, the prospect and scope of hospitalization must be explained with almost total candor. Parental emotional support and attachment will, in essence, remain the only consistency in the child's life upon which he can depend, and deviation from the truth will subvert efforts to maintain ego functioning. The child can more adequately deal with disruptions and substitutions in his routines if he is apprised beforehand of the impending hospitalization, the procedures to be employed, and the postoperative limitations which he will experience. Further, he must be made to understand that the final outcome of hospitalization will include a return home.

Since not all instances of hospitalization can be anticipated, a distinction must be made between procedures and priorities involved. I perceive three major categories of hospitalization: episodic, elective, and chronic.

Episodic hospitalization is generally one in which there is little advance knowledge of illness. This is best typified by emergency treatment where speed in providing medical intervention takes priority over psychological preparation for the procedure. In such an instance, since preventive measures generally cannot be taken to forestall stress reactions from the trauma, postoperative support services must be made available. These services would include a *post hoc* explanation to the child as to the procedure that occurred and what events will follow, why the procedure was necessary, and an attempt to dispel fears of punishment. Methods of stress relief, such as recreational and play therapy, should be made available to the child as soon as he is physically capable of participating in them.

Elective hospitalization allows the physician and family the prerogative of choosing the time of admission. The illness in these circumstances is not immediately life-threatening and time can be taken to prepare the child emotionally for the ensuing changes in his routines. Under these circumstances, psychosocial disadvantage, age of child, and other factors likely to place the patient at emotional risk can be considered in scheduling the hospitalization. Neglecting to consider such conditions places the child in an unnecessary and potentially dangerous position with regard to his emotional adjustment.

41

J. was a 3-year-old male child admitted to a small local hospital for the removal of his tonsils, an elective procedure. Two months prior to his hospitalization, J.'s family had adopted an infant male child. At J.'s age, the fear of abandonment is still present and, combined with the necessary separation of hospitalization, he was particularly at risk for a stress reaction. To further catalyze the separation anxiety, poor (if any) preadmission preparation was done. J.'s mother reports that he was given a "shot" to relax him, and immediately taken to the operation room, still screaming. J.'s mother was not permitted to accompany him while he was still quite awake.

Immediately after returning home, J. refused to interact with adults other than his parents and refused to leave his parents' side in new situations. The following months were marked with night terrors as well as the continued fear of adults. Two years after this incident, J. still refuses to separate from his parents or to talk to strangers. When he does talk, it is with an observable stammer.

An elective surgery that should have been postponed, due to the risk factors of the newly adopted child and J.'s abandonment fears, was compounded by a barbaric lack of preparation for the surgical procedure. The result is a disturbed, phobic child, with speech dysfluency two years posthospitalization. It might be suggested that, in general, elective surgery be postponed until after preschool years. When time is not an option, however, the child should be prepared for the actual admission as well as operative and postoperative procedures. To dispel fears of abandonment, he must further be assured that he will be returning home after hospitalization. The fear of a new and strange place must also be considered in preparing the child for hospital admission.

Today many hospitals provide books and brochures to children before they enter the hospital, to make the hospital experience seem like an adventure. A major New York City hospital provides a brochure written in the form of one long riddle that spurs the child's curiosity; the answer finally turns out to be the name of the hospital to which he will be admitted.[14] These booklets probably make the child more familiar with the routines to be encountered and therefore minimize the threat of the unknown.

Preparation for the actual admission can include a series of steps to dispel fears of abandonment. Just as a parent plays peek-a-boo with an infant, leading to the infant's expectation that the parent will return after disappearing from sight, similar procedures can be employed with the preschool child. A "peek-a-boo" preparation can begin with a number of visits of both parent and child to the hospital and then a return home. Once the child is admitted to the hospital, he can visit the x-ray room, operating room, etc. with his parent, physician, technician, or nurse, then returning to the hospital room. In both instances, the child experiences a return to a more secure environment. Barlow[4] reports that a hospital invited a group of children who were to be hospitalized for a party prior to their formal admission. After the party the children were given a conducted tour of the facilities, particularly of the facility for those services they were subsequently to receive.

The operative or therapeutic procedures to be experienced should also be introduced to the child patient. Many hospitals provide the physician, nurse, technician with "scripts" enabling them to better explain the impending procedure; for example, "You are going upstairs where a cardiac catheterization will be done. A cardiac catheterization is . . . ." and end, "Do you have any questions?" This leaves the door open for the child to ask questions and, possibly, to dispel some of his fears.

Preparation may also include allowing the child to perform the prospective procedure on a doll, or possibly even on a willing nurse (short of surgery). This might include mock administration of anesthesia, whose effects children often perceive as death and therefore fear, giving an injection, or bandaging the respective area that is to receive treatment.

Preparation for the postoperative period is also essential. The child may go through admissions and medical procedures without incident, and then wake in a recovery room and be frightened severely by postoperative procedures, such as the intravenous mechanism or postoperative oxygen being administered.

C. was a 17-year-old male with spina bifida, scoliosis, and other multiple anomalies for which he had been receiving treatment since birth. On what was approximately his tenth hospitalization for another bout with surgery, all went well until he woke in the recovery room to find a mask over his face. C. had not been informed of this possibility prior to surgery, and he started thrashing in his bed enough to shake all the postoperative equipment around him. Later C. said, "If they only told me before, I wouldn't have been so scared."

Chronic hospitalization involves the patient in numerous returns to the hospital, often for prolonged periods. The chronically hospitalized child experiences marked disruption in his routines, including absence from school which often precludes the establishment of friendships with peers and failure to attain age-appropriate academic skills. It is with this group of hospitalized patients that greatest long-term effects are observed. Many of the chronically hospitalized are orthopedically disabled; such a condition adds to the psychological risk factor, because the interaction of the disability and the prolonged separation may result in psychological disturbance.

The chronically hospitalized child requires particular and intensive support. Both psychological services and a well-rounded recreational and educational program must be made available. One of the most frequent complaints made by hospitalized adolescents is to the lack of educational preparation which leads to their perception that they are behind when reentering school. Their complaints also focus on the lack of sufficient activity, particularly during weekends. If possible, allowances should be made so that under certain circumstances even the long-term patient may leave the hospital to attend his regular educational or vocational placement.

B. is a physically disabled adolescent male who has had multiple and extended periods of hospitalization. Most recently, admission was made for extensive evaluation and further therapeutic intervention for an orthopedic disorder. Total inpatient treatment would have removed B. from the vocational educational placement he had been attending, and would have disrupted ties with classmates. Rather than upset this aspect of his functioning, adjustment was made to allow B. to leave the hospital in the afternoon to attend his vocational program and then return to the hospital at night and for the following morning's evaluation procedures. This practice required the cooperation of the hospital's medical staff as well as the local school system, but has apparently paid off in B.'s adjustment to the prolonged hospitalization.

HOSPITALIZATION

Consideration of risk factors in preadmission, admission, and preoperative preparation facilitate adaptation just so far. Further consideration must be made for the child's stay (as in the case of B). Disruption of routines and separation from parents, siblings, and friends must still be dealt with, as well as the child's acceptance of limitations placed upon him by his illness.

For the young patient, a number of strategies can facilitate his adjustment and minimize his potential for subsequent posthospitalization disturbance.

In an early study, Prugh[24] et al. observed that when hospital programs maintained rigid visiting schedules for patients, greater disturbance in the child during hospitalization and posthospitalization periods occurred as compared with those hospitals that allowed a greater frequency of visits. Not only the frequency but the length of the visit appears to play an important role in the adjustment during hospitalization, although how the time is utilized appears less significant. Even through children may seem to pay little attention to their visitors, frequent visiting should be encouraged.[18] Visits also should not be restricted to parents, but extended to siblings as well as other close friends. The presence of brothers and sisters appears to be consoling to the hospitalized child.

Recently many hospitals have turned to "rooming in" procedures as standard for the preschool hospitalized child. These procedures allow the mother or father to stay with the child through the night, and often also during diagnostic procedures and therapeutic intervention periods when the risk of stress is high. Allowing and even encouraging the parents to remain with the child during these times may have positive therapeutic effects as long as the medical staff sets limits concerning what parents may and may not do. Often parents can assist nurses with procedures, thus effecting their accomplishment even with the most anxious or reluctant child. The emotional support of the parent's presence can not be overstated, ". . . for any child . . . needs the mother's reassurance in the strange, disconcerting atmosphere of the hospital during what is often a frightening and painful episode. With the mother present, the child will rest, sleep and feel better."[29] In a corresponding way, allowing the mother to remain in the hospital affects her attitudes toward her child and in itself may present an ancillary intervention with immeasurable effects. These procedures also may facilitate parental adjustment to the child upon the child's return home.

J. is a 10-year-old male who underwent a tibial derotation and osteotomy to correct an orthopedic impairment. After surgery and an uneventful recovery, J.'s mother indicated that this was the first time she had been allowed to "room in" with him throughout his hospitalization. He had been hospitalized for similar orthopedic surgery on two prior occasions. Further questioning was directed at assessing the difference in visitation practices that J.'s mother had experienced. She volunteered that his need for medication to control pain appeared to be less and his hospital stay was shortened when she was permitted to "room in." Many explanations can be offered in attempting to explain this report. It is even possible that J. required no less medication than during previous hospitalization. However, it is significant that J.'s mother saw a positive change in J. in response to her presence.

The child may feel more comfortable in a strange surrounding if he is permitted to transplant a piece of the familiar from a more secure setting to his new quarters. Just as the young child sometimes insists upon bringing a favorite toy or object from home to his first school setting, the same may be encouraged in the preschool child who is entering the hospital. The child who is to remain in the hospital for an extended period of time, might bring along a favorite chair, lamp, or other small piece of furniture that he likes. Needless to say, clearance from the hospital should be obtained before any suggestion of this sort is even made to the child.

If it is not possible for the mother to room in with her toddler or infant, making a cassette tape of her voice and playing it to the child at frequent intervals may have a reassuring effect to the child.[4]

Across all age levels, children must be provided with activities to meet their specific developmental needs. This practice is receiving added support by hospital accreditation agencies in their attempts to develop and require individual program plans (IPP) for the long-term hospitalized child.[20] The activities must include recreational, therapeutic, and educational interventions and should accommodate the interest levels of each child. The IPP further should reflect any exceptional needs that the patient may have as a result of developmental delay, physical disability, or emotional lability.

Such patient needs can best be established not by guesswork, but rather by allowing the child to voice his opinion on matters which directly affect him. Many children are indeed able to voice their discontent, and a great deal can be learned from their statements regarding the failure of hospitals to satisfy their emotional needs.

When questioning the chronically hospitalized adolescent, a frequent complaint centers around the frequency and quality of educational services. I have often heard statements indicating discontent with the infrequency of tutoring, and with the tedium of the way subjects are taught. These complaints may be equally applicable to the nonhospitalized educational milieu under certain circumstances, but they are more significant for an individual confined to a single setting who must rely upon his experiences in that setting for educational growth as well as for emotional support.

Even younger children have an idea of those experiences which would make a hospitalization more palatable: they generally focus on the simple desire to be treated as a person!

M. is a 5-year-old female spastic quadriplegic whose cognitive functioning is within normal limits. She had been hospitalized on three occasions: at 1 year, 3½ years, and 5 years of age. During each hospitalization she underwent surgery for her heel cords. When questioned about what she did in the hospital, she said "It was boring. Lots of kids . . . didn't let you out of your bed. Never told us why they kept you in bed. They should have put phones in the kids' rooms. Parents can. We couldn't call our friends. I was there for my birthday. They had some nerve what they did to me. They gave me a shot when I was sleeping. My mother said she was going to come and see me. My mother left and I thought she wasn't going to see me."

An explanation of why M. was hospitalized, of what she might expect during her hospitalization, and assurance that her mother was going to visit, leave, and return would have made M.'s stay more acceptable. Nor was her evident need for peer interaction met sufficiently. Moreover, performing certain procedures while a child is asleep may lead to fears of going to sleep and of the dark, which are often found during the hospitalization and posthospitalization period. Hospitalization that overlaps the child's birthday and special holidays might also be avoided, especially in cases of elective surgery.

A similar report of a hospital experience is offered by R., a 13-year-old male who was hospitalized for a broken leg which did not mend properly.

R. was hospitalized for 2½ months. "At first it was boring. They wouldn't let me out of my room for two months 'cause I was in traction. It was terrible. I never should have went (sic) there. The nurses were good . . . there were only three kids in the hospital Christmas. It was boring. There for Thanksgiving, Christmas, and Halloween. I hate the presents. They don't know how to give presents. They give crayons and coloring books. When I got out I couldn't come to school 'cause I had a body cast. They shouldn't give a cast like that to no one. I hate when they give blood tests. They stick needles all over my body. I was afraid of that screw going in my leg. (They) have to put screws in to bring bone together . . . My parents had to leave. They put on a sheet so I wouldn't see it but there was a light . . . and all the blood gushing."

In both cases, the patients' developmental needs were certainly neglected. Socialization and peer interaction were evidently stifled, and activities were provided irrespective of needs. The irrelevance is unobtrusively stated by R. when he refers to the crayons and coloring book which would have been more appropriate for a younger child, but certainly not for a teenager. It is also evident that when a painful and frightening procedure is employed, exclusion of the parent does not add to the emotional security of the child.

Both children expressed their disturbance over the limitations imposed upon them by their illness. Proper preparation, as well as alternative activities during their confinement, would have made the limitations less aggravating.

The perceived effectiveness of the interventions employed also contributes to the hospitalized child's adjustment. If the child can see progress in overcoming his illness and can anticipate its course, he is more likely to cooperate with procedures although they may be somewhat uncomfortable. However, this consideration in part depends upon the nature of the illness.

The "visibility" of the illness plays a role in the acceptance of limitations and in the feeling that it is receiving the attention it should. Orthopedic patients, for example, are more likely to accept restrictions placed upon them than are cardiac patients, because of the visible nature of orthopedic disorder and the tangible presence of the devices facilitating recovery.[6] This is not to say that the child's adjustments to prosthetic and orthotic devices are without incident.[3,9,11] It is much easier to explain the need for restricted activity to the child who is casted and whose mobility is obviously compromised, than it is to explain the same need to the child who cannot "see" his illness. The more care taken to anticipate the child's social and emotional needs, the more the hospitalized child will be able to cope with this traumatic rearrangement of his life.

Nevertheless, adjustment to the hospital is often incomplete and the young patient will demonstrate aberrant reactions and perceptions, which are based upon the limited experience of youth and on a limited ability to integrate contemporary experiences into a preestablished framework. Fears and anxieties associated with former occasions sometimes are revived when the child enters the hospital; past experience with doctors, hospitals, and separation will affect the child's reaction to the present situation. Often, the child's sensitivity to the parents' reaction and his identification with the parent will result in a negative advance response.

In addition to his fears of abandonment, the child may perceive hospitalization as punishment for "bad actions," or "bad thoughts." Particularly, children from about the age of 4 may see surgery or similar intervention as mutilation—or as some will have it—castration. The patient may react by screaming, throwing a tantrum, or through withdrawal, regression, denial, or the employment of other protective defenses. When these defenses fail, decompensation and severe emotional withdrawal may be evidenced. The more overt behaviors are easily identified and dealt with accordingly. Others may evolve to what is perceived by the unwary professional as healthy adjustment to the hospitalization, in that the child may become quiet, acquiescent, and cooperative. Just as in a classroom setting, it is often the loud, disruptive child who receives the needed psychological assistance while the quiet, withdrawn child is psychotherapeutically ignored and left to his own resources, being apparently settled.

Young children go through stages in which they initially exhibit typical stress reactions such as crying, and finally become more acquiescent. This acquiescence is, however, nonetheless pathological because the fears and anxieties are not dispelled, but are maintained in a fashion in which they have become less accessible to intervention. These patterns of "settling in" may persist throughout the hospitalization and may be seen upon readmission or subsequent contact with future health service providers. A striking example is that of the very young child with a history of hospitalizations who shows not even the slightest overt reaction to separation for a therapeutic procedure.

On a number of occasions, I have observed children who leave their parents to take any outstretched hand and who follow the requests of a virtual stranger without even the slightest glance back, but who then fail to establish any visual contact with the therapist or physician. Such behavior is more disconcerting to the professional than that of the reluctant child who attempts initially to thwart separation.

If the child is to have his fears dispelled, the clinician must establish an atmosphere of trust, preferably through a therapeutic alliance. Intervention through any channels available to the child is indeed vital to healthy adjustment. Psychological intervention in a form accessible to the child's developmental level may include play therapy, art therapy, or even the modeling of other more healthy children. When the child is limited by his illness and cannot actively engage in play, the clinician sometimes can play for him by manipulating the environment in accordance with the child's interests and abilities.[23] Erickson[16] points out that adults, when traumatized, tend to solve their tension by talking it out, and that it is play which is often the child's "talking out." If possible, the child should be given an opportunity to discuss and explore his fears; however, this is a difficult if not impossible approach with many young hospitalized children.

A Note on the Handicapped Child

The handicapped or developmentally delayed child, because of the nature of his disorder, is at special risk in regard to adverse effects and stress of hospitalization. The disabled child is more likely to have multiple hospitalizations for extended periods of time, a situation which has been shown to be related to adverse residual effects. Repeated separation from the primary care-giver prevents the child from forming a secure attachment; in turn, the absence of this bond leaves the child with little support when he is displaced from home to the threatening environment of the hospital. The child's need for multiple therapies to meet his developmental delay further precludes attachment to any one significant person. In addition, impaired mechanisms for communication, physical manipulation, and the like, may make it more difficult for the child to reduce levels of anxiety and stress through talking things out and through play. Lack of stimulation resulting from immobilization calls for modifications in the child's hospital environment within the limits imposed by medical treatment. Morgenstern[22] suggests that the "monotony of a constant environment can partly be met by periodic changes in the position of the bed, either within the ward or far from the ward to the playroom." Even the child who requires immobilization need not view his environment from a supine position. Circumstances may permit the use of prone boards, standing braces, or standing tables to permit the immobile child an upright or quasi-upright position. Such a position is more conducive to manipulation of toys and learning materials; it frees his hands and arms to some degree while furnishing the necessary physical support to maintain the upright posture. In addition, changing the child's position from prone to supine to upright tends to minimize descubiti (bed sores) which often result from confinement to one position for a prolonged period of time. Casting, in the treatment of orthopedic disability, need not render the child immobile or prevent his interaction with stimuli, including individuals in his environment. When a child is permitted to explore his world, activities may be made available within limited or confined space so that his proximity to other children functioning under similar circumstances will foster increased socialization.

Children with central nervous system damage or similar developmental delays often manifest impaired sensory functioning. Caution should be employed in not inundating the sensorily impaired child with stimuli in all modalities, since an optimum level exists for any given child.

In developing toys for the very young hospitalized child, stress should be placed upon the need to expose these children to objects that provide "adequate tactile, visual, auditory and kinesthetic stimuli."[31] Additional emphasis should be placed upon other criteria which require toys to be "nontoxic, nonflammable . . . too big to swallow . . . not small enough to be stuffed into casts and durable." The role of toys in alleviating acute distress in children can not be overstressed.[26]

Further considerations for the child's comfort and emotional security must focus on adjustment to prosthetic and orthotic devices, as well as upon possible impairment of body image and the potential insults to the development of a healthy ego. There is strong reason, therefore, to encourage rooming in procedures for the parents of the handicapped hospitalized child, as well as to reduce the number of therapists intervening in the child's care. The use of the parent as therapist whenever such procedures can be taught helps to strenghthen the strained bond between parent and child. The parent's presence may also assist the child to communicate his needs, thus dispelling fears of abandonment. The disabled child who appears deficient in communication skills may have a gestural system which is familiar to the parent. The parent's participation in interpreting this system may help to allay frustration in meeting the child's emotional and physical needs. While these considerations may be relevant to every child, they are especially important for the disabled child in meeting the demands and pressures imposed by his hospitalization.

Hospitalization is indeed a disrupting and threatening experience even for the older, more experienced adult patient. Rationalization often fails to serve a palliative function, and emotional strain may overwhelm even the most well-defended individual. With more limited coping skills, less elaborate problem-solving schema, and greater vulnerability, the young child is at particular psychological risk. While adequate and adept preparation for an ensuing hospital experience is no absolute guarantee against psychological discomfort, it may greatly reduce the probability of acute psychic trauma.

REFERENCES

1. Ainsworth, M. D. S., & Bell, S. M. Attachment exploration, and separation: Illustrated by the behavior of one-year-olds in a strange situation. *Child Development*, 1970, *41*, 49–67.

2. Ainsworth, M. D. S. Patterns of attachment behavior shown by the infant in interaction with his mother. *Merrill-Palmer Quarterly*, 1964, *10*, 51–58.

3. Aitkin, G. T, & Frantz, C. H. Prosthesis for the juvenile amputee. *American Journal of Disabled Children*, 1955, *89*, 137–143.

4. Barlow, J. Meeting the developmental needs of hospitalized children: Infants, toddlers, preschoolers. Paper presented at the meeting of the Association for the Care of Children in Hospitals, New York, 1976.

5. Barowsky, E. I. Transdisciplinary assessment and habilitation of the atypical infant. *Pediatric Psychology*, 1975, *3*, 12–14.

6. Bergmann, T., & Freud, A. Children in the Hospital. New York: International Universities Press, 1965.

7. Bowlby, J., Ainsworth, M. D. S., & Bell, S. M. Attachment exploration and separation: A follow-up study. *British Journal of Medical Psychology*, 1956, *29*, 211–247.

8. Bowlby, J. The nature of the child's tie to his mother. *International Journal of Psychoanalysis*, 1958, *39*, 350–373.

9. Brooks, M. B., Beal, L. L., Ogg, H. L., et al. The child with deformed or missing limbs, his problems and prosthesis. *American Journal of Nursing*, 1962, *62*, 88–92.

10. Caldwell, B. M. The effects of psychosocial deprivation on human development in infancy. *Merrill-Palmer Quarterly*, 1970, *16*(3).

11. Chittenden, R. F. Problems related to prosthesis in childhood. *Applied Journal of Orthopedics and Prosthetics*, 1956, *8*, 197–208.

12. Cooke, R. E. Effects of hospitalization upon the child. In J. Haller et al. (Eds.), *The hospitalized child and his family*. Baltimore: Johns Hopkins Press, 1967, pp. 3–18.

13. Decarie, T. G. *Intelligence and effectivity in early childhood*. New York: International Universities Press, 1965.

14. Dickinson, L., Frankel, E., & Shufer, S. *Where is a place that . . . ?* New York, Lenox Hill Hospital.

15. Douglas, J. W. B. Early hospital admissions and later disturbances of behaviour and learning. *Developmental Medicine and Child Neurology*, 1975, 17, 456–480.

16. Erickson, E. *Childhood and society*. New York: Norton, 1950, p. 222.

17. Fraiberg, S. H. *The magic years*. New York: Scribner's, 1959, p. 51.

18. Gellert, E. Reducing the emotional stresses of hospitalization for children. *American Journal of Occupational Therapy*, 1958, *12*(3), 125–129; 155.

19. Haller, J. A. Preparing a child for his operation. In J. Haller et al. (Eds.), *The hospitalized child and his family*. Baltimore, Johns Hopkins Press, 1967, pp. 19–32.

20. Joint Commission on Accreditation of Hospitals: *Standards for community agencies: Serving persons with mental retardation and other developmental disabilities*. Chicago, 1973.

21. Madden, M. Reactions of young preschool children to hospitalization. Unpublished masters thesis, Hunter College, City University of New York, 1976.

22. Morgenstern, F. S. Facilities for children's play in hospitals. *Developmental Medicine and Child Neurology*, 1968, *10*, 111–114.

23. Petrillo, M., & Sanger, S. *Emotional care of hospitalized children*. Philadelphia: Lippincott, 1972.

24. Prugh, D., et al. A study of the emotional reactions of children and families to hospitalization and illness. *American Journal of Orthopsychiatry*, 1953, *23*, 70.

25. Quinton, D., & Rutter, M. Early hospital admissions and later disturbances of behaviours: An attempted replication of Douglas' findings. *Developmental Medicine and Child Neurology*, 1976, *18*, 447–459.

26. Rutter, M. Maternal deprivation reconsidered. *Journal of Psychosomatic Research*, 1972, *16*, 241–250.

27. Spitz, R. A. Hospitalism: An inquiry into the genesis of psychiatric conditions in early childhood. In O. Fenichel et al. (Eds.), *Psychoanalytic studies of the child* (Vol. 1). New York: International Universities Press, 1945, pp. 53–74.

28. Spitz, R. A. Hospitalism: A follow-up report. In O. Fenichel et al. (Eds.), *Psychoanalytic studies of the child* (Vol. 2). New York: International Universities Press, 1946, pp. 113–117.

29. Williams, E. D., & Jelliffe, D. B. Mother and child health: *Delivering the services*. New York: Oxford University Press, 1972.

30. Winnicott, D. W. *The capacity to be alone in maturational processes and the facilitating environment*. London: Hogarth, 1965.

31. Wolinsky, G. F., & Kolher, N. A cooperative program in materials development for very young hospitalized children. *Rehabilitation Literature*, 1973, *34*, 34–41.

PSYCHOLOGICAL ISSUES IN CHRONIC ILLNESS AND HANDICAP

Edward Sperling, M.D.

With the virtual conquest of infectious diseases of childhood, and with improved neonatal care for infants at risk, chronic illness and disability have become the most important problem in pediatrics. This is true not only because of the large numbers of children involved but also because of the profound and long-lasting effects of such conditions upon the child and his family. The birth of a child with congenital anomalies, the discovery of diabetes in a young child, the development of paraplegia following a childhood accident, are deeply shocking events that will occupy these children and their families for the rest of their lives. Depression, rage, anxiety, and despair are ever-present threats, straining the coping capacities of these children and their families to their limits. And yet many, probably most, of these handicapped children grow up to be as well adjusted psychologically as their physically healthy counterparts.[17]

Such a happy outcome is not easily won, however. Personality resources of child and family must play a major role. But even the most resourceful family needs the skillful support and guidance of a compassionate caretaker in dealing with children with chronic illness and handicap. In order to best fulfill this role, the physician, nurse, rehabilitation worker, and other professional caretakers should be thoroughly acquainted with the various pathways these children and their families traverse and with the various outcomes at which they arrive. This chapter aims to survey this terrain, discussing first, the prevalence of chronic illness, and then its psychological effects. How these effects are influenced by the child's stage of development and by the nature of the illness or handicap will be reviewed, and some illustrations of parental and professional efforts to help chronically ill children will be given.

MAGNITUDE OF THE PROBLEM

Without including mental deficiency, it is estimated that, depending upon strictness of definition, 5% to 20% of children suffer from chronic illness and handicap.[22] In one of the largest surveys of its kind, Pless and Douglas[20] report on a study of children (N = 5,362) randomly selected from all the children born in Great Britain during the first week in March 1946 (N = 15,130). The random samples were followed from birth until the age of 15 years, with information periodically obtained from mothers, doctors, schools, and the children themselves. In addition, all the children were tested for IQ level. In this study, chronic illness is defined as an illness which lasts over three months in any given year or which requires one month or more of continued hospitalization. Moreover, the illness must interfere with "the child's ordinary activity to some degree."

Using this definition, the prevalence of chronic illness was found to be 112 per 1000. The three most frequent types of illnesses were respiratory (20%), neurological (14%), and musculoskeletal (11%). (Mental deficiency was not included in this survey.) Males outnumbered females 1.4 to 1, compared to 1.1 to 1 in the general population. The severity of illness was distributed as mild (54%), moderate (34%), and severe (12%). Different surveys using varying sampling procedures and different definitions yield a prevalence rate of 5–20%, depending largely upon the severity of illness included in the definition; however, an average of 10% can serve as roughly accurate. At the same time it should be remembered that many of these illnesses, e.g., diabetes and cystic fibrosis, are lifelong. In the Great Britain survey, it was discovered that, regardless of age of onset, the illness was still present at age 15 in more than 60% of the children.

EFFECTS OF CHRONIC ILLNESS AND HANDICAP

Having indicated the extent of chronic childhood illness in the population at large, the question arises as to the effect of chronic illness and handicap on the psychological development of the afflicted child and his family. Ideally, the answer to this question should derive from longitudinal studies in which children with chronic diseases are matched with suitable controls; it is well known, however, how difficult it is actually to complete such studies. In their comprehensive survey of chronic childhood disorders, Pless and Pinkerton state, "In striking contrast to the abundance of studies describing problems of adjustment in childhood, however, there is paucity of evidence to help settle the important question of adult outcome. This lack of evidence reflects the enormous difficulty in mounting prospective or longitudinal studies; but it may also reflect a curious lack of interest on the part of pediatricians in the long-term results of their care. Whatever the case, the omission remains."[21, p. 162] In a thoughtful article regarding research on families with handicapped children, Hewett adresses the question of whether later maladjustment in the handicapped child is caused by the handicap or by the parents. Referring to readers of such research literature, she states, "If they read more than one book or paper they will discover confusing differences in the ways in which studies have been conducted or even more confusion and conflict in the results."[12, p. 34]

Three large surveys of children's development give us a rough guide as to the effect of chronic illness on psychological adjustment.[22] The previously cited National Survey of Child Health and Development followed more than 5,000 children from birth to the age of 15 years, with periodic examinations and assessments. The Rochester Child Health Survey examined a 1% random sample of all children under 18 years of age living in Monroe County, New York (N, ages 6–16 = 1,756). Information was gathered in a semistructured household interview supplemented by a battery of psychological tests given to each child and by information from parents and teachers. Both of these studies revealed a consistent but statistically nonsignificant excess of psychological difficulties among those with chronic illnesses, when compared with controls.

The third survey, the Isle of Wight study, examined all children from the ages of 10 to 12 years living on the Isle of Wight (N = 3,271). This survey revealed psychiatric disorders in 17% of the children with chronic illness, compared with 7% in the healthy population.

In reviewing these three surveys, Pless and Roghmann conclude, "Based on these findings, about one child in ten will experience one or more chronic illnesses by the age of 15, and up to 30% of these children may be expected to be handicapped by secondary social and psychological maladjustments. Possibly half of this latter malfunctioning can be attributed to the physical disorders."[22]

Pless and Pinkerton[21] have summarized a large body of literature concerning the consequences of chronic illness during adolescence and adult life. Chronically ill adolescents present a mixed picture. Referring to studies by Collier[9] and others, Pless and Pinkerton point out that a number of studies of adolescents with diabetes found them not to differ significantly from matched healthy controls with respect to a number of personality traits, and that their overall academic achievement and adaptive behavior were within normal limits.

Some studies are cited to illustrate that siblings of handicapped children may be more severely affected psychologically than the handicapped child. Shere and Kastenbaum[32] found that the nonaffected sibling of a handicapped twin may more frequently be emotionally disturbed than the affected twin. Similarly, Demb and Ruess[11] found that although the national average rate of high school dropouts is 30%, the rate for children with "clefts" (lip, palate, or both), is 25% while the rate for their siblings is 42%! The dropout rate was similar within families, thus pointing to an interaction between the condition and family characteristics rather than to the physical condition per se as a causative factor in the dropout rate.

If school achievement is used as an indicator of adjustment, once again the picture is mixed. In 1966, Klapper and Birch reported a followup study of children with cerebral palsy. In this study, 155 children, 2–16 years of age, were initially assessed in 1947–48; of these, 89 were followed up in 1962–63 by home interviews and psychological testing. Although the educational level of the 89 adolescents and young adults was consistent with their intellectual levels and social backgrounds, their occupational and social achievement lagged behind. To quote the authors, "The typical individual at followup, therefore, was a young adult with a high school education, a menial job, financially dependent, unmarried, living at home with his family and minimally involved in community activities and interpersonal relationships."[13] While these youngsters achieved adequately in school, other groups of children with cerebral palsy[5] and with epilepsy[28] were significantly behind their healthy peers.

Studies such as the ones discussed above yield conflicting and seemingly contradictory results, because findings are highly dependent upon the nature of the study, the particular population being studied, and other like factors. Despite these limitations, some of the more general findings are remarkably consistent and well established.[21] These are:

1. Children with chronic illness generally will have rates of maladjustment higher than those of comparable peers.

2. Certain features of the illness—its age of onset, its course and severity, its visibility, the degree of handicap it imposes—will affect the overall adjustment of the child.
3. Personality attributes of the child—his maturity, intelligence, charm, sense of humor, special talents—will play a major role in how well the child manages with his illness.
4. Family resources—stability, warmth, commitment, and flexibility—all of which naturally interdigitate with the personality of the child, will play a major role in the long-range outcome.
5. Support systems available to the family—the quality and affordability of medical care; the extended family, friends, and community resources—will weigh heavily in ameliorating suffering and in the ultimate adjustment to the illness.

We can add that the chronicity of illness and disability constitute a severe trial to the child and family, adding an extra dimension of anxiety, grief, and effort to the pain and discomfort imposed by illness itself.

An Atmosphere of Stress

The onset of a chronic illness or the development of a handicap profoundly alters the life of the afflicted child. The threat to life, the loss of function, the changes in appearance (cosmetic changes) call forth intense reactions of anxiety, grief, rage, and despair. Becoming less physically attractive or less able causes profound feelings of becoming less worthy. Threats to survival, to body integrity, and to self-esteem marshall defenses and coping devices which may or may not be adaptive. The patient becomes a "survivor" or a "cripple" or a "freak" and thus feels alienated from other people. Similar feelings of anxiety, rage, and despair are aroused in the parents. They must draw upon defenses and develop coping styles that will, in turn, influence their own equanimity, their care of the child, and their interaction with professional caretakers. Doctors, nurses, and other therapists respond to the illness and handicap with their own emotional responses, empathic or defensive, as they interact with the afflicted child and family.

In essence, an important chronic illness creates a cycle of *severe stress* with an attendant stressful atmosphere that must be dealt with by the child, family, and professionals. Such an atmosphere of stress constitutes its own world, in which reality takes on a different aspect—more somber, charged, threatening, and unpredictable. The helping nurse can suddenly become an instrument of pain. The cooperative parent may be transformed into an explosive antagonist. A reasonable child can become a protesting and rejecting patient. A trivial lapse in hospital routine may loom as an extraordinary breach of professional care.

During the first two days following the birth of a premature malformed infant, the father visited his child in the premature intensive care unit, maintaining a quiet, stoic, but friendly attitude toward the staff. On the third day, he found a blood pressure cuff lying in the infant's crib and leaning against its cheek. He burst into a rage and threatened to sue the staff for negligence.

This atmosphere of stress may be thought of in two phases: acute and chronic. The acute phase, with its dramatic impact and high intensity, appears when the disease is first discovered; when hospitalization, important medical or surgical interventions, or potentially toxic chemotherapy are instituted; or when there is an upsurge in the intensity of the illness. The chronic phase appears during the day-in, day-out strain of coping with the ongoing symptoms of illnesses such as diabetes, cystic fibrosis, asthma; or of handicaps such as paraplegia. Both phases constitute a fluctuating but ever-present, largely invisible but potentially disruptive world of stress. The nature of this volatile atmosphere should be thoroughly understood by the professional person so that he may not only find his own way but also serve as guide for the child and family in their strange and frightening encounters with illness and handicap.

The chief variables in this world of stress are the developmental stage of the affected child, the nature of the illness or handicap, the coping resources of the child and family, the nature of the medical caretaking network, and the support structure available to the child and family in the community. In what follows, each of these variables will be discussed in turn.

AGE AND DEVELOPMENTAL CONSIDERATIONS

Infancy. The important psychological issues in this earliest era have to do with parent-child bonding. In recent years our views about the development of infants and their ability to respond to their environment have undergone considerable change. A decade or two ago, infants in the first few weeks and months of life were thought to function almost exclusively on a subcortical level, to be mainly involved with sleeping, eating, and maintaining internal homeostasis. We now see infants as able to make visual and auditory discriminations even during the first few days of life, and as entering into a subtle but elaborate pattern of interaction with the caretaking adult. (See Rexford, Sander, and Shapiro[25] for a recent overview of work in this field.)

Our views of motherhood have also undergone some transformation. The maternal response to the infant has been scrutinized and found to be more variable and complex than is implied by the term *maternal instinct.* Some recent work has indicated that bringing the mother and newborn together during the first few days of the infant's life may alter the mother's response to that child for months, perhaps years.[14] A related finding has to do with parents and children born with a life-threatening condition such as extreme prematurity or illness. This is an area of burgeoning investigation, however, and the long-term results are not yet known.

We are becoming more sensitive to the parental trauma of giving birth to a child whose development is at risk; we are learning to pay special attention to psychological approaches to such parents.[4,14,15,30] One of the chief lessons we have learned is the importance of the first communication to the parents concerning the illness or defect. The timing and nature of this communication make a deep impact on the parents and influence their ability to adjust to the child as well as influencing their feelings toward their medical caretakers. Of course, if a child is born with a cleft palate or with spina bifida, the defect will be obvious from the beginning and cannot long be hidden from the mother. But when the defect is not so visible, e.g., Down's syndrome, parents may not become aware of the condition for months or even years. When mothers of such children are surveyed, they generally express the importance of being told the truth as early as possible. Carr[8] cites an example of a mother who became aware that her child was abnormal just after the hospital pediatrician had left the hospital after completing his weekly rounds. Since the nurses were not empowered to give her this information, the mother had to wait for a week before she could get a straight answer to her questions. In addition to the element of timing, mothers express the need to have such information expressed in a clear but warm and sympathetic manner by a person who is open to being questioned and who will continue to be available for further information and advice.

We have learned that, right from the beginning, parents should be encouraged to be as physically and emotionally close to their infants as is feasible, even when the infants need the care of a neonatal intensive care unit. Obviously, however, each person must be dealt with as an individual; some mothers, for example, may be more comfortable separated from their newborn. Nevertheless, it should be kept in mind that the highly artificial arrangements which modern Western medical care has decreed are just that. Barnett, Leiderman, and Grobstein[3] have investigated behavioral patterns in 220 cultures and found that there is no cultural practice anywhere except in the premature and high-risk nurseries of the Western world which routinely and completely separates a mother from her infant during the first few days after birth.

Toddler and preschool years. By learning to walk and to talk, the child takes giant strides—the metaphor is meaningful—toward becoming a separate person, physically and psychologically. He gradually emerges from the sensorimotor stage[18] and can begin to divorce thought from action. He develops a rudimentary sense of time, space, intentionality, causation, personal relationships, and the future. By the age of 2 years he has a vocabulary of 200-300 words and can understand many more,[10] although his reasoning is crude, fragmented, dominated by egocentrism and animism,[19] and prone to false conclusions. His fantasy life is full of violence.[2] The young afflicted child tends to assume that his illness or handicap is a punishment brought on by his bad behavior. Adults are seen as omnipotent beings who, besides meting out punishments such as needles and operations, could magically cure him if they so wished. This magical, unpredictable, and arbitrary view of the world infuses the atmosphere of anxiety surrounding illness and medical procedures with its own volatile quality.

The need of young children to have their parents close to them, especially during periods of stress such as hospitalization, has been well documented[24,33] and is widely known, if not always practiced. In coping with chronic illness, wherein hospitalizations and medical procedures are repeated, prolonged, and recurrent throughout many years of the child's life, the need to have a loving and protective caretaking adult near at hand is all the more multiplied. What is not so readily appreciated is the necessity for the parent to understand how the child's development is affected by the illness so that the parent can bolster the child's sense of mastery, and can arrange for suitable compensatory experience for the child. Parents and physicians alike tend to underestimate the need and the capacity of a 2- to 3-year-old child to be prepared for medical procedures, separations, and the like.

The tendency to underestimate the needs and capacity of young children is dramatically illustrated by Shere and Kastenbaum,[32] who studied the interaction between mothers and their young children who had cerebral palsy. Thirteen children between the ages of 2½ and 4½ years, unable to speak or walk, were studied. The children were tested psychologically; the mothers were interviewed carefully and extensively. The mother-child interaction was studied during a minimum of six home visits per child of two or three hours' duration. These visits were followed by a guidance program of five "lessons" and five "practica" spread out over a five-month period.

One of the most striking findings was how uniformly the mothers encouraged nearly complete psychological passivity in their children. In contrast to their healthy siblings, these children when left alone were typically placed in front of the television with no toys within reach. Also, they were not encouraged to play with toys or with members of their families. Instead, all efforts were bent toward encouraging the children to overcome their physical incapacities: for example, by holding a desirable toy at some distance so that the child would try to move towards it. The subsequent guidance program allowed some of the mothers to stimulate their children to play and to explore materials, thereby encouraging a more mature level of interaction.

The school years. J. S. Bruner has written, "We begin with the hypothesis that any subject can be taught effectively in some intellectually honest form to any child at any stage of development."[7, p. 33] This dictum holds true particularly for the child of school age. During these years, the child leaves the egocentric world of the preschooler—a world in which he tends to measure everything in reference to himself—to enter the world of objective standards, the world of logical classes, the realm of peers, a world in which he is judged by what he can produce, athletically, artistically, and scholastically. Children now know more about the body and how it works (see Chapter 2). Well developed school-age children can understand a good deal about the causation of illness and handicap, the necessity for treatment, as well as something about prognosis. Under the impact of fear and pain, their understanding may temporarily break down and need bolstering, but in the long run it is a valuable asset.

An 8-year-old boy suffered a 40% burn over his trunk and extremities. During most of his two months of hospitalization he was mainly depressed, apathetic, and complaining. As his burn and grafts healed, he began to discuss going home and to think about his future adjustment. He anticipated that the hardest moment for him would be his first day back in school and he worried about being self-conscious. By thinking ahead and discussing his thoughts, he was able to prepare himself for a critical time.

Adolescence. The impact of illness or handicap can be most sharply seen in adolescents. Before this time, the child's self-image, self-esteem and basic adjustment to life are largely dependent on his family, particularly his parents. A young handicapped child, if he is loved and esteemed by his family, can generally cope with the pressure of the outer world—cooperation with peers, accomplishment in school—as important as these may be. But while the adolescent's adjustment is, as well, heavily dependent on the support of his family, a distinct difference appears. This difference lies in the basic task of adolescence: the task of gradually giving up his home of origin and loosening parental ties while, at the same time, forging his own independent personality and life. The adolescent knows that his parents do not always know best, and that he has to find a way of coping that suits him individually. His peer group now takes on a new importance, since in the not-too-distant future, he will be living amongst his peers— perhaps even married to one of them—rather than in his parental home. Moreover, his emerging sexuality accentuates his interest in his body, which even if healthy, becomes the subject of intensive scrutiny from all conceivable angles. The adolescent, then, in this developmental sense, must face his illness alone—a fact that adds poignancy to his struggle with his physical condition. Schowalter, Ferholt, and Mann[29] have written a moving paper on an adolescent's decision to die, that dramatically highlights this issue.

Of course, the way an adolescent reacts to his illness may be intimately bound up with the typical struggles of this stage of development. The diabetic may go off his diet to be "one of the boys," or to defy his parents or their surrogate (his doctor), or to arouse parental concern. He may ignore his illness as a way of trying to preserve a view of himself as being no different from anyone else.

A boy who suffered from epilepsy insisted on being part of the lighting crew of his high school drama group. This job involved climbing ladders, a risk which he steadfastly overlooked despite his parents' objections. After having examined this issue in psychotherapy, he was able to give up this activity.

NATURE OF ILLNESS AND HANDICAP

While all chronic illness and handicap share certain features—notably the imposition of a state of chronic stress upon the child and family—the nature of the illness makes its own contribution to the quality of the psychological experience of both child and family.[21]

The anatomical location of the illness itself is an important factor psychologically. For example, while emotional sequelae are more frequent for all chronically ill children as compared with normal, those with central nervous system involvement are even more at risk. Seidel, Chadwick, and Rutter,[31] studied all crippled children (5–15 years of age) of normal intelligence who were available through lists of handicapped children in three London boroughs ($N = 75$). They found that psychiatric disorder was twice as common in those children whose crippling was caused by disease of the central nervous system, compared with those with peripheral damage. Since the groups were well matched in terms of physical incapacity and social background, it was concluded that the increased vulnerability to mental problems was due to the brain damage.

A cosmetic disturbance, such as a disfiguring burn or the replacement of a limb by a visible prosthesis, sets up adverse reactions not only in the afflicted person but also in persons in the environment.[26,27] Richardson, Goodman, Hastorf, et al.[27] demonstrated the reactions of children to pictures of mildly handicapped children. There was remarkable uniformity in the ranking of these pictures whether or not the child doing the ranking was himself handicapped. In order of preference, the pictures were ranked as follows: (1) a child with no handicap, (2) a child with crutches and a brace on one leg, (3) a child sitting in a wheelchair with a blanket covering both legs, (4) a child with one hand missing, (5) a child with a slight facial disfigurement on one side, and (6) an obese child.

It is interesting to note that the intensity of illness and degree of handicap do not correlate directly with psychological disability. As McAnarney, Pless, Statterwhite, et al.[16] have demonstrated for children with juvenile arthritis, and Bruhn, Hampton, and Chandler[6] for adolescents and adults with hemophilia, those who are marginally affected seem to be at greatest psychological risk. If the disability is so severe that neither the child nor society expects competition to be possible or necessary, it seems easier for the ill person to accept his condition and to make a more reasonable adjustment. In describing the adjustment of children who were congenitally deformed because of maternal thalidomide ingestion, Pringle[23] found a stronger correlation between family attitudes and emotional adjustment in the child than between degree of physical disability and emotional adjustment.

An illness with a genetic component, such as hemophilia or diabetes, will foster guilt feelings in the parents. Illnesses in whose treatment the youngster must play an active role—diabetes with its regime of diet, activity, and injections is a prime example—serve as irresistible battlefields for all the strife inherent in growing up, particularly when one is at an unfair disadvantage in being physically chronically ill.

RESOURCES OF CHILD AND FAMILY

The term *coping* refers to all the adaptational resources which an individual marshals in order to maintain his psychological equilibrium and level of functioning in the face of a major psychological threat. (See Adams and Lindemann[1] for a recent overview.) These resources include cognition, motor activity, emotional expression, and defenses[17]—the term *defense* having a narrower meaning than the term coping, and referring here to unconscious, more automatic, rigid responses to real or imagined threat. To quote Mattson, "Many studies on long-term childhood disorders report a surprisingly adequate psychosocial adaptation of children followed to young adulthood. . . . The nature of the specific illness appears less influential for a child's successful adaptation than such factors as his developmental level and available coping techniques, the quality of the parent-child relationship, and the family's acceptance of the handicapped member."[17, p. 805]

As in all other aspects of their lives, children's attitudes toward themselves are largely modeled after the appraisals of significant others, most notably their parents. If the parents can accept and work with the illness and handicap with some degree of equanimity, the child is likely to follow suit. As noted at the beginning of this chapter, chronic illness taxes the capacity even of well-integrated families to the utmost. Despite this, as the surveys cited demonstrate, the majority of chronically ill children do not manifest any significant degree of psychopathology. The hazards are there, however; there is room for parents to feel guilty, to become overly solicitous toward the ill child to the detriment of his own ego functioning as well as to the relative neglect of his siblings and parents. More pathological parents may reject the child totally, although as Hewett[12] points out, parents who place their children in hospitals or residential schools are not necessarily rejecting them.

Adams and Lindemann,[1] in a thoughtful paper, dramatically illustrate the interplay between disability and coping styles by comparing the outcome of traumatic quadriplegia in two young men. The first was an 18-year-old single white male who was in excellent health until he suffered a fracture of the sixth cervical vertebra with subsequent quadriplegia. The patient and his family developed a coping style predominated by denial; that is, the disability was never accepted and dealt with in realistic terms. This patient's course was characterized by feelings of depression, as well as hypercritical, hostile, and demanding attitudes toward the many agencies involved with his care. After several years he was living at home, reportedly very unhappy, possessed of vague plans, with nothing accomplished toward his independence, and apparently still clinging to the idea that he might again walk. The other patient, a 17-year-old single white male, also in good health until he fractured his sixth cervical vertebra, was able, with his family, to face his disability early on and to make suitable adjustments. While sharing and verbalizing their hope that their son would again walk, his parents began adjusting behaviorally to their son's condition by placing ramps in their home and widening doorways to accommodate a wheelchair. This patient ultimately graduated from college and began teaching at a college level. The first patient and his family viewed his disability as a sickness from which he would eventually recover; the second patient saw himself as permanently different in ways which called for suitable adjustments.

MEDICAL CARETAKING NETWORK

Although they sometimes resemble conglomerates rather than networks, medical care facilities are complex social institutions where people in various caretaking roles coordinate their efforts to further the patient's welfare. Chronic illness and disability challenge doctors and their associates in special ways; by their intrinsic nature, they frustrate the need of doctors to cure their patients, and certainly threaten omnipotent wishes. Moreover, this happens in a context in which the doctor and patient are repeatedly brought together over a long period of time, a situation that encourages strong feelings to develop on both sides. The physician, in addition, is aware of the patient's more realistic dependency upon him; and all of these factors add up to that part of the stress atmosphere which impinges upon the caretaker. The physician, too, being mortal, must fall back upon his own coping devices and defenses, not all of which are productively adaptive.

Alice, a 14-year-old girl, suffered from a neuromuscular illness of unknown etiology that resulted in generalized weakness and difficulty in swallowing. She would occasionally aspirate food and develop pneumonia. At home, the youngster would lie in bed all day watching television and insisting that her mother not leave her side for even a moment. This same pattern was repeated in the hospital, but with the additional factor of Alice's refusal to relate to any of the hospital staff. She was silent and morose, and unwilling to participate in the child life program even from her bedside. All diagnostic tests, including muscle biopsy, were inconclusive. Reluctant to send her home, yet not having a therapeutic approach to her condition, the staff developed an attitude of smoldering resentment and despair toward her. Both sides were entrenched in a stalemate; it was only after a pediatric liaison team conference that this constellation was explicitly recognized and that the staff saw how much they had withdrawn from the mother and child. Alice's depression and clinging were seen as signs of her conviction that she was hopelessly ill and unable to progress in her life. Since it was not clear how much of her weakness was due to prolonged inactivity and disuse atrophy of her muscles, a rehabilitation approach was developed in which her day was scheduled between exercises, school work, and recreation. With firm guidance from a social worker, Alice's mother was able to leave the child's bed for counseling interviews. Alice responded to this more optimistic renewed interest in her by gradually participating in activities and relating to the staff.

While chronic illness challenges the staff, it also permits and calls forth strong feelings of caring and caretaking.

Tony, a 14-year-old boy, suffered from asthma from the age of 8 years. He also suffered from a chronic depression which dated back to the age of 2 years when his mother placed him with an aunt. He lived with this aunt for the next three years since his mother had felt too overwhelmed with her other children to care for him during that time. When, at 5 years of age, he was returned to his mother, he began a battle with her which has continued to the present. Each winter for the past several years, Tony would appear in the emergency room in an acute asthmatic crisis, insisting upon being admitted. It was obvious that he saw the hospital as a second home wherein he sought periodic respite from his battles with his mother. On the ward, however, although he was well liked, he tended to be mischievous, to provoke other adolescent patients into petty stealing and aggressive behavior, and to be generally disruptive to ward routine. In between hospitalizations, both he and his mother refused to accept outpatient psychotherapy. This cycle of repeated hospitalizations was broken only after a young male house officer acted as a "big brother" toward Tony, visiting him at home, taking him out on excursions, and maintaining regular contact with him.

COMMUNITY RESOURCES

The care of a chronically ill or handicapped child, in summary, is a time-consuming, expensive, emotionally draining experience for all involved. It is no wonder that the patient and his family require multiple support systems. Specialized pediatric clinics, specialized hospitals (such as those for asthmatic children or those for the rehabilitation of a variety of medical conditions), special classes within the educational system, residential schools, interdisciplinary teams, group sessions for handicapped children, and group counseling for parents of such children—these are some of the services the community must provide. Their very multiplicity creates problems for parents who must run from one agency to another and try to keep straight all the advice and prescriptions. The need for one professional person to provide continuity and coordination of care is apparent. There is equally the need for the child to mingle with and be accepted by both handicapped and normal children; for the parents to share experiences, become more sophisticated caretakers, more effective lobbyists for their children through parents' organizations; and for government agencies, professionals, and employers to provide appropriate employment opportunities for handicapped children grown up.

REFERENCES

1. Adams, J. E., & Lindemann, E. Coping with long-term disability. In G. V. Coelho, D. A. Hamburg, & J. E. Adams (Eds.), *Coping and Adaptation.* New York: Basic Books, 1974.
2. Ames, L. B. Children's stories. *Genetic Psychology Monographs,* 1966, *73,* 337–396.
3. Barnett, C., Leiderman, P., Grobstein, R., et al. Neonatal separation: The maternal side of interactional deprivation. *Pediatrics,* 1970, *45,* 197–205.
4. Benfield, D. G., Leib, S. A., & Reuter, J. Grief response of parents after referral of the critically ill newborn to a regional center. *New England Journal of Medicine,* 1976, *294,* 975–978.
5. Bowley, A. H. A follow-up study of 64 children with cerebral palsy. *Developmental Medicine and Child Neurology,* 1967, *9,* 172.
6. Bruhn, J. G., Hampton, J. W., & Chandler, G. C. Clinical marginality and psychological adjustment in hemophilia. *Journal of Psychosomatic Research,* 1971, *15,* 207–213.
7. Bruner, J. S. *The Process of Education.* New York: Random House, 1960.
8. Carr, J. Mongolism: Telling the parents. *Developmental Medicine and Child Neurology,* 1970, *12,* 213–221.
9. Collier, B. N. Comparison between adolescents with and without diabetes. *Personnel and Guidance Journal,* 1969, *49,* 679.
10. DeHirsch, K. A review of early language development. *Developmental Medicine and Child Neurology,* 1970, *12,* 87–97.
11. Demb, N., & Ruess, A. L. High school drop-out rate for cleft palate patients. *Cleft Palate Journal,* 1967, *4,* 327.
12. Hewett, S. Research on families with handicapped children—An aid or an impediment to understanding? In D. Bergsma & A. E. Pulver (Eds.), *Developmental Disabilities: Psychologic and social implications.* (Conference, The Johns Hopkins Medical Institutions School of Hygiene and Public Health) New York: Alan R. Liss, 1976.
13. Klapper, Z. S., & Birch, H. G. The relation of childhood characteristics to outcome in young adults with cerebral palsy. *Developmental Medicine and Child Neurology,* 1966, *8,* 645–656.

14. Klaus, M. H., & Kennell, J. H. *Maternal-infant bonding.* St. Louis: C. V. Mosby, 1976.

15. Leifer, A. D., Leiderman, P. H., Barnett, C. R., et al. Effects of mother-infant separation on maternal attachment behavior. *Child Development,* 1972, *43,* 1203–1208.

16. McAnarney, E. R., Pless, I. B., Statterwhite, B., et al. Psychological problems of children with chronic juvenile arthritis. *Pediatrics,* 1974, *53,* 523–528.

17. Mattson, A. Long-term physical illness in childhood: A challenge to psychosocial adaptation. *Pediatrics,* 1972, *50,* 801–811.

18. Piaget, J. *The origins of intelligence in children.* New York: International Universities Press, 1952.

19. Piaget, J. *The construction of reality in the child.* New York: Basic Books, 1954.

20. Pless, T. B., & Douglas, M. B. Chronic illness in childhood: Part I. Epidemiological and clinical characteristics. *Pediatrics,* 1971, *47,* 405–414.

21. Pless, I. B., & Pinkerton, P. *Chronic childhood disorder—Promoting patterns of adjustment,* London: Henry Kimpton Publishers, 1975. (Distributed by Year Book Medical Publishers, Inc., Chicago.)

22. Pless, I. B., & Roghmann, K. J. Chronic illness and its consequences: Observations based on three epidemiologic surveys. *Journal of Pediatrics,* 1971, *79,* 351–359.

23. Pringle, M. K., & Fiddes, D. O. *The challenge of thalidomide.* London: Longman Group Ltd., 1970.

24. Provence, S. A., & Lipton, R. C. *Infants in institutions.* New York: International Universities Press, 1963.

25. Rexford, E. N., Sander, L. W., & Shapiro, T. *Infant psychiatry: A new synthesis.* New Haven: Yale University Press, 1976.

26. Richardson, S. A. Attitudes and behavior toward the physically handicapped. In D. Bergsma & A. E. Pulver (Eds.), *Developmental Disabilities: Psychologic and social implications.* (Conference, The Johns Hopkins Medical Institutions School of Hygiene and Public Health, 1976.) New York: Alan R. Liss, 1976.

27. Richardson, S. A., Goodman, N., Hastorf, A. H., et al. Cultural uniformity in reaction to physical disabilities. *American Sociological Review,* 1961, *26,* 241–247.

28. Rutter, M., & Graham, P. Psychiatric aspects of intellectual and educational retardation. In M. Rutter, J. Tizard & K. Whitmore (Eds.), *Education, Health, and Behavior.* London: Longman, 1970.

29. Schowalter, J. E., Ferholt, G., & Mann, N. M. The adolescent patient's decision to die. *Pediatrics,* 1973, *51,* 97–103.

30. Seashore, M. J., Leifer, A. D., Barnett, C. R., et al. The effects of denial of early mother-infant interaction on maternal self-confidence. *Journal of Personality and Social Pathology,* 1973, *27,* 369–378.

31. Seidel, U. P., Chadwick, O. F. D., & Rutter, M. Psychological disorders in crippled children: A comparative study of children with and without brain damage. *Developmental Medicine and Child Neurology,* 1975, *17,* 563–573.

32. Shere, E., & Kastenbaum, R. Mother-child interaction in cerebral palsy: Environmental and psychosocial obstacles to cognitive development. *Genetic Psychology Monographs,* 1966, *73,* 255–335.

33. Spitz, R. A. Hospitalism: An inquiry into the genesis of psychiatric conditions in early childhood. *The Psychoanalytic study of the child,* 1946, *1,* 53–74.

ADDITIONAL READING

Battle, U. The role of the pediatrician as ombudsman in the health care of the young handicapped child. *Pediatrics,* 1972, *50,* 916–922.

Bergsma, D., & Pulver, E. (eds.), *Developmental disabilities: Psychologic and social implications.* (Conference, The Johns Hopkins Medical Institutions School of Hygiene and Public Health, Baltimore, 1976.) New York: Alan R. Liss, 1976.

Bothe, A., & Galdston, R. The child's loss of consciousness: A psychiatric view of pediatric anesthesia. *Pediatrics,* 1972, *49,* 252–263.

Burton, L. *The family life of sick children.* Boston: Routhledge and Kagan, 1975.

Collier, B. N. Interpersonal traits of secondary school adolescents with or without diabetes. *Rehabilitation Counselling Bulletin,* 1969, *13,* 190–196.

Creer, T. L., & Christian, W. P. *Chronically ill and handicapped children: Their management and rehabilitation.* Champaign, Ill.: Research Press, 1976.

Downey, J. A., & Low, L. *The child with disabling illness: Principles of rehabilitation.* Philadelphia: W. B. Saunders, 1974.

Freeman, R. D. Psychiatric problems in adolescents with cerebral palsy. *Developmental Medicine and Child Neurology,* 1970, *12,* 64–70.

Goldie, L. The psychiatry of the handicapped family. *Developmental Medicine and Child Neurology,* 1966, *8,* 456–462.

Hopkins, E. W. The chronically ill child and the community. In M. Debuskey (Ed.), *The Chronically Ill Child and His Family.* Springfield, Ill.: Charles C. Thomas, 1970.

Korsch, B. M., Gozzi, E. K., & Francis, V. Gaps in doctor-patient communication. *Pediatrics,* 1968, *42,* 855–870.

Maddison, D., & Raphael, B. Social and psychological consequences of chronic disease in childhood. *Medical Journal of Australia,* 1971, *2,* 1265–1270.

Stainhauer, P. D., Mushin, D. N., & Rae-Grant, Q. Psychological aspects of chronic illness. *Pediatric Clinics of North America,* 1974, *21,* 825–840.

Tizard, J. The experimental approach to the treatment and upbringing of handicapped children. *Developmental Medicine and Child Neurology,* 1966, *8,* 310–321.

Travis, G. *Chronic illness in children: Its impact on child and family.* Stanford University Press, 1976.

Wertheimer, N. M. A psychiatric follow-up of children with rheumatic fever and other chronic diseases. *Journal of Chronic Diseases,* 1963, *16,* 223–237.

Wolfish, M. G., & McLean, J. A. Chronic illness in adolescents. *Pediatric Clinics of North America,* 1974, *21,* 1043–1049.

TERMINAL AND LIFE-THREATENING
═════════ILLNESS IN CHILDREN═════════

Margaret C. Heagarty, M.D.

For centuries the subject of death has been considered the proper concern of poets. Within the past decade, however, physicians and behavioral scientists have joined their more artistic colleagues in the investigation of this ultimate crisis of human existence. Changes in medical practice and in social norms have prompted the development of clinical interest in this previously neglected subject.

Each generation perceives death differently, and such a perception is forged from an amalgam of the values, norms, and experiences of the times. While generalizations are always risky, certainly the marked increases in the longevity of our population have escalated the emotional premium we place upon life and death. Health professionals of past generations, with the limitations of their clinical resources, often had little more than sympathy and understanding to offer their patients and families at the time of death. Contemporary professionals, armed with the clinical and technological advances of modern medicine, less frequently face the reality of death, particularly in children and young adults.

The field of pediatrics clearly illustrates this shift in clinical practice. In 1940, health professionals could predict that 47 of every 1000 infants would die before reaching the age of 1 year. By 1973 this infant mortality rate had fallen to 17.7 per 1000.[17] This decrease in the infant mortality rate has been associated with a decline in the birth rate; in 1910 the birth rate stood at 30.1 per 1000, by 1940 it had fallen to 19.4 per 1000, and in the 1970's it has hovered at the level of 14.9–15.0 per 1000.[18]

These two demographic trends, the fall in the death rate and the fall in the birth rate of children, are the result of many technological, scientific, and cultural changes. Mastery of infectious diseases, advances in contraceptive techniques, rising standards of living—all have played a role. But whatever the demographic, medical, or social causes, the fact is that parents, health professionals, and society view children differently. With fewer births and with childhood death a rare event, the emotional impact of the death of an individual child has heightened. Health professionals must understand this impact and find ways to help themselves, the child, and his family cope with it.

As a result, considerable interest and some research has developed concerning the emotional aspects of the dying child and the concomitant mourning process of his family; and while more remains debated than settled, the general sensitivity of the profession to these issues has improved considerably.

Three elements must be considered in any discussion of the dying child: the child, the family, and the health professionals. An understanding of each of these elements is essential for the appropriate resolution of the tragedy of the death of a child.

CHILDREN'S PERCEPTION OF DEATH

The child, by definition, is a developing organism; therefore, one must begin any consideration of the child's view of death with an understanding of child development. Two theorists, Jean Piaget and Erik Erikson, provide a framework upon which to build some insight into the development of a child's perception of death.

Piaget and Erikson both dissect development into age-related stages and provide complementary views of the child. Piaget's theories explain the child's cognitive development,[11] while Erikson deals with the child's emotional and personality development.[5] Each stage of cognitive and emotional development can be correlated with the level of the child's perception of death.

During the first 2 years of life the infant gradually develops a primitive sense of internal representation, the sense that objects have an existence outside himself. Since this preverbal stage of cognitive development does not include the ability to conceptualize, death as an idea has no meaning to the infant. During this period, through the consistent gratification of his needs by his mother or another mothering figure, the infant develops the ability to trust others in his environment. Absence or withdrawal of this consistent nurturing figure results in the appearance of symptoms of anxiety, fear, or depression. Infants with serious or terminal illnesses that require prolonged hospitalizations may develop such symptoms because of the separation from their mothers.

Between the ages from about 2 to 7 years, the child's cognitive style is characterized by egocentrism, correlational logic, realism, and animism. Children of this age consider their viewpoint as the only one possible (egocentrism). They are able to deal with only one specific at a time; they cannot manage abstractions but, instead, reason from one specific to another. In terms of logic, such children tend to reason that two events occurring together are caused by one another (correlational logic). To a child of this age, thoughts and events are equally realistic (realism) and inanimate objects are invested with emotions, feelings, and personalities (animism).

The child's emotional development likewise proceeds during this time. During the toddler years the child develops increasing autonomy, independence, and self-confidence. As his need for instant gratification lessens, he begins to achieve some measures of self-control and will power. In the immediate preschool period, the child develops some awareness of sexual differences, of birth, and of death. Children of this age have a rich and elaborate fantasy life through which they work out many of their conflicts and fears. The play of such children demonstrates these fantasies and, characteristically, it is not bound by realities of time or place. It is spontaneous, often imitates adult roles, and shows obvious concerns for fearful and threatening situations. In general, boys tend to fear physical injury and girls isolation and abandonment.[9]

While the details of Freud's description of the Oedipal conflict remain uncertain and controversial, children of this age do begin to differentiate their sex roles and to identify with the parent of the same sex. They also begin to develop a conscience, a sense of right and wrong. At this stage of cognitive and emotional development, the preschool child commonly will see himself as the cause of outside events and blame himself for them. The child's thinking may follow this type of sequence: "I thought it, I made it happen, I am to blame for it."

While there has been little investigation of children under the age of 5 years concerning their beliefs about death, knowledge of the preschool child's cognitive level suggests that such children have no concept of the universality and irreversibility of death. When a group of healthy 6- and 7-year-old children were asked "What makes things die?" they replied, "A bird might get real sick and die if you catch it . . . ; "They could eat the wrong foods like aluminum foil. . . ." "They eat poison and stuff; pills. You'd better wait till your mother gives them to you. . . . Drinking poison water and stuff like going swimming alone."

This same group when asked "How do you make dead things come back to life?" responded, "You can't revive them unless you take them to the emergency room and get them doctored up. Then they'll be okay."; "If you know a lot of science, and give them some pills, you can do it."[7]

These responses reflect the cognitive style of young children as well as their rudimentary concept of death. It is during these years that the child first begins to ask questions about such emotionally charged issues as sex, birth, or death, and the parent responding to preschool children's questions must appreciate their level of development. Commonly, the young child personally encounters death for the first time when a grandparent dies. Questions about death should be answered directly, simply, and without denying the child's emotional reaction. The parent should be made aware of the amount of fantasy characteristic of a child of this age so that any distortions or fantasies in the child's thinking about death can be corrected.[3,1]

While the fatally ill preschool child has no adult concept of death, both his emotional and his physical condition must be treated in the course of the illness. The frequent and prolonged hospitalizations usually associated with fatal diseases of childhood tend to accentuate the fears of physical injury and of emotional isolation and abandonment characteristic of a child of this age. For this reason, every effort should be made to avoid hospitalization whenever possible and to make certain that arrangements for frequent parental visiting and for rooming-in are available in the hospital.

The preschool child, with his rich fantasy life and with the magical quality of his thinking, may view his illness as punishment for something he did wrong. In addition, sensitive to the feelings and emotions of the adults around him, the child may feel guilty for causing their obvious distress. If such fantasies and fears are not detected and managed, the child will suffer devastating, incapacitating, and unnecessary anxiety and emotional pain.

The child of school age slowly develops the ability to perform more complicated mental tasks, to understand the relationship of objects in serial order, and to reason from specific instances to general principles. Major changes in such a child's emotional development occur in the areas of increased independence, self-awareness, and socialization. The typical child of this age is task-oriented, industrious, and enjoys the mastery of tasks or problems for their own sake. School becomes the focus of the child's life; interpersonal relationships with peers of the same sex become extremely important.

By this age the child has the cognitive skills to understand that every living thing dies eventually. He is also beginning to develop some ideas about the irreversibility of death.[2,10] Studies reveal that children of school age with fatal illnesses quickly realize that they have no ordinary disease. While they may not have a fully formed adult concept of death, they do show increased anxiety and concern about their illness.[13,14]

One study,[3] using projective techniques, asked children with fatal illnesses to tell a story about a picture given them.

A six-year-old child with leukemia told this story about a picture of a woman entering a room with her hands to her face.

This is about a woman. She's somebody's mother. She's crying because her son was in the hospital, and died. He had leukemia. He finally had a heart attack. It just happened . . . . he died. Then they took him away to a cemetery to bury him and his soul went up to heaven.

A seven-year-old child with cystic fibrosis told this story about a picture of a child in the hospital.

The little boy had to stay in the hospital because the doctor wanted it. He had a shot in the back; a big needle. He was scared of shots, and didn't want it. And the doctor did it hard. His lungs are gone—he can't breathe. His lungs got worse and he didn't get well. He died and he was buried with a big shovel.[18]

A pediatric surgeon caring for a seven-year-old child with carcinoma of the liver observed to the pediatrician, "Of course, he doesn't know how sick he is." On the way to the hospital, the child and his family had to drive past a cemetery; as they passed this spot, this little boy regularly asked his mother, "When I die, can I have a gravestone like that one?"

For obvious reasons, many parents and health professionals tend to deny the extent of the dying child's awareness of his eventual death. Most children of this age do not ask direct questions about death, but talk about their disease indirectly. Although many parents, quite simply, cannot bear to listen to or talk with their child about such issues, the health professional caring for the child should be comfortable enough to allow the child to talk, directly or indirectly, about his concerns. If all of the adults around the dying child are unable to deal with the child's feelings and fears, the child's sense of isolation and abandonment is unnecessarily heightened.

In helping the dying child, the act of listening is more important than the act of saying anything to the child. Only by listening carefully can the professional detect the child's specific fears and fantasies which, once uncovered, can be dealt with directly. The young school child often fears a specific diagnostic or therapeutic intervention more than the abstract event of death. In general, most professionals caring for dying children accentuate the positive aspects of the child's life. If the child asks directly about death, the professional should first establish what the question means to the child and then respond to it directly, but always in a fashion that leaves the child with some hope for the future, if only the immediate future.

The preadolescent and adolescent is capable of the adult mode of thinking. He can reason from a general principle to a specific instance, can work out a problem in his head, and can use abstractions. Children of this age are capable of such a logical sequence as, "If all men can die, I can die." To an adolescent, death has both a personal and general reality. Fatally ill teenagers are aware of their own eventual death and of its finality.

In addition to the obvious physiological and physical changes of puberty, adolescence is a time of enormous emotional development. The typical adolescent struggles to define the boundaries of his own identity apart from that of his parents and family; such a struggle includes a mastery of his impulses and of his rapidly growing body with its increased physical capacities. Additionally, the adolescent must cope with awakened sexual impulses and with budding relationships with the opposite sex.

The dying adolescent carries two burdens. Not only must he deal with the emotional stress of the normal adolescent emotional development, he must also bear the ultimate stress of his own death. With minor differences relating to his stage of emotional development, the adolescent endures reactions to his impending death similar to those described in the adult patient.[8]

"I don't believe it. It can't be true. I'll wake up from this bad dream soon." All of us, when confronted with tragedy, use denial as a mental device to protect ourselves from an unacceptable reality. The adolescent confronted either directly or indirectly with the fact of a fatal illness will almost certainly deny the possibility of eventual death, and may deny the existence of the disease itself. This initial stage of denial is healthy and constructive unless it is prolonged or interferes with the patient's medical care. In the face of what seems to be irrational denial, health professionals may be tempted to confront the patient with the final prognosis of the disease. Such confrontations are unnecessary and can be destructive. If given enough time, most patients will gather their psychological defenses to face the next phase in the evolution of the process.

"Why me? It's not fair." Anger inevitably follows the initial denial of personal tragedy. For the future-oriented adolescent struggling to enter the adult world, the anger may be intense. This rage at the unfairness of his fate may be transformed into extreme hostility toward those around him: his parents, family, and the health professionals caring for him. The health professional must understand that the adolescent's anger and hostility are normal, legitimate reactions to his fate; without such insight, the health professional may find himself responding punitively to the fatally ill adolescent's hostility. In addition, the professional must be prepared to interpret the adolescent's anger and hostility to his parents, his family, and to the hospital staff responsible for the care of the patient.

"If I don't miss a single dose of chemotherapy, maybe I will last long enough to go to the senior prom." Once the first phases of denial and anger pass, dying patients begin to limit their horizons and to bargain for smaller gains. (The process resembles the small child's reaction to parental discipline. After initial anger the child will try to bargain and cajole his parents: "If I go to bed on time every night this week, will you let me do it?") So also the dying adolescent may bargain for extra privileges and time. "If I take all my medicine and don't cry when the doctors hurt me, maybe the disease and its symptoms will go away for a little while." This normal process of bargaining for limited goals helps the adolescent come to terms with the reality of a shortened life span.

Inevitably, the dying adolescent grows sad. Actually, the depression found in fatally ill patients is of two varieties. The first type is a reactive depression, which usually results from the loss of some part of the body important to the patient's self-image. As part of their stage of emotional development, healthy adolescents are particularly sensitive to real or imagined defects in their body images. Thus, at this stage, the fatally ill adolescent becomes extremely vulnerable to a serious depression caused by the real loss of a part of the body as a result of surgical therapy for the disease. This reactive depression, in addition to profound sadness, is associated with deep feelings of guilt and shame. The health professional should anticipate the possibility of such a reactive depression in any adolescent submitted to radical surgery for potentially fatal disease. Moreover, his parents and family should be warned to expect a period of serious depression in the child. This reactive depression will resolve if the adolescent has a trusting relationship with an adult to whom he can talk openly about his feelings. As in other phases of this tragic process, members of his family, because of their own grief, may be unable to fill this role; the task falls to the health professional to help the adolescent to work through and resolve his depression.

The second type of depression seen in dying patients is best described as an anticipatory mourning of the loss of family, friends, and life itself. This anticipatory depression over the loss of one's own future signals the beginning of the final stage, the acceptance of one's own death. Adolescents suffering from this type of depression often make those caring for them extremely uncomfortable and anxious. In their own anxiety, both family and professionals tend to try to cheer the patient with bright, patently absurd comments. Such attempts deny the inescapable reality and rob the adolescent of his rightful dignity as he grieves for the loss of all he loves and enjoys.

Perhaps a more serious reaction to the depressed adolescent lies in the weakening of the important relationships in his life. Depressed patients make those around them sad; avoidance is a natural reaction to such patients. Parents and family begin to visit the hospital less regularly; physicians and nurses on the hospital floor spend less time in the adolescent's room. By this time, the adolescent needs, most of all, simple comfort and warmth. Merely sitting quietly for a few minutes with the patient may be more useful than any words. A quick hug, a hand held for a few minutes, a pat on the shoulder tells him someone cares and understands.

Finally, after this long travail, as death approaches the adolescent finds some peace and equanimity. With this acceptance of imminent death, the patient loses interest in his surroundings, turns inward, and surrenders to the inevitable. Adolescents who reach this stage should not be viewed as "giving up the fight" but as being prepared to accept death calmly.

PARENTAL REACTION TO THE DEATH OF A CHILD

Parental reactions to the death of a child parallel those of the adolescent with a fatal illness. Although basically similar, these reactions may vary, depending upon whether the child dies suddenly and unexpectedly or after a prolonged terminal illness.[6]

When a physician must tell parents that their child has a potentially fatal disease, he should expect the understandable reactions of shock and disbelief. During this first discussion of the child's disease, these emotional reactions usually interfere with the parents' comprehension of any subsequent conversation about the child's treatment or prognosis. For example: Parents of a child with leukemia usually suspect that the child has a serious condition before they are referred to a pediatric hematologist; nevertheless, from the moment the physician confirms this diagnosis, the parents hear little else until they have assimilated the diagnosis and have begun to deal with it. During this first interview the physician should certainly offer the parents hope for the child, but should always be aware that the parents cannot now grasp detailed technical explanations and instructions. Actually, in this situation, the physician's style is more important than the content of what he says. He must present himself as a sympathetic and competent professional who understands the parents' pain and grief and who will deal not only with the medical details of the disease but also will help the parents with its emotional sequelae.

After the initial shock passes, the parents of a dying child often use denial as an emotional defense for coping with this tragic reality. Such a defense mechanism can be viewed as constructive unless it interferes with the medical management of the disease. During this period the parents may wish to seek another medical opinion in hopes of finding someone who will provide a different diagnosis and prognosis. A physician caring for a fatally ill child should raise this issue routinely, and should offer to provide another opinion through a professional consultation. Such a maneuver relieves the parents of the uncomfortable dilemma of wishing to keep the trust and respect of their own physician while wishing to validate the diagnosis by seeking another physician's advice. This strategy may also prevent parental "shopping" from medical center to medical center for a different diagnosis, a process which can interfere with the proper medical care for the child. It should be noted that most parents, even as they deny the full implications of their child's disease, cooperate with the diagnostic and therapeutic interventions required for his care.

Parental guilt, anger, and depression follow this initial phase of denial. It is a first principle of pediatrics that all parents of sick children tend to feel guilty, and that all parents need to be reassured that they did not cause the illness by something they did or did not do for the child. In parents of dying children this guilt is intensified. Parents will ruminate endlessly over the events of the child's life preceding the diagnosis, questioning and searching for sins of their own which explain the child's fate. Health professionals, unaware of this phase of parental mourning, often unwittingly reinforce and exacerbate this guilt by careless and insensitive remarks. Such statements as "Why didn't you bring him in sooner?" uttered by health professionals out of their own frustration and stress as they deal with the dying child, do nothing more than make "guilty" parents feel more guilty.

Guilt projected outward becomes anger. In the search for a reason for this tragedy, a parent of a dying child may angrily blame anyone nearby, including the other parent and the health professionals caring for the child. Thus, the tragedy of a child's death may rupture the relationship between a husband and wife at the time when their need for one another is most intense. The management of the dying child should include an awareness of the impact of the situation upon the relationships within the family. All health professionals should be alert to the possibility of mutual blame and anger between parents, with its resulting trauma to their relationship, and should attempt to intervene before the bond between the parents is destroyed by misplaced guilt and anger.

Parents also become angry with and blame the health professionals caring for their child. These are the parents who are labeled "difficult" by the hospital staff; they seem always angry and impossible to please. The health care team can do nothing right, the hospital food is inadequate, the intern asks too many questions, they have to wait too long to see their physician. All of these, of course, are surface manifestations of the parents' rage over the injustice of their child's fate. When the health professional understands that this anger is not directed against him as an individual but is a symptom of the normal mourning process that these parents must endure, he is better able to cope (and to help others cope) with this parental anger.

As the child's disease gradually evolves toward its unfortunate end, parents and family come to accept the child's death. With such an acceptance of the inevitable comes the beginning of an emotional detachment from the child, a reinvestment in other segments of their life and in other relationships within and outside the family. These feelings of emotional detachment coupled with the normal (if often unstated) desire for the child's death to occur soon, makes most parents feel guilty. This detachment may also appear to some health professionals as callous parental indifference to their child. But both parents and health professionals should understand that these feelings represent normal and constructive coping mechanisms. If the parents' reinvestment in outside activities and relationships leaves the child too isolated, the physician may need to help the parents to continue some emotional investment in their child. The hospital personnel may now be required to substitute, in part, for the parental relationship so as to prevent the child's loss of important emotional ties at a time when they are badly needed.[4]

While parents and family may have had a prolonged period of mourning at the moment of their child's death, they must resolve their residual feelings of loss, guilt, anger, and depression before they can pick up the threads of their lives. If this grieving process is successful, the family will eventually take up their lives with renewed competence and health.

The child's physician should schedule a visit with the parents about 4 to 6 weeks after the child's death. During this visit, the physician can answer any remaining questions about the cause of the death and review the findings of the postmortem examination. More importantly, this visit gives him the opportunity to assess the level of the parents' grief and to detect any pathological reactions requiring psychiatric intervention.

After the death of a child, parents often tend to overprotect their remaining children. In extreme cases, parents who have not resolved their grief may unconsciously select one of their remaining children (usually younger) to replace the lost child; on occasion, parents may actually conceive a child who is designated as the replacement for the dead child. Such children, reared in the idealized image of the dead child, are not allowed to develop their own personality and identity. The physician caring for such a family should be alert to counsel the parents about these possibilities.[12]

While there has been little systematic study of the effect of the death of a child upon his siblings, a few generalizations seem reasonable. Older children are likely to show the same progression in the grief reaction as do their parents. Younger children, without the cognitive skills to understand death, may develop unrealistic and guilty fantasies about the cause of their sibling's death; if left uncovered, these fantasies may result in the appearance of serious emotional symptoms. Finally, parents deeply involved with the care of a fatally ill child may neglect their other children to such an extent that the siblings feel completely rejected and unloved.

HEALTH PROFESSIONALS AND THE DYING CHILD

Most health professionals, particularly those dedicated to the care of children, enter their profession for the satisfactions of helping patients recover from illness and maintain health. To these professionals, the death of any patient, but especially that of a child, represents the ultimate frustration of their career goals.

In the course of their professional maturation, pediatric health professionals must learn to face and to accept the fact of a death of a child. Although the evolution of this professional development varies with the life history, personality, and values of the individual professional, the process must include the recognition and acknowledgement that a child's death has an emotional impact not only upon the family but also upon the medical team caring for the child.

The competent health professional must make some emotional investment to provide medical care for any child; this investment is accentuated in the instance of a fatally ill child. When the child dies, the professional shares, albeit to a lesser degree, the feelings of loss and depression seen in the parents and family. In addition, the professional may find himself overwhelmed with feelings of guilt and anger at the loss of the child. Nevertheless, until the professional recognizes these as normal reactions to tragedy, his ability to assist the family in their own grief is limited.

Professionals who have not resolved this issue tend to behave like the parents of their dying patient. When a child is dying on a hospital ward, the staff often find themselves fighting with one another over trivial matters. The physician, using the "scientific approach" to defend against the inevitable, sometimes orders unnecessary and drastic diagnostic and therapeutic interventions. Individual members of the care team may indulge in relentless, guilty self-examination of their care of the patient.

Finally, as the child's impending death can no longer be denied, and in an effort to defend themselves against the feeling of loss, the hospital staff become so detached from the child and his family that they spend less and less time with them. These behaviors, found on any pediatric unit, are symptoms of the stresses placed on professionals confronted by death in children.[15]

While there remains no simple formula for handling these understandable stresses, certainly the first requisite is the awareness of their existence. Until a health professional becomes human enough to recognize his own feelings, he cannot become professional enough to help his patients and their families through the final crisis of life.

REFERENCES

1.   Aradine, C. R. Books for children about death. *Pediatrics*, 1976, *57*, 372–378.
2.   Childers, P., & Wimmer, M. The concept of death in early childhood. *Child Development*, 1971, *42*, 1299–1301.
3.   Crase, D. R. Death and the young child. *Clinical Pediatrics*, 1975, *14*, 747–750.
4.   Easson, W. M. The family of the dying child. *Pediatric Clinics of North America*, 1972, *19*, 1157–1165.
5.   Erikson, E. *Childhood and society*. New York: W. W. Norton, 1963.
6.   Friedman, S. B. Psychological aspects of sudden and unexpected death in infants and children. *Pediatric Clinics of North America*, 1974, *21*, 103–111.
7.   Koocher, G. P. Talking with children about death. *American Journal of Orthopsychiatry*, 1974, *44*, 404–411.
8.   Kubler-Ross, E. *On death and dying*. New York: Macmillan, 1969.
9.   Lewis, M. *Clinical aspects of child development*. Philadelphia: Lea and Febeiger, 1971.
10. McIntire, M. S., Angle, C. R., & Struempler, L. J. The concept of death in Midwestern children and youth. *American Journal of Diseases of Children*, 1972, *123*, 527–532.
11. Melnick, S. D. Piaget and the pediatrician. *Clinical Pediatrics*, 1974, *13*, 913–918.
12. Poznanski, E. O. The "replacement child": A saga unresolved parental grief. *Journal of Pediatrics*, 1972, *81*, 1190–1193.
13. Spinetta, J. J., & Maloney, L. S. Death anxiety in the outpatient leukemia child. *Pediatrics*, 1975, *56*, 1034–1037.
14. Spinetta, J. J., Rigler, D., & Karon, M. Anxiety in the dying child. *Pediatrics*, 1973, *52*, 841–845.
15. Tietz, W., & Powars, D. The pediatrician and the dying child. *Clinical Pediatrics*, 1975, *14*, 585–591.
16. Waechter, E. H. Children's awareness of fatal illness. *American Journal of Nursing*, 1971, 7, 1168–1172.
17. Wegman, M. E. Annual summary of vital statistics—1973. *Pediatrics*, 1974, *54*, 677–681.
18. Wegman, M. E. Annual summary of vital statistics—1974. *Pediatrics*, 1975, *56*, 960–966.

PREPARING CHILDREN PSYCHOLOGICALLY FOR PAINFUL MEDICAL AND SURGICAL ══════════PROCEDURES══════════

Lloyd O. Eckhardt, M.D.
Dane G. Prugh, M.D.

Introduction

The psychological preparation of children for the stress related to painful medical and surgical procedures is a complicated task. This challenge is compounded by the ever-changing cognitive and emotional responses that spring from the child's level of physical, cognitive, psychosexual, and psychosocial development. The child's genetic endowment, his developmental capacities, the degree of supportiveness offered by his family environment, his past experiences, and his psychological defenses will play major roles in determining the nature of the outcome of his reaction to stressful stimuli.

It would appear from the studies of Bergman and Freud[5] and Vernon, Foley, Sipowicz, and Shulman,[26] that children from middle infancy to the middle or later preschool period (approximately 8–10 months to 3–4 years of age) are the most vulnerable to such painful procedures. This group no longer feels totally supported and protected by its parents, and is most vulnerable to separation anxiety. In addition, these children's cognitive development is not sufficient to enable them to comprehend fully the meaning of or need for such painful procedures. These procedures, therefore, are often poorly understood and/or misinterpreted. Anna Freud notes that "according to the child's interpretation of the event, young children react to pain not only with anxiety but with other affects appropriate to the content of the unconscious fantasies, i.e., on the one hand with anger, rage and revenge feelings, on the other hand with masochistic submission, guilt or depression."[9] Painful procedures may be viewed as punishment for real or imaginary transgressions. Fears of bodily mutilation or even of annihilation may arise, especially when painful procedures are performed on the head, eyes, or genital organs.

Part of this work was supported by a training grant, MH-7740-05, from the National Institute of Mental Health, Bethesda, Maryland.

In addition to anxiety and specific fears, many hospitalized children, especially older infants and preschool children, show a ubiquitous pattern of emotional regression. Such regression may take the form of the reappearance of thumb sucking; a return to the bottle; more demanding, clinging, negativistic, or aggressive behaviors. Learned patterns of behavior such as speech, walking, and bowel or bladder control may also be given up temporarily. Such regression appears to stem partly from the direct effect of the hospital experience on the child's ego and partly from the temporary retreat to earlier, more familiar modes of satisfaction or the surrender of more highly developed functions in an adaptive withdrawal and regrouping of forces to defend the developing ego against further disruption. Prugh and Eckhardt[19] have also noted patterns of depressive reactions, conversion reactions, misinterpretations, perceptual motor lags, and dissociative reactions in children who are exposed to painful medical and surgical procedures. Schmitt and Kempe[21] have observed that, in the absence of normal reactions to painful surgical and medical procedures, the physician is wise to consider the possibility that the nonreacting child may have been exposed to repeated abusive or painful experiences and therefore is no longer capable of responding normally. (See also Chapter 3.)

THE APPROACH TO PREPARATION

Preparing the child for painful medical and surgical procedures must include a careful assessment of the previous adaptive capacities of both the child and his parents. The child's capacity to master anxiety, especially through play, as well as his current and past emotional resources and coping capacities should be evaluated. As noted previously, the level and degree of stability of his adaptive capacity will depend on his prior level of physical, cognitive, psychosexual, and psychosocial development. Also, the nature of prior and present family equilibrium will strongly influence his understanding of the psychological meaning of the painful medical or surgical procedures as well as their actual or fantasied connections to current or past stressful experiences. The child's parents will have their own concerns and fantasies, which are related to their current life situation and to their past experiences with such procedures. Obviously, their reactions will be strongly influenced by the nature and quality of their relationship with their child. Assessment of the above factors will help the physician to form an alliance with the child and his parents, and to proceed to the next step in the necessary psychological preparation.

Considerations in Relation to Developmental Level

For the preschool child and the child of early school age, explanations should be simple and brief. They should be repeated as many times as necessary, and the child should be permitted to ask as many questions as he needs to in order to clarify misconceptions about the procedures or about parts of the body which will be affected. Toy doctor or nurse kits may be helpful in helping the child play out his feelings and achieve a sense of mastery over the coming experience. Simple drawings are often useful adjuncts to verbal discussions. Older children and adolescents may be able to profit from more detailed anatomical discussions and drawings related to the upcoming procedures or surgery. A controlled study by Vaughn[25] in England has demonstrated that such preparation is effective in minimizing deleterious emotional reactions in children.

Information should be so communicated to the child that he can utilize it on his own level to deal with an otherwise unknown situation that is causing him much apprehension and fear. (Even adults show some similar feelings under such circumstances.) Likewise, if the physician avoids critical, judgmental attitudes toward the parents and their child, he can help them minimize their guilt and self-recrimination, while fears and fantasies can be shared and thus more fully understood. Such a posture will help to strengthen the therapeutic alliance.

Methods Used Prior to Hospitalization

If the child should require hospitalization, the physician and the parents need to discuss the hospitalization and any medical or surgical procedures that will take place prior to the hospitalization. Parents and children may be given booklets and story-books[10,14,23,27] to faciliate their understanding, but these are not an adequate substitution for an open discussion with the doctor. Families from various ethnic backgrounds may have special belief systems about illness, hospitalization, and operations, and staff members from similar backgrounds can be of great help. With families from Hispanic or other backgrounds an interpreter may at times be necessary, and a booklet about going to the hospital should be available in the appropriate language.[2] Once the parents feel more comfortable and knowledgeable about coming events, they can discuss them with their child. Then the parents, child, and doctor can meet to talk over specific questions.

Parents and children may also profit from a prehospital or emergency room visit if such a visit or tour can be scheduled.[15] Azarnoff,[3] in California, and others have done this routinely for elective procedures. Such a visit can help to familiarize everyone with the environment and with the equipment that is going to be utilized. A recent, unpublished, controlled study by Parmalee[16] has shown that such tours, together with the use of booklets and discussion of coming procedures, can be beneficial, particularly with children of late preschool and early school age.

Preschool children should not be prepared for elective procedures more than a week or so in advance; this length of time allows for questions and for mobilization of appropriate defenses without allowing too much time for the buildup of excessive anxiety. With children under 4 years of age, however, the only really effective preventive measure, as indicated long ago by Robertson[20] in England and demonstrated more recently by Fagin[8] in a controlled study in this country, is overnight stay or "living-in" by the parent. With older children and adolescents, a longer preparation time is more appropriate.

Methods Used at the Time of Hospitalization

When the child is admitted to the emergency room or hospital, the doctor or staff should take the time to explain to the child and his parents the medical or surgical procedures that are going to be performed; someone must take the responsibility for seeing that this is done. Younger children should be given brief, rather concrete explanations, whereas older children can benefit from more detail. Toy equipment can be utilized in a play program to demonstrate procedures before they are performed.[1,4,7,17] Puppet shows and "puppet therapy" on either an individual or group basis, can help to prepare the child for surgery or more extensive procedures.[6] Special equipment, including masks for anesthesia, traction, intravenous setups, and the like, can be demonstrated in these play sessions. If other units, for example, intensive care, physical therapy, or occupational therapy, are going to be part of the child's treatment program, the child and his parents should have an opportunity to visit these areas and to ask questions about the particular role they will play in his hospital stay.

Painful Medical Procedures

Painful procedures such as venipunctures, injections, catheterizations, lumbar punctures, and the like, create anxiety for almost all children. The person performing these procedures should state truthfully, without minimizing or exaggerating, that some pain will occur. The person should tell the child when and where it will hurt, and should encourage the child to express his feelings. A standardized play kit has been developed by Erickson[7] for use by nurses or other staff members, to help children play out their feelings about such procedures, both before and after they are performed. Very young children cannot be expected to cooperate unassisted and firm but kindly restraint is necessary. One explanation for such restraint is "in order to help you hold still"; the message thus conveyed to the young child is that the doctor and nurse are working together to get the procedure finished with as little pain as possible. Older children can often make use of an explanation of the procedure to gain a sense of mastery and control over the anticipated painful procedure.

Preparation for Surgery

Preparation for surgery should include those techniques previously discussed in relation to painful procedures plus special attention to pre– and postsurgical procedures. Plank[18] has observed that children who have had troubled relationships with their mothers since early childhood, or who have grown up without fathers, are particularly vulnerable to surgery. Preoperative medication and anesthesia induction and recovery states—"funny" feelings, smells, and so forth—should be thoroughly explained. Vernon et al.[26] have observed that preschool children feel much more secure if a parent or a familiar nurse accompanies them to the anesthesia room and is present during the induction and recovery period. Some children need reassurance they will not awaken before the surgical procedures is completed. In a personal communication, Frain has emphasized that if local anesthesia is to be used, children need similar reassurance that pain will not occur during the procedure and that there will be a complete return of sensation following the procedure.

A short discussion of postoperative pain and any necessary restriction on activity should also be presented prior to the surgical procedure. Some children may mistake the onset of unconsciousness as impending death; they need to know that the "forced sleep" is temporary, and will be followed by complete awakening and survival. It is also helpful to explain the differing functions of the mask used to administer the anesthetic and the mask which provides oxygen during the recovery period. Children of late preschool and early school age, for whom fears of mutilation are paramount, should be told that "nothing else" will be done or "taken out" at the time of surgery. (In the past, boys hospitalized for a tonsillectomy or adenoidectomy occasionally underwent a circumcision, "thrown in," without being told about this preoperatively.)[12] Older children often fear loss of control during anesthesia, and they may need reassurance that they did not do or say anything of which they might be ashamed while under the anesthetic.

In a controlled study, Jackson,[11] an anesthesiologist, had children admitted to the hospital the day before surgery; she then personally prepared and accompanied children to the operating room. Her study demonstrated that fewer preoperative emotional problems and postoperative complications (such as vomiting) resulted from this approach. She also showed that significantly less anesthetic was required, thus allowing a greater margin of safety for children with cardiorespiratory or other special medical problems. Jessner and Pavenstedt[13] also believe this practice to be helpful for children of school age, since it allows them to become familiar with the hospital setting. However, Jessner does not feel this approach is helpful for preschool children, because they have a more limited sense of time. Levy[14] recommends that preschool children have a basal anesthetic or preoperative medication administered in their rooms so they may go to sleep and awaken in the presence of their mothers; such a technique eliminates battles on the way to the operating room. If the child's condition permits, this approach may also help the parent who is anxious about accompanying the child to the anesthesia room. Considerable staff support may be required to deal with problems surrounding anesthesia, and no parent should be pushed to participate in any potentially disturbing preparatory approach. In addition, it should be noted that some parents may be upset at the sight of their child recovering from anesthesia.

Special postoperative procedures involving tracheostomy, placement of a pacemaker, deep suctioning, and the like, are more difficult for both younger and older children to understand. If these procedures are going to be performed, special preoperative attention should be given to help the child understand any questions or problems related to such procedures. This approach helps the child to avoid excessive preoperative anxiety, and reassures him that the staff will continue to try to do everything possible to help him master postoperative problems.

CONTRIBUTIONS OF MENTAL HEALTH PROFESSIONALS

Children who have a premorbid history of psychosocial problems, who develop psychological problems secondary to painful medical procedures or surgery, or who develop problems because of the reactivation of a previous traumatic event related to painful procedures or surgery, may need to consult with a specialist in the mental health field. A child psychiatrist, clinical child psychologist, or social worker can often help the physician, nurse, or other hospital staff members understand the reasons for and the meaning of the particular psychological problem or behavior that is interfering with optimal management of the medical or surgical condition. The mental health specialist can also offer brief, focal psychotherapy to the patient and his family in order to help reduce particularly intense anxiety and conflicts that may arise. Brief daily visits with the child and his family have been found to be more efficient than extended, less frequent sessions. For very anxious, or severely disturbed children of school age, a preparative approach similar to that recommended by Levy[4] for preschool children has been combined with preoperative psychotherapy and successfully employed by one of the authors (D.G.P.).

Schowalter and Lord[22] describe group meetings between patients and staff or a mental health worker that can provide a setting for sharing information, fears, and fantasies surrounding potentially painful procedures, as well as about anesthesia and pre- and postoperative experiences. A supportive, educational approach is used and the major focus is directed at the reactions of the group members to such procedures. (See Chapter 7 for a discussion of multiple applications of hypnosis, including its use in painful burns and in surgical procedures.) The utilization of behavior modification techniques for specific problems is widely acknowledged. Antianxiety medications may be indicated to reduce excessive anxiety, and can facilitate (but should not supplant) the implementation of the other methods that have been discussed. It should be remembered that the preschool child is often paradoxically stimulated by barbiturates.

THE ROLE OF THE PHYSICIAN AND OTHER HEALTH PROFESSIONALS

At every level of preparation, the physician can rely on the child's natural need and wish to confide and share his feelings. For younger children, it is the parents' positive relationship to the doctor that enables the child to displace his confidence from his parents to his doctor and to communicate freely without experiencing a conflict of loyalty. Although older children still utilize their parents' trusting relationship with the doctor, they can more easily form an independent alliance with him. Within this setting of trust and understanding, the physican, parent, and child work together to help prepare the child psychologically for painful medical and surgical procedures. Fragmentation of the preparation program and poor patient compliance can be greatly reduced if the physician in charge acts as leader in the planning and implementation of this extremely important and complicated task.

In so doing, he must integrate the contributions of nurses, health associates, recreational and occupational therapists, and other persons involved in the care of the child. He must draw upon the principles of the five C's—communication, continuity, consultation, collaboration, and coordination—to make such help most effective to the child and his family. In hospital settings, a ward management conference, regularly scheduled and chaired by the pediatrician in charge of the ward, can support the implementation of such principles. A similarly coordinated approach to preparation can be achieved in an outpatient clinic or in the office of the practicing physician.

CASE STUDIES

A 4½-year-old boy who had received a transfusion prior to the puppet show had developed fears that the hospital would run out of blood. A puppet story about the blood bank and a later trip to the blood bank area were most reassuring.

A 6-year-old girl who had many tubes of blood drawn, feared she would soon run out of blood. A short puppet story about how the body replenishes blood raised questions that helped the girl understand this phenomenon; consequently, she no longer feared to have her blood drawn.

A 5½-year-old boy watched the puppet boy receive a shot before surgery, and then watched a mask placed over its face. The puppeteer carefully explained that the mask would not hurt, and would provide a sweet-smelling substance that would help the little boy puppet go to sleep. The patient played eagerly with the mask, placing it repeatedly on the puppet's face and then on his own. He left the show area feeling much better.

It was later learned that the preoperative medication and anesthetic induction had gone very well. However, when the boy woke up in the recovery room, the recovery nurse began to place a mask on his face to administer oxygen. When the boy screamed out in alarm, the nurse then explained what was going to happen. It was learned later that the boy was afraid that something had gone wrong, and that the postoperative oxygen mask was to be used to administer more anesthetic to put him back to sleep.

Before the puppet show, the puppeteer should assess how much the patients to be present know about why they are in the hospital, what part of their body is "sick," what other members of the family have told them, and what questions they may have about what is going to happen to them. The show may then focus on the issues and questions that seem to be of most concern to the patients. Following the show, the patients can be asked questions about what they learned and can use the puppets and other play material actively, in order to replay any segments that were unclear or especially useful in helping them master their anxiety.

A 5-year-old girl who feared that she might drown from the intravenous fluids, played extensively with the toy I.V. setup until she could finally give the doll an I.V. She then realized that the I.V. fluids could be accurately controlled and would not harm her.

A 9-year-old boy was referred to the child psychiatry consultant on the pediatric service because of chronic intense anxiety and apprehension about any new event, as well as a number of specific fears, including that of dying. He was to be operated upon for a patent ductus arteriosus and the pediatric surgeon was worried about the child's reaction to the surgery. He was seen by the child psychiatrist in weekly interviews over a 3-month period, with psychotherapy focused on his fears of surgery and death. It was arranged that he would receive sodium pentothal as a basal anesthetic in his room with his mother present. In addition, the psychiatrist assured the boy that he would accompany him to the operating room, and would remain throughout the operation. While they were in the anesthesia room, the patient on the operating table, with another congenital cardiac abnormality, died suddenly of a vasovagal crisis, and the surgeon felt emotionally unable to operate on the boy. When the boy awoke, he was told that another patient (with a different kind of heart abnormality, and with special complications) had died, and that his surgery must be postponed. Although the psychiatrist was now worried about the boy's reaction to the postponed surgical experience, with a repetition of the preoperative psychotherapy and with anesthetic induction in his room, he underwent surgery without serious emotional ill effect.

REFERENCES

1. Adams, M. S. A hospital play program: Helping children with serious illness. *American Journal of Orthopsychiatry*, 1976, 46, 416–424.
2. Azarnoff, P. *It's your body* [Es tu cuerpo]. Los Angeles: University of California, Los Angeles Hospital, 1973.
3. Azarnoff, P. The preparation of children for hospitalization. Los Angeles: National Institute of Mental Health, 1975.
4. Azarnoff, P., & Flagel, S. *A pediatric play program.* Springfield, Ill.: Charles C Thomas, 1974.
5. Bergmann, T., & Freud, A. Children in the hospital. New York: International Universities Press, 1966.
6. Cassel, S., & Paul, M. The role of puppet therapy on the emotional response of children hospitalized for cardiac catheterization. *Journal of Pediatrics* 1967, 71, 233.

7. Erikson, E. Play interviews of four year old hospitalized children. *Monographs of the Society for Research in Child Development*, 1958, *33*, 7.

8. Fagin, C. M. Rooming in and its effects on the behavior of young children. Ann Arbor, Mich.: University Microfilms, Inc., 1964.

9. Freud, A. The role of bodily illness in the mental life of children. *The Psychoanalytic Study of the Child*, 1952, *7*, 69–75.

10. Green, C. Doctors and nurses: What they do. New York: Harper and Row, 1963.

11. Jackson, K. Psychologic preparation as a method of reducing emotional trauma of anesthesia in children. *Anesthesiology*, 1951, *12*, 293.

12. Jessner, L., Blom, G. E., & Waldfogel, S. Emotional implications of tonsillectomy and adenoidectomy of children. *The Psychoanalytic Study of the Child*, 1952, *7*, 126–147.

13. Jessner, L., & Pavenstedt, E. Dynamic psychopathology. New York: Grune & Stratton, 1959.

14. Levy, D. M. Psychic trauma of operations in children and a note on combat neurosis. *American Journal of Diseases of Children*, 1945, *69*, 7–25.

15. Love, H., Henderson, S., & Steward, M. Your child goes to the hospital. Springfield, Ill.: Charles C Thomas, 1972.

16. Parmalee, A. H. Mimeographed report from the Mental Health Services Division, National Institute of Mental Health, 1977.

17. Petrillo, M., & Sanger, S. Emotional care of hospitalized children. Philadelphia: Lippincott, 1970.

18. Plank, E. Working with children in hospitals (2nd ed.). Cleveland: Western Reserve University Press, 1971.

19. Prugh, D., & Eckhardt, L. Children's reactions to illness, hospitalization, and surgery. In A. Freedman, H. Kaplan, & B. Sadock (Eds.), *Comprehensive textbook of psychiatry* (2nd ed.). Baltimore: Williams & Wilkins, 1975.

20. Robertson, J. Young children in hospitals. *New York: Basic Books*, 1958.

21. Schmitt, B., & Kempe, C. The pediatrician's role in child abuse and neglect. *Current Problems in Pediatrics* 1975, *5*, 5.

22. Schowalter, J., & Lord, B. Utilization of patient meeting on an adolescent ward. *Psychiatry in Medicine* 1970, *1*, 197.

23. Simpson. Come inside the hospital. London: Studio Vista, 1973.

24. Stein, S. B. A hospital story. New York: Walker, 1974.

25. Vaughn, G. F. Children in hospitals. *Lancet*, 1957, *1*, 1117–1120.

26. Vernon, D., Foley, J., Sipowicz, R., & Schulman, J. L. *Psychological responses of children to hospitalization and illness.* Springfield, Ill.: Charles C Thomas, 1965.

27. Wolinsky, F. G. Materials to prepare children for hospital experiences. *Exceptional Children*, 1971, *37*, 527.

THE USE OF HYPNOTHERAPY IN A PEDIATRIC SETTING

G. Gail Gardner, Ph.D.

Although hypnotherapy has been used clinically for the relief of pediatric problems at least since the time of Mesmer in the latter half of the eighteenth century,[41] physicians have widely varying views about the value of this treatment modality. Some categorically reject hypnosis as worthless and even harmful, others believe that it can be useful in certain situations, and a few others indiscriminately use it to the exclusion of other valuable approaches.

Negative attitudes toward hypnosis generally derive from some combination of lack of knowledge and unfortunate past experiences with stage hypnotists or other lay persons who, although well intentioned, do not have sufficient background in any professional area (medicine, psychology, dentistry) to employ hypnotherapy judiciously. Moreover, indiscriminate use of hypnosis by a few professionals, combined with their often exaggerated advertising claims, further decreases the willingness of the responsible professional to use hypnosis.

In pediatric settings, the problem is further compounded by confusion about whether children are hypnotizable at various ages, and how hypnotic techniques suited for adults can be modified appropriately for children. Also, the question of parental consent arises since parents, too, have many misconceptions about hypnosis. (These issues have been discussed in detail in previous publications, and need not be discussed here except briefly.) Children generally are better hypnotic subjects than adults;[9,10,32,33,34,35,37] although this finding has not been fully explained, several hypotheses have been suggested.[11,14] If clarification and education regarding hypnosis are provided for parents, their misconceptions can change to enthusiasm.[16] Even many pediatricians with skeptical attitudes would be interested in learning more, were a suitable opportunity available.[17]

Thus, given a qualified hypnotherapist, the question of the feasibility of hypnosis becomes a meaningless issue. This chapter, therefore, will first survey some situations in pediatric practice in which hypnotherapy has been found helpful; the latter part of the chapter will offer some guidelines for the evaluation of a hypnotherapist and for sources of training information.

HYPNOTHERAPY IN WELL-CHILD CARE

During routine pediatric visits with well children, observations and interviews with the child and parents often reveal minor problems which most pediatricians tend to ignore. When such problems are brought to their attention, they often respond by offering casual reassurance that the child will outgrow the problem eventually and that, since it probably will not lead to significant physical problems, it does not warrant the time and expense of further investigation and treatment. On the contrary: while the problem may seem unimportant to the pediatrician, it may be extremely important to the child and his family, and often with good reason. For example, a 10-year-old child who wets his bed is likely to encounter teasing, name-calling, and rejection by family and peers. He must cope with parental annoyance at the frequent changing of sheets and pajamas; he probably is not allowed to stay overnight with friends whose parents do not have proper mattress covers; he may even be denied the privilege of joining organized children's groups at summer camps or weekend outings. It takes but a little imagination to foresee the possible emotional problems, such as strained parent-child relationships, peer avoidance, low self-esteem, and even reluctance to attend school. For the pediatrician to reassure himself that there is no organic cause for the enuresis is not sufficient, because the psychological sequelae are too damaging to be ignored or dismissed; instead, the pediatrician needs to look for a solution to the problem. The 8- or 9-year-old child who still requires night lights and prolonged rituals because of bedtime fears, the 6-year-old child who stammers, the child with extensive food idiosyncrasies, the child who panics during academic tests—all these children will suffer erosion of self-esteem which, in turn, will inhibit their capacity to master progressively complex developmental tasks.

If one agrees, then, that minor problems in the well child may eventuate in major sequelae, the importance of early intervention is obvious. (It should be emphasized that hypnotherapy is only one of several possible treatment approaches. Since an evaluative review of the relative effectiveness of possible treatments for pediatric problems is far beyond the scope of this chapter, discussion of each problem area will include references to available literature concerning the utility of hypnosis, though generally not comparing it with other approaches. The "state of the art" in clinical child hypnosis simply has not yet advanced to that degree of sophistication.)

Generally, the advantages of hypnotherapy are that it is a method easily accepted and used by most children, that children are active participants in the treatment process, that progress usually occurs quickly, and that results are usually lasting. Symptom substitution is rare. The chief disadvantage of hypnosis is that it requires motivation and some degree of effort from the child; for example, it will probably be ineffective if the child is not concerned about his problem or if he derives significant secondary gain from it. Although the length of time required is often considered a disadvantage in using hypnosis, the technique usually saves time in the long run, especially if the child is taught self-hypnosis. (This will become more apparent in specific discussions that follow.)

Other cautions relate more to the hypnotherapist; he must be aware of the bounds of his competence in using this deceptively simple but potent technique.

Careful wording is essential. Thus, a psychologist asked to assist in managing postsurgical pain must be sophisticated enough not to suggest that the patient will have no pain at all, for such pain may be the only evidence of a complication that requires rapid attention. Likewise, the physician must know that certain childhood symptoms may serve to bind severe anxiety or depression, and, therefore, it may be dangerous to proceed with symptom removal before evaluating the child's overall emotional status.[24]

Habit Disorders

A hypnotherapeutic approach to habit disorders generally follows a dictum of behavior modification: An approach is likely to be more effective if it is positive rather than negative. Thus, the pediatrician using hypnosis emphasizes how the child can alter the habit to achieve a more positive experience. Also, most children react more favorably when they actively participate in solving the problem rather than when they must submit passively. In hypnosis, the child may be asked to first visualize himself gaining control over the habit and then, with the habit eliminated, enjoying happy experiences that now become available to him. If the child can see himself as having actually mastered the problem, then the assumption that he is a helpless victim of his habit weakens automatically. Put it another way: The child needs (a) to be convinced that he has a problem and (b) to let go of the idea that the problem has him!

If the child is not motivated to change the habit, the pediatrician can often enhance motivation by pointing out to the child the connection between his habit and various unpleasant life experiences, and by showing him how his habit denies him certain pleasant experiences that would otherwise be available. If there is secondary gain, such as obtaining attention or expressing hostility, it may be possible for the child to find more adaptive ways of dealing with these underlying issues. Sometimes a solution will be obvious; either times it is necessary to recommend psychotherapy for the child or the parents, or both. Since it is impossible to cover the whole range of specific habits, some of the more common ones seen in pediatric practice are now described.

Enuresis and encopresis. Hypnotherapeutic treatment of enuresis and encopresis, habit disorders that are often related, has been described in detail by Baumann and Hinman[4] and Olness.[38,39] These pediatricians emphasize the need for appropriate medical workup to rule out any underlying organic cause. They report rapid and lasting success. Their techniques are similar, although Olness puts greater emphasis on the child's use of self-hypnosis and the noninvolvement of the parents in the treatment process. Obviously, there are a tremendous number of hypnotherapeutic approaches to any problem; from several approaches with which he is familiar and comfortable, the skilled and experienced therapist selects the specific ones he thinks will be useful in a particular case.

Thumbsucking and toothgrinding. Thumbsucking is especially annoying to parents who know that it can lead to serious malocclusion. Yet they also know that their child derives intense pleasure from it and has no motivation to change. Exhortations to "be a big girl," offers of nail polish, and threats or use of gloves or bitter medicine on the thumb often are of little value. Frustration grows when the parents realize that the child is probably unaware of the behavior, engaging in it when engrossed in a story or when going to sleep. Toothgrinding produces similar frustrations. Fortunately, a young child's ability to conceptualize sufficiently so that he becomes motivated to change these habits is often underestimated. Hypnosis can be used (often in conjunction with a reward system) to increase the child's awareness of the habit and to encourage his willingness to substitute a less harmful behavior.

Clinging to blankets and other transitional objects.   While it is appropriate for a small child to find special comfort in a blanket, a teddy bear, or some other object, such behavior becomes a source of embarrassment and shame for an older child. Although it is thought rare to find a child of 12 years or more who still sucks on a baby bottle or uses some other objects designed for infants, the incidence of such problems may be far greater than is readily apparent. These children become masters at hiding their behavior, and may admit it only under severe stress, such as a long hospitalization where privacy is minimal. Hypnotherapeutic treatment in these cases, essentially, is the same as that for thumbsucking. With older children, it is to the therapist's advantage that the child is motivated to change, but sometimes the advantage is countered by the duration of the habit and the child's entrenched conviction that his particular object is the only pathway to a complete sense of security.

Nailbiting and hairpulling.   Nailbiting and hairpulling are often easier to treat than some habits previously mentioned. The child usually has less emotional investment in maintaining the habit and can quickly appreciate the results of change. In addition to awareness training and future-oriented imagery, the hypnotherapist can use interference techniques, such as suggesting that the child will imagine a stop sign as soon as he is aware of nailbiting. The child can then enjoy the feeling of stopping the behavior as it comes more and more under his control.

Tics, stammering, and voice problems.   Although tics and stammering are often a manifestation of significant emotional disturbance, they sometimes may be simply a functionally autonomous residual of a problem that has already been resolved and, occasionally, they may be nothing more than habitual imitation of another person. In hypnotherapy, the child's sense of awareness and control may be enhanced by asking him to show the therapist an exaggerated form of the tic or stammer. The child then gets the idea that if he can make it worse, he can also make it better. Falck states that the reestablishment of confidence is essential in such treatment.[13] Laguaite likewise emphasizes control issues in her report of hypnotherapy for children with deviant voices.[29]

Drug abuse.   Baumann[3] has described hypnotherapeutic treatment of adolescent drug abusers. In one of a very few studies of hypnosis-treatment subjects vs. no-treatment controls, he found no significant differences for marijuana smokers. Adolescents who used certain more dangerous drugs were more likely to benefit from treatment, presumably because of greater motivation to stop the habit. In treating drug abuse, it is sometimes helpful to teach the patient to have a "hypnotic high," in order to feel as well or even better than when using the drug. This "high" produces the desired feeling, and avoids the medical and legal complications of actual drug usage. This method may also be useful in legitimate drug usage; for example, a cancer patient may achieve significant pain relief, and remain alert and able to relate to his family, rather than being "knocked-out" on actual medication.

Fears and Phobic Reactions

As in the case of habits, the possible variations of fears and phobic reactions are great indeed. The parent who has been told that childhood fears are "normal" and will be outgrown probably helps the child avoid the feared object or event as much as possible, until the child soon develops his own avoidance skills. While this approach usually yields satisfactory immediate effects, the long-term results can be disastrous. An obvious example: Every dentist has regretfully performed multiple tooth extractions on terrified patients who have avoided dentistry for several years—probably since childhood—with the consent of their parents.

Even in less obvious situations, the avoidance strategy can be damaging. The child with fear of darkness may develop complex bedtime rituals that strain not only the electric bill but also his relations with siblings, parents, and peers. Fear of strangers or of leaving parents rapidly and severely limit a child's capacity for normal socialization. Fear of animals may confine a child to his house. The tragedy of the avoidance strategy is that parents and other people who assist in the child's avoidance unwittingly communicate the message that the fear is valid, and thus strengthen it. Simultaneously with repeated avoidance, the child has no opportunities for corrective experiences, and no chance to gain any sense of mastery. The fear may then generalize, adding further constraints.

Fears and phobias are among the few psychological problems for which there is a specific treatment with a high success rate: desensitization. This technique has several variations, but often involves the patient's achieving strong feelings of comfort and safety in hypnosis and then using imagery techniques to pair the feeling of safety with the experience of the feared object or event. Sometimes the therapist may go on to help the patient cope with the fear by real-life experiences, either with or without hypnosis. Hypnotherapeutic techniques may also encourage more rapid understanding of social dynamics, as for example in the treatment of "school phobic" children.[30]

Nightmares and Sleep Disturbances

Although all children have occasional nightmares, some children have them with such frequency that they interfere with sleep patterns and sometimes cause further development of daytime fears. Nightmares tend to be considered as something over which a sufferer has virtually no control, except, perhaps, through psychotherapy. This attitude of helplessness is probably the main reason that parents reinforce and increase the likelihood of nightmares by providing the nightmare-prone child with middle-of-the-night snacks and stories, or by allowing him to sleep with one or both parents. Yet there are hypnotherapeutic techniques that can sometimes provide relief in one or two sessions. One method is a variant of the desensitization procedure: It pairs the dream content (or the stimulus for the dream if that is known) with hypnotic suggestions of safety. Other techniques employ the capacity of the patient to have a hypnotic dream. While in hypnosis, for example, the child is asked to redream his nightmare but this time to proceed with it to a happy ending. The therapist then follows with the suggestion that the child can do the same thing when he is actually sleeping. Since the therapist is willing to confront the nightmare, the child, too, gains courage. Jacobs has described treatment by hypnosis for several other sleep problems.[22]

Learning Disabilities

Many learning problems are associated with a presumed central nervous system dysfunction that results in true deficits in conceptual or perceptual ability, memory storage and retrieval, fine motor coordination, and other skills essential for learning; but some children have difficulty mastering schoolwork because of a problem in the emotional sphere, often consisting of anxiety about measuring up to high standards first set by teachers, parents, or siblings and then introduced by the child himself. Depression, unwillingness to accept new information, aversion to achieve on request, concern about family disharmony or some other nonschool-related stress—all may lead to school failure, but anxiety over adequacy of performance seems most common. This is true not only for intellectually normal children but also for children with primary learning disabilities. In the latter case, however, an already difficult situation is further complicated. When significant amounts of attention and energy are siphoned off into anxiety, obviously there is less available for investment in the learning process.

In cases of performance anxiety, hypnotherapeutic strategies that emphasize relaxation, mastery, and personal value are especially useful. The child in hypnosis can have a strong image of concentrating well and successfully completing his work. Such imagery will weaken negative self-image and decrease anxiety.[20,21,23] If the child then does improve his schoolwork, his success becomes self-perpetuating. However, as with other problems, the pediatrician must decide whether complex emotional conflicts requiring psychotherapy exist, or whether a more direct approach can be employed.

HYPNOTHERAPY IN ACUTE CARE PROBLEMS

It is a rare pediatrician who can suture a laceration and make the procedure into a positive experience for the child. Even giving a tetanus shot for a minor wound often results in a struggle of brute force. Not infrequently, the child's anxiety triggers an angry response in the doctor or nurse, and thus the trauma increases. In this sort of atmosphere, one shudders even at the thought of having to debride a burn, to place a naso-gastric tube, or to cope with postoperative care after emergency surgery.

Equal stress can be associated with behavioral and psychiatric emergencies in which the pediatrician may be the first professional involved. Such emergencies might include the youngster who has just been beaten or sexually molested, the child who has just witnessed a terrible accident or a death, the child whose parent has suddenly left home, the girl who has just been rejected by her boyfriend and seems intent on suicide.

How can the pediatrician go beyond merely managing this sort of emergency to the point of helping the child derive something positive from the experience? Hypnotherapy is one technique which has been found helpful.

Minor Accidents

When a child with a laceration is brought to a busy pediatric office or emergency room, the most likely sequence is a brief attempt at reassurance, followed by holding the child down, trying to ignore his screams, and doing whatever has to be done as rapidly as possible. The saving in time is illusory. The child learns that doctors and nurses are people who hurt and people who do not listen. As a result, when the child comes in later for a simple checkup, the examination may take much longer because of his refusal to cooperate. A more serious possibility is that some children will try to ignore or deny medical problems in an effort to avoid repetition of earlier trauma at the doctor's office. The following example illustrates how hypnotherapy can help avoid such an unfortunate sequence.

A 4-year-old boy was brought to the emergency room for treatment of a laceration in his thigh. A nurse suggested that she get some people to help hold down the child. The pediatrician (trained in hypnosis) said, "No. Holding him down will only scare him." Using a method of hypnotic imagery, she then asked the boy what he liked to do best, and he answered, "Play with my cat." The pediatrician elicited further details about the cat, and encouraged the child to develop imagery of playing with the cat, as she prepared her suture tray. When all was ready, she said to the child, "OK, you go on playing with your cat while I fix your leg. What's the cat doing now? (Playing with the ball.) Really? Look, the ball rolled away. Can the cat get it? (Yes, he went under the chair and rolled the ball back to me.) Wow! You and your cat really know how to have fun. . . ." During this interchange, the pediatrician put four sutures in the child's leg without any local anesthesia. As the astonished nurse looked on, the pediatrician complimented the boy for his skill in thinking about happy things, helped him off the table, and walked with him to his mother to whom the child said, "That is the silliest doctor I ever saw."

Others have published similar accounts.[7,12]

Although some might view these cases as simple distraction, it is the writer's belief that the children are in a true altered state of consciousness (hypnosis) in which there is narrowing and shifting of attention with concomitant alterations in sensation and awareness, including partial dissociation of the wounded area. (For a careful and thorough discussion of recent experimental work and theoretical development concerning hypnosis for pain relief, see the excellent book by Hilgard and Hilgard.[19])

Major Medical and Surgical Problems

The problem of helping the child cope with more prolonged and complicated painful procedures, such as those involving serious burns or postoperative care after major surgery, is often more challenging because of the greater complexity of the situation, the large number of nurses and doctors involved (some of whom may have negative attitudes toward hypnosis), and the concomitant stress of prolonged isolation or activity restriction. In such cases, the assessment of psychodynamic issues, such as the possibility that the child feels that he is to blame for the problem and therefore deserves the punishment of pain, becomes more important.

In surgical situations, both the surgeon and the anesthesiologist can utilize hypnosis to minimize preoperative anxiety, reduce the amount of chemoanesthesia, modify postoperative pain, and facilitate return of normal body functions such as hunger, urination, and ambulation.[2,5,8,36]

The writer recalls the case of a severely burned 11-year-old girl whose pediatric surgical team worked closely with a psychologist skilled in hypnotherapy. The child quickly learned to substitute hypnosis for preoperative injections. She used hypnosis to control pain, itching, hunger (both decreasing hunger before surgery and increasing hunger afterwards), periodic severe anxiety and depression, and to facilitate ambulation. An interesting example of using hypnosis to restore normal body function occurred several weeks after the accident, when, for the first time, the surgeons left the child's right hand unbandaged. The staff were pleased with this evidence of progress, but when the child first saw her hand—scarred, grafted, and blackened from repeated applications of silver nitrate—she was literally horrified by its appearance. She begged, "Oh no, get it away from me! I don't want to see it! I don't want it!" The psychologist and attending nurse, respecting the child's need for immediate defense, covered her hand with the sheet; yet they communicated acceptance by continuing to stroke and hold her hand. The psychologist then gave posthypnotic suggestions, taking care to respect the temporary need for dissociation by referring to "that" or "the" hand rather than "your" hand. She said "Yes, that hand doesn't look very good right now (implying that the future might be different), but you may find, little by little, that it looks better and feels better. And you may soon find that the hand wants to do more and more. It hasn't been able to do much during these weeks when it was bandaged. Soon it can want to learn to do things again." The next day the child used a felt-tipped pen to circle preferred items on the breakfast menu. Although the psychologist had offered to circle the items for lunch and dinner, the child asked if she could complete the menu herself, and promptly did so. This event, of course, was then incorporated into further suggestions for acceptance and mastery. The following day the child spontaneously practiced writing the alphabet, including extra practice on letters she felt were poorly executed. Thus she reintegrated her hand as part of herself and used it to further her recovery.

Other hypnotherapeutic approaches to working with severely burned children have been reported by Bernstein[6] and LaBaw.[26] Both stress the need for early intervention and prevention of additional complications in an already complicated situation.

Psychiatric Emergencies

In most psychiatric emergencies, the pediatrician will elect to refer the child to a psychiatrist or psychologist; yet he must still deal with the immediate problem, since referral may take hours or even days. The pediatrician may choose to sedate the child, upset or hysterical from an acute emotional trauma such as witnessing a gruesome accident, suddenly finding that a parent has left home, or being molested. Pharmacological sedation, however, is of temporary benefit only; hypnotherapeutic methods, on the other hand, may not only quiet the child but also be particularly useful in helping to orient him toward an ability to cope with the situation. What happens is that, in hypnotherapy, the child rapidly begins to focus on a solution rather than to limit himself to contemplating the problem. In addition, he may become better motivated to form a positive alliance with a therapist who can help him work through the trauma to a lasting solution.

When confronted with a youngster who is acutely depressed and possibly suicidal, the pediatrician should think carefully before recommending immediate psychiatric hospitalization. For the child obviously intent on suicide, hospitalization is indicated. But short of that, psychiatric hospitalization may only exacerbate feelings of helplessness, hopelessness, and passivity. In many cases, brief hypnotherapy can be combined with reassurance so as to mobilize the child's ego in the direction of active coping. Hypnotic imagery techniques can be combined with a request to the child that he participate in planning referral to a mental health specialist or in arranging for close followup care with the pediatrician. When the pediatrician's first reaction is not to refer and flee but rather to work with the child, he conveys a sense of hope and confidence, an emotional store from which the youngster can borrow in order to replenish his own ego resources.

HYPNOTHERAPY IN PROBLEMS OF
CHRONIC AND TERMINAL CARE

In working with children with chronic and fatal illness, the pediatrician must deal not only with repeated medical and surgical procedures (or both) but also with psychological sequelae. To a greater extent than in acute situations, it is important to help the child find ways of accepting diagnostic and treatment procedures, since these may occupy a significant portion of his time. For example: Chronic renal dialysis is a situation wherein perceived bodily invasions and assaults combine with uncertainty to produce serious emotional problems for many children. Unable to have faith in permanent recovery, many children verbalize correctly that one thing after another seems to go wrong, and that the general trend is downhill. Even when there is no real physical deterioration, the impact of major limitations may increase as the child gets older.

Major Congenital Defects

Although the child with a problem such as spina bifida or severe cerebral palsy will probably be treated by several specialists, a pediatrician presumably will coordinate the various services. It is no simple feat, however, to elicit optimal cooperation from the child too young or too limited intellectually to appreciate the potential gain. Obviously a combination of well-coordinated efforts is here required, including work with the family as well as with the child. For certain children, hypnotherapy can be an important contribution to their adjustment.

LaBaw, for example, has reported that group hypnotherapy can decrease frequency and severity of bleeding episodes in hemophiliac children.[25,27] Lazar has used hypnosis to facilitate motor function in a mildly retarded, cerebral-palsied child.[31] These are excellent examples of the interplay between psychological and physical factors in the development of these handicapped children. Commonly seen problems of poor self-image with associated depression or acting-out may respond to hypnotherapy, especially when techniques are employed that help the child deal with underlying anger and guilt, feelings he may not have confronted because of their unacceptability to others.

Major Acquired Chronic Problems

The child who is severely and permanently disabled after an accident or who develops diabetes may experience so many changes in his life that he does not even feel like the same person. Previous major sources of self-esteem, for example, excellence in football or physical attractiveness, may suddenly vanish. Just as an amputee mourns the loss of his limb, children with other kinds of permanent loss often go through a period of mourning for the lost self, and rejection—usually by denial—of the new self. For example, a 4-year-old girl, whose spinal cord was severed, with resulting paralysis below her neck, became deeply depressed on major holidays during the next year because she repeatedly convinced herself that she would magically recover, often by means of a gift such as a tricycle that demanded use of the functions she had lost. The diabetic child who resists learning necessary self-care routines may be engaging in a similar kind of thought process, knowing that the new learning implies affirmation of the changed self. A major task, which can be facilitated through several of the hypnotic techniques already described, is the establishment of a new identity that integrates the changed functions with a basic sense of continuity and personal value within the child. Again, early intervention may contribute significantly to the success or failure of the child's efforts to master future developmental tasks. Depending upon his concept of himself as a meaningful person in his environment, the child with acquired blindness, for instance, may become a beggar or a teacher.

Published reports of hypnotic intervention in children with major, acquired, chronic, nonfatal physical problems include a case of multiple warts which were refractory to dermatological treatment,[40] a case of psychogenic epilepsy,[15] and several cases of asthma.[1]

It is well known that hypnosis has been used adjunctively in the psychotherapeutic treatment of children who develop enduring and disabling primary emotional problems. Such use is not discussed in this chapter, since these children are likely to be followed by a mental health specialist rather than by a pediatrician. However, it is important to dispel the notion, held by many pediatricians, that hypnosis is useful only for symptom removal. On the contrary: Hypnotic techniques can be and have been employed by many persons in dynamic or analytically-oriented treatment.[42] Hypnotherapeutic techniques can be integrated with all aspects of psychoanalysis, including free association, dream interpretation, analysis of resistance, and analysis of transference. Indeed, certain patients may make marked gains in hypnoanalysis when previous work in psychoanalysis has been of little or no value.

Terminal Illness

In the last decade, interest in the problems of dying persons (including children) has increased greatly. Therapists report the use of hypnotherapy to alleviate terminal pain and fear so that heavy sedation can be reduced or eliminated, enabling the patient better to relate to his family.[18,28] With the aid of hypnosis, some dying children have continued to engage in age-appropriate activities until a few hours before death. For the children and their families, hypnotherapy supports and enhances ego functions, even when the children are fully aware of their condition. Thus, even dying allows opportunity for a sense of mastery.

DISCUSSION

The aim of this paper has been to review the application of hypnotherapy to a broad spectrum of pediatric problems in order that the pediatrician may become more aware of its possible uses and advantages. (It must be noted that the price of breadth in these few pages is the absence of depth. The reference list points the way to further exploration for the interested reader, although it is in no way a complete bibliography of the literature on hypnosis with children.)

There has been no attempt to describe the many techniques of hypnotic induction appropriate for children of different ages, or to discuss hypnotherapeutic approaches to be used once induction has been achieved. The writer believes strongly that such skills cannot be obtained from books, but must be learned in workshops and seminars taught by professionals for professionals. Such courses are available from the Society for Clinical and Experimental Hypnosis (SCEH) and the American Society of Clinical Hypnosis (ASCH) as well as in several medical schools and graduate programs in clinical psychology. (More information may be obtained from local and national societies in medicine, psychology, and dentistry.)

Because of its complexities (which could only be alluded to in this chapter), use of hypnotherapy should be limited to qualified professionals. Though hypnotic induction methods are easily learned, hypnosis is not a therapy in itself; it is, rather, a technique to be used adjunctively within the context of medicine, psychotherapy, or dentistry. When hypnosis is used by lay persons, their lack of basic professional training may increase the likelihood of harm to the patient or subject. (For this reason, the state of Oregon has now passed legislation making it illegal to use hypnosis for entertainment purposes, and other states are considering similar legislation.)

As a general rule, when patients ask to be referred for hypnosis, it is best to caution them to go to qualified physicians, psychologists, or dentists, and to avoid lay hypnotists listed in the "yellow pages" or in the classified section of the local paper. Lay hypnotists may be well meaning and sometimes quite skilled, but, by definition, their lack of professional training in medicine, psychology, or dentistry precludes their effective treatment of patients with problems in these areas. The patient who cannot locate a qualified hypnotherapist through a local medical, psychological, or dental society can contact the headquarters of either SCEH or ASCH, both of which maintain national directories.*

REFERENCES

1. Ambrose, G. *Hypnotherapy with children.* London: Staples Press, 1961.
2. Antitch, J. L. S. The use of hypnosis in pediatric anesthesia. *Journal of American Society of Psychosomatic Dental Medicine,* 1967, *14,* 70–75.
3. Baumann, F. Hypnosis and the adolescent drug abuser. *American Journal of Clinical Hypnosis,* 1970, *13,* 17–21.
4. Baumann, F., & Hinman, F. Treatment of incontinent boys with non-obstructive disease. *Journal of Urology,* 1974, *111,* 114–116.
5. Benson, V. B. One hundred cases of post-anesthetic suggestion in the recovery room. *American Journal of Clinical Hypnosis,* 1971, *14,* 9–15.
6. Bernstein, N. R. Observations on the use of hypnosis with burned children on a pediatric ward. *International Journal of Clinical Experimental Hypnosis,* 1965, *13,* 1–10.
7. Clawson, T. A., Jr., & Swade, R. H. The hypnotic control of blood flow and pain: The cure of warts and the potential for the use of hypnosis in the treatment of cancer. *American Journal of Clinical Hypnosis,* 1975, *17,* 160–169.
8. Cullen, S. C. Current comment and case reports: Hypno-induction techniques in pediatric anesthesia. *Anesthesiology,* 1958, *19,* 279–281.
9. Cooper, L. M., & London, P. Sex and hypnotic susceptibility in children. *International Journal of Clinical Experimental Hypnosis, 1966, 14,* 55–60.
10. Cooper, L. M., & London, P. The development of hypnotic susceptibility: A longitudinal (convergence) study. *Child Development,* 1971, *42,* 487–503.
11. Cooper, L. M., & London, P. Children's hypnotic susceptibility, personality, and EEG patterns. *International Journal of Clinical Experimental Hypnosis,* 1976, *24,* 140–148.
12. Erickson, M. H. Pediatric hypnotherapy. In J. Haley (Ed.), *Advanced techniques of hypnosis and therapy: Selected papers of M. H. Erickson, M. D.* New York: Grune & Stratton, 1967.
13. Falck, F. J. Stuttering and hypnosis. *International Journal of Clinical Experimental Hypnosis,* 1965, *12,* 67–74.
14. Gardner, G. G. Hypnosis with children. *International Journal of Clinical Experimental Hypnosis,* 1974, *22,* 20–38.
15. Gardner, G. G. Use of hypnosis for psychogenic epilepsy in a child. *American Journal of Clinical Hypnosis,* 1973, *15,* 166–169.
16. Gardner, G. G. Parents: Obstacles or allies in child hypnotherapy? *American Journal of Clinical Hypnosis,* 1974, *17,* 44–49.
17. Gardner, G. G. Attitudes of child health professionals toward hypnosis: Implications for training. *International Journal of Clinical Experimental Hypnosis,* 1976, *24,* 63–73.
18. Gardner, G. G. Childhood, death, and human dignity: Hypnotherapy for David. *International Journal of Clinical Experimental Hypnosis,* 1976, *24,* 122–139.
19. Hilgard, E. R., & Hilgard, J. R. *Hypnosis in the relief of pain.* Los Altos, Cal.: Wm. Kaufman, 1975.

---

* The American Society of Clinical Hypnosis, 2400 East Devon Ave., Suite 218, Des Plaines, Ill., 60018. The Society for Clinical and Experimental Hypnosis, 129-A Kings Park Drive, Liverpool, N.Y. 13088.

20. Illovsky, J. An experience with group hypnosis in reading disability in primary behavior disorders. *Journal of Genetic Psychology*, 1963, *102*, 61–67.

21. Illovsky, J., & Fredman, N. Group suggestion in learning disabilities of primary grade children: A feasibility study. *International Journal of Clinical Experimental Hypnosis*, 1976, *24*, 87–97.

22. Jacobs, L. Sleep problems of children: Treatment by hypnosis. *New York State Journal of Medicine*, 1964, *64*, 629–634.

23. Jampolsky, G. G. The use of hypnosis and sensory motor stimulation to aid children with learning problems. *Journal of Learning Disabilities*, 1970, *3*, 570–575.

24. Kaffman, M. Hypnosis as an adjunct to psychotherapy in child psychiatry. *Archives of General Psychiatry*, 1968, *18*, 725–738.

25. LaBaw, W. L. Regular use of suggestibility by pediatric bleeders. *Haematologia*, 1970, *4*, 419–425.

26. LaBaw, W. L. Adjunctive trance therapy with severely burned children. *International Journal of Child Psychotherapy*, 1973, *2*, 80–92.

27. LaBaw, W. L. Auto-hypnosis in hemophilia. *Haematologia*, 1975, *9*, 103–110.

28. LaBaw, W. L., Holton, C., Tewell, K., & Eccles, D. The use of self-hypnosis by children with cancer. *American Journal of Clinical Hypnosis*, 1975, *17*, 233–238.

29. Laguaite, J. K. The use of hypnosis with children with deviant voices. *International Journal of Clinical Experimental Hypnosis*, 1976, *24*, 105–121.

30. Lawlor, E. D. Hypnotic intervention with "school phobic" children. *International Journal of Clinical Experimental Hypnosis*, 1976, *24*, 74–86.

31. Lazar, B. S. Hypnosis as a tool in working with a cerebral-palsied child. *International Journal of Clinical Experimental Hypnosis*, 1977, *25*, 78–87.

32. London, P. Hypnosis in children: An experimental approach. *International Journal of Clinical Experimental Hypnosis*, 1962, *10*, 79–91.

33. London, P. *The children's hypnotic susceptibility scale*. Palo Alto, Cal.: Consulting Psychologists Press, 1963.

34. London, P. Developmental experiments in hypnosis. *Journal of Projective Techniques in Personality Assessment*, 1965, *29*, 189–199.

35. London, P., & Cooper, L. M. Norms of hypnotic susceptibility in children, *Developmental Psychology*, 1969, *1*, 113–124.

36. Marmer, M. J. Hypnosis as an adjunct to anesthesia in children. *American Journal of Diseases of Children*, 1959, *97*, 314–317.

37. Morgan, A. H., & Hilgard, E. R. Age differences in susceptibility to hypnosis. *International Journal of Clinical Experimental Hypnosis*, 1973, *21*, 78–85.

38. Olness, K. The use of self-hypnosis in the treatment of childhood nocturnal enuresis. *Clinical Pediatrics*, 1975, *14*, 273–279.

39. Olness, K. Autohypnosis in functional megacolon. *American Journal of Clinical Hypnosis*, 1976, *19*, 28–32.

40. Surman, O. S., Gottlieb, S. K., & Hackett, T. P. Hypnotic treatment of a child with warts. *American Journal of Clinical Hypnosis*, 1972, *15*, 12–14.

41. Tinterow, M. M. *Foundations of hypnosis from Mesmer to Freud*. Springfield, Ill.: Charles C. Thomas, 1970.

42. Williams, D. T., & Singh, M. Hypnosis as a facilitating therapeutic adjunct in child psychiatry. *Journal of American Academy of Child Psychiatry*, 1976, *15*, 326–342.

PLAY PROGRAMS
IN PEDIATRIC SETTINGS

Elizabeth Crocker, M.Ed.

Introduction

Play is a universal phenomenon. All vertebrates, including humans, engage in play and game behavior that involves exploration of and interaction with things, people, and the environment. These behaviors, prevalent in all cultures, stimulate and foster cognitive, social, emotional, and physical development.

In spite of the above statements about the universality and importance of play, two situations continue to be a reality in North America. First, if randomly selected people are asked to define the word *play*, they are likely to give a variety of answers (vague or otherwise) that may or may not be compatible with one another;—in other words, some confusion exists in people's thinking about play. Such a situation, in part, leads to the second situation: It is not uncommon to find people who, in passing, will pay lip service to the importance of play, but when it comes to spending money for play programs, will indicate their true feeling that play is "nice but really a nonconstructive and frivolous activity." Until there is a common understanding of the meaning and value of play, those who advocate planned play programs and those who control budgets will probably continue to talk at cross purposes.

This chapter proposes, therefore, to try to explain what play is, what things interfere with play, and what happens when humans cannot play. Such a discussion will provide a background for a rationale for planned play programs as well as a brief look at the implications for play programs in various pediatric settings. The last part of the chapter will explore some of the necessary and practical considerations in setting up and operating play programs in such settings. (While the focus of this chapter will be on children and play, it should be noted here that most of what is said about children is true also for adults; but adults play more covertly, so their needs are not as obvious.)

WHAT IS PLAY?

Theorizing about play is not a new activity. Many classical theories continue to be popular and to receive much support. In spite of their variety, however, many theories of play cannot be generalized to include the broad range of activities that are known as play; several have serious logical shortcomings and lack empirical substantiation.

Classical Theories of Play

The surplus energy theory suggests that play is what children do when they have surplus energy—except that we know that children will continue to play even when exhausted. The preparation theory implies that children play to develop competencies and to absorb knowledge necessary for later life—but today lives are so complex and changeable that it is impossible for a child to know what to prepare for. Besides, what does hopscotch have to do with preparation for life? Relaxation is the explanation for the focus of another theory of play—but would it make sense to say that young children relax all day when they appear to be busily engaged in a myriad of bustling activities? The popular psychoanalytic or cathartic theory of play suggests that children's play is an acting out of accumulated or deep-seated feelings of tensions, such as insecurity, frustration, fear, aggression, bewilderment or confusion. While some of children's play may represent various tensions or an active replay of what they have experienced passively, much of their play appears to be happy and more related to natural and joyous curiosity than to troublesome past events.

However, much of what the classical theorists have had to say about play holds true in certain situations; children's play sometimes does appear to burn up surplus energy or prepare, or relax, or relieve. The writer believes, however, that none of these theories are eclectic enough to explain all the different types and contexts of play behavior, and that a more inclusive understanding of the dynamics and importance of play has come from the theorists of recent decades who have studied the relationships between exploration of the environment's various stimuli and play behavior.

Importance of Stimulation

In 1949, Hebb's book, *The Organization of Behaviour*,[17] explained the importance of experience for the development of intelligence. Since then, many researchers and theorists also have stressed the importance of environmental stimuli for normal growth and development. The consensus of enrichment/deprivation studies points clearly to the need for experiences (sensory input from environmental interactions) if the animal or human is to develop appropriately. For example: Rats who have received stimulation develop larger brains; if kittens are deprived of visual input, their vision cells atrophy (irreversibly) and die; Dennis[9] showed that infants deprived of stimulation do not develop normally physically or socially in spite of apparent general health.

More recent researchers have demonstrated the relationship between developmental gains and provision of additional tactile, visual, auditory, and kinesthetic stimulation.[4,25] Other research has suggested that if infants are separated from the significant people in their lives and thus from the corresponding individualized and appropriate stimuli, their eating behaviors will be disturbed and they may "fail to thrive."[27] Still others have shown how important is the existence of environmental stimuli in terms of encouraging exploratory behavior;[20] it seems sensible that a dull environment or repetitive, unvarying stimulation would not be conducive to the growth of curiosity or exploration.

Exploratory Behavior, Competence/Effectance Motivation

Not only must a child have a rich environment, but he must also be able to explore and interact with it. It is through exploration and interaction with the environment that one learns about self, and about understanding and coping with people and with the world. Exploratory behavior, competence/effectance motivation, and play have received increasing research attention in the last few decades. Animal studies have shown that rats will cross an electric grid and undergo the resultant shock just for the opportunity to explore. Exploratory behavior has been referred to as the means of fulfilling the competence/effectance drive of the human organism; that is, the organism strives to interact competently and effectively with the environment (competence) and to have an effect on the environment (effectance). Piaget[22] refers to the child's joy in acting as a cause of events (dropping things, splashing water, banging pots) as well as to his repetition of these acts in order to assimilate and accommodate them in his intellectual repertoire. Some of these exploratory and interactive activities have often been referred to as "just play"; in fact, they are developing the organism's learning, sense of competence/effectance, sense of self, and role of self in relation to the environment.

Optimum Arousal: Play

Both White[26] and Ellis[12] have referred to the organism's need for optimum arousal. Such a need is postulated from the organism's striving to maintain or elevate arousal to avoid boredom, or striving to reduce arousal in situations of unpleasant overstimulation. Play, once viewed as a trivial, nonutilitarian activity, is now felt to be an arousal-elevating or arousal-depressing behavior as well as a child's way of learning how to interact effectively with the environment. The ingredients of play are now seen as activity, exploration, investigation, manipulation, and problem-solving; it is now thought that the purpose of these behaviors is to move to a state of optimum arousal.

Play, therefore, can be seen as behavior that is motivated by an intense desire to learn and to be challenged by things that are new, complex, somewhat uncertain, and responsive. We can also see that as a child continues to deal with and learn from appropriate levels of stimuli he becomes more complex and, therefore, able to learn more. Conversely, if levels of stimulation are inappropriate (too complex, too uncertain, too new, or overabundant) we learn that a child will withdraw or regress in behavior, will not explore, and will be less likely to learn.

The rate of a child's intellectual development is greater during his first four years of life than during the rest of his life; so the impact of a child's early environment and its stimuli greatly affects later cognitive abilities. Play behavior, which is a child's way of interacting at optimal levels with his environment, and of seeking stimuli, is therefore critical for normal growth and development. Given the rate of development in the early years, it can be suggested that even short-term exposure to a stimulus-poor environment or to a situation where a child is not free to explore, may impair or retard a child's development.

The Significance of Play

Research has clearly shown that the playful behavior engaged in by the young is critical for development.[12] The infant's play is indeed serious business. If he did not while away his time pulling strings, shaking rattles, examining wooden parrots, dropping pieces of bread and celluloid swans, when would he learn to discover visual patterns, to catch and throw, and to build up his concept of the object? When would he acquire the many other foundation stones necessary for cumulative learning? "Infancy . . . is a time of active and continuous learning during which the basis is laid for all those processes, cognitive and motor, whereby the child becomes able to establish effective transactions with his environment and move toward a greater degree of autonomy."[26]

From White's eloquent description of infant play and its relationship to learning, we can begin to review the consequences of play—or lack of play—opportunities. For the purposes of this discussion, the word *play* will refer to those behaviors which involve exploration, manipulation, and investigation of the environment and its stimuli, which lead to the raising or lowering of arousal levels toward the optimal.

Opportunities for play behavior enable a child (a) to seek appropriate levels of stimuli that lead both to cognitive development and a sense of well-being, of being involved; (b) to interact with people, which fosters social development as well as language development; and (c) either to avoid or cope with unpleasant, stressful situations by changing the focus of energies, retreating, or developing sociodramatic or fantasy play to express anxieties and tensions.

Sometimes children cannot play, either because of inappropriate levels of stimulation (too much or too little, depending on the child's age and situational context) or physical or psychological inability to interact with the environment. Whether a situation causes play behavior to diminish or cease or whether a child is otherwise restricted from engaging in play behavior is often a subtle distinction; in either case the implication of "no play" is detrimental. The consequences of inhibited play may include (a) depression, leading to physical and emotional health problems (disturbances in eating, sleeping, body temperature; extreme crying; listlessness; stereotypic behavior); (b) impaired or retarded growth, development and learning; atrophy of cells and muscles; inhibition of language development; limited cognitive development; or (c) stress and disorientation (from either too little or too much stimulation) leading to physical and emotional health problems.

The price of "no play" is high. It is important, therefore, to understand what can interfere with or inhibit play, so that such situations and conditions can be prevented or changed.

What Inhibits Play?

1. *Immobility.* If children are immobilized, the outlets for their behavior are limited and they are unable, totally or partially, to interact with the environment and its stimuli. Certain injuries, traction, or cast restrictions for fractures and orthopedic repair can limit the extent to which the environment can be explored. Actual physical placement of a child can also create a type of immobilization; for example, a child in a stroller cannot "get at" all the stimulating things in a store, and a child in a crib cannot "get at" the things he may see.

2. *Dull or Repetitive Environment.* Experiments which have placed people in stimulus-deprivation chambers have shown these situations to be so physically and emotionally intolerable that subjects have begun to hallucinate.[28] If there is nothing in the environment to look at, listen to, manipulate, or investigate, then a child has nothing to explore or play with. While he may try to create some stimuli by babbling, moving about, or singing, after a while this too becomes boring. If the stimuli remain constant and repetitive, then their novelty wears off, and interest in exploring or responding to them wanes.

3. *Overstimulating Environment.* Some situations can be overwhelming for certain

children. For example: A young child who has been raised in the tranquility of the countryside, who has come into contact with only a limited number of people at any one time, may find a large, urban shopping center at Christmastime overstimulating. In such a situation (too much noise, too many people, too much movement, too much to see), a child can "freeze" or emotionally withdraw, and be unable to explore and to play.

4. *Fear.* The emotion of fear is usually in response to situations that are very strange, unknown, or that induce a feeling of aloneness and insecurity. One research study[13] suggested that a high degree of anxiety or fear correlates with avoidance of anxiety-relevant objects and with an inhibition of exploratory behavior. Research has also shown that, although a strange environment can make a child afraid, he is better able to overcome the fear if he is in the presence of a familiar and trusted person.[24] Similarly, a child in a familiar environment who is separated from familiar people, may feel frightened and insecure for a period of time. The simultaneous combination of separation and a strange environment is likely to induce considerable fear and, therefore, to inhibit exploratory behavior until the fear is overcome.

This first section has attempted to (a) outline some of the theoretical and research background for an explanation of play behavior; and (b) provide a background for a consideration of the implications of play in pediatric settings. While certain classical theories of play are suitable to explain or describe play in some situations, this writer has suggested that the optimum arousal theory more generally and appropriately describes the reasons for and the nature of much of children's play behavior. In this context, play has been shown to be critical for cognitive, social, emotional, and physical development. One can conclude, therefore, that it is important to facilitate children's play and to understand what types of situations may interfere with play behavior.

IMPLICATIONS OF PLAY FOR PEDIATRIC SETTINGS

It is generally accepted that illness and hospitalization constitute a crisis in the life of a child and his family. Not only is a child likely to feel unwell or to suffer pain, but when hospitalized, he enters a very unusual place. Kunzman[18] compared a child's normal home environment with the hospital environment: At home a child is exposed to consistent nurturing persons, family associates, regular play with peers, changes in environmental stimuli, school and extracurricular activities, and independence appropriate to growth and development level; in a hospital, a child is exposed to many people in a caretaking role, limited family associations (in some hospitals more than in others), a strange environment, unfamiliar hospital routines, limited (or no) play with peers, limited changes in environmental stimuli, limited (or no) school and extracurricular activities, and a loss of independence. By reflecting on this comparison and by recalling the factors that may interfere with children's play—immobility, dull or repetitive environment, overstimulation (it is estimated that children are exposed to 52 new people in the first 24 hours of hospitalization), and fear caused by separation and a strange environment—it becomes easy to understand how hospitals can be traumatic for children.

Although hospital care primarily concerns itself with what is "wrong" with a child and works to correct that particular infirmity, it is also important to remember what is "right" with a child and to provide activities in which he can continue the normal growth and development patterns that would be occurring were he not hospitalized. The thrust of development does not stop just because of hospitalization; and if special facilities and programs are not provided in hospitals, such development may be retarded or regressive.

Fortunately, as theory and research in the field of child development have increased, hospitals have changed so as to make children's experience of them less traumatic. Many hospitals now have more liberal (or even unrestricted) visiting hours so that children can have more contact with family members; programs to prepare children for hospitalization have been developed to offset the impact of unfamiliarity; and play programs have become part of many pediatric units so that children can be exposed to those environmental stimuli and normal activities that foster growth and development.

Prevalence of Play Programs in Pediatric Settings

To some degree, children will play in spite of where they are. However, their play is likely to be safer and more constructive if they have access to space, materials, time, and a play "opportunist"—someone who can foster group and individualized activities suitable for the children's needs to explore, manipulate, and investigate.

PLAY PROGRAMS FOR INPATIENTS

In a survey of hospitals in Canada and the United States conducted in 1966,[15] it was found that 76% of responding pediatric hospitals and 61% of responding general hospitals with pediatric units had child life programs. (The term *child life program* generally refers to a recreational [sometimes educational] program designed to meet the social, emotional, cognitive, and physical activity needs of children in hospital. Child life programs are also known by names such as "play therapy," "recreation," "patient activity," and "therapeutic play.") In 1974, it was determined that of the seven (now eight) pediatric hospitals in Canada, six had play programs for at least some of the pediatric inpatients. Attention was then directed to general hospitals with pediatric units, and an indepth study of 30 general hospitals with pediatric units of 20 beds or more was carried out in the summer of 1974.[7]

This study determined the following:

1. Although 80% of the hospitals had playrooms, many were not in use because of distance from the nursing station or because of lack of supervisory staff (volunteers, nurses or play staff).
2. Only 10% of the hospitals had play programs. One was staffed by volunteers and two were staffed by specialists in child development.
3. Only 13% of the hospitals had a budget for toys and other play materials.
4. Only 13% of the hospitals had any type of program to enable children to keep up with their school work.

Those who work in pediatric hospitals may take services such as organized play programs for granted. However, the evidence shows that very few general hospitals with pediatric units have provided space, materials, or play opportunists. There appears to be, therefore, a "pediatric paradox": On the one hand, we know that provision for play or arousal events should be considered part of total care, part of furthering the normal health, growth, and development of children; and on the other hand, we know that the great majority of general hospitals' pediatric units are not meeting this responsibility.

PLAY PROGRAMS FOR OUTPATIENTS

In 1977, a survey of 150 hospitals throughout the United States and Canada revealed that 62 of them had activity centers in their outpatient departments;[8] however, no specific studies have been done to determine the actual incidence of professionally staffed play programs in outpatient clinics or emergency waiting rooms. Anecdotally, however, it is known that, while such programs have been fairly uncommon, there is now a trend to set them up in pediatric hospitals, at least. While child life programs for inpatients are usually staffed by specifically trained and salaried personnel, it is not uncommon for play programs in clinics to be staffed by volunteers and students.

PLAY PROGRAMS IN DOCTORS' OFFICES

Every place and every moment is a potential situation for play. Doctors' offices, where children and families often have to wait, are similar in situation to hospital outpatient clinics. Some pediatricians are now setting up their office waiting rooms as a kind of playroom, but most general practitioners have not made this move—a move certainly warranted when one realizes that most children do not go to a pediatrician but to a general or family practitioner.

The benefits that accrue from providing constructive outlets for play behavior, be it in a doctor's office, clinic, or hospital ward, are numerous. Not only can children benefit, but medical staff and parents can find it useful; they may observe children at play, and they will find children more relaxed and cooperative during examinations and treatments.

Benefits of Play Programs in Pediatric Settings

We know that understimulation and overstimulation can cause stress; we know that stress can cause both physiological and psychological problems. We know, too, that through play children can try to manipulate stimulation toward the optimal level, thereby reducing stress. However, unless children have access to planned or supervised play programs in pediatric settings, their own attempts at exploration or manipulation may not be appropriate.

Possibly the following examples will seem quite familiar.

1. Scene: Hospitalized infant in a crib with no toys and no people around to entice into social interaction.

Action: The infant begins to tear his disposable diaper into small pieces, scattering some on the floor and eating others.

Interpretation: The infant is saying, "There's nothing interesting to do here. I'm bored. I don't know how to push the call button to get someone to come and play with me, and I can't find anything else to do."

2. Scene: Crowded outpatient clinic. Parent has tried to keep 2-year-old child in his stroller but the crying and protestation is not worth it. The room has nothing in it except magazines, chairs, and people.

Action: The toddler toddles around, and is ignored by the adults who are trying to lose themselves in the magazines. He discovers a "sand box" (an ashtray) and decides to make a castle on the floor. He spills the contents in the process.

Interpretation: The child is innocently exploring the environment and finds something interesting. There are no alternatives.

In both situations, the children probably receive attention for their play but the attention may not be positive, thus, possibly, leading to greater stress.

Both situations could have been quite different if there had been planned play programs to involve the children's energies. One small study reported in *Play in*

Hospital[16] showed that children in hospital cry less when they can play or interact with people. Based on anecdotal experiences of hospital workers and reports of parents, it is believed that children's adjustment to hospital is more positive, with fewer postdischarge behavior problems, when children's stress has been reduced through attention, information, and play.

Planned play programs in hospitals, clinics, or doctors' offices provide some or all of the following benefits:

- Children continue normal activities that foster curiosity, learning, growth, and development.

- Children find the hospital less strange if they can play with familiar things, or play out familiar roles.

- Children express their concerns and confusions and receive accurate, reassuring information. (Role-playing and puppet play are very successful for this.)

- Children have safe outlets for their natural energies and anxieties.

- Children avoid boredom and pass time through constructive activity.

- Children have a sense of autonomy and independence through play: They can make choices about what they want to do, feel like part of them is still intact, and feel that they can still do things.

- Children meet other children and give each other much needed companionship and support; they often know how it "really feels" and can share that feeling with others.

- Children become more relaxed and cooperative for treatments and procedures if they have a chance to rehearse through play.

- Children are reinforced in the knowledge that hospitals are caring places.

- Children integrate or work out upsetting experiences, because play can be cathartic for pentup feelings.

- Children at play make their parents feel comfortable; parents can learn both from observation of and participation with their children at play.

- Children show the medical staff what their behaviors are when they are having fun and are not frightened; such observation of normal behavior and development levels can aid in diagnosis and selection of therapeutic approach.

- Children at play foster their physical health without realizing it. For example, blowing bubbles after a heart operation is fun, not therapy; playground activity is fun, not physiotherapy.

- Children will be distracted from the reasons for their hospitalization, because play can be an antidote for pain.

- Children are challenged and helped to mature through play.

- Older children learn to cope, to be brave, and to face hospitalization as an adventure; a play opportunist can provide support during this growing-up experience.

Children need every opportunity to participate in daily living and exploration with all their available emotional, intellectual and physical energies. Children in hospitals, particularly those who are very young, in isolation, those experiencing complex or painful treatments, or hospitalized for a long time, have acute needs both for appropriate stimulation and for emotional expression and support. Planned play programs in pediatric settings can help to meet these needs, provide these opportunities, and thus yield worthwhile returns.

SETTING UP PLAY PROGRAMS IN PEDIATRIC SETTINGS

A number of factors must be considered when setting up play programs for inpatients and outpatients in a hospital setting. Thought and planning should be directed toward staff; location, indoors and outdoors, and design of play space; programs, and materials.

STAFF

Most hospitals with well established play programs have specific job descriptions and qualification requirements for their play staff. The *Directory of Child Life Activity Programs in North America* published by the Association for the Care of Children in Hospitals[8] gives the names and addresses of such hospitals together with additional information concerning numbers and training of staff. If a hospital plans to set up a play program, it is suggested that hospitals of comparable size be contacted for information about staffing.

Three factors are important in selecting staff for play programs: personality, training, and experience. Working with children and families in pediatric settings obviously requires the personality traits of liking children and being able to relate well to people of all ages; in addition, however, play staff should be flexible, spontaneous, and (in certain cases) assertive. Flexibility is necessary because one often has to change plans quickly in order to accommodate new situations that arise in hospital routines; spontaneity is frequently needed in responding to urgent, often unforeseen needs of children and families; the ability to be an assertive spokesman for children and their families helps to ensure that their total needs are not overwhelmed by hospital habits or routines.

Because of budget constraints, to discuss training and experience desirable for play staff is often to discuss the unobtainable. Ideally, however, play staff for pediatric settings should have a thorough grasp of child growth and development, child psychology, the significance of various types of play and creative expression, techniques of stimulation and supervision, and the impact of hospitalization and illness on children and their families. Very few places in North America offer such comprehensive training in a university program; consequently, when selecting staff, one should look for someone with as many of these attributes as possible who is also eager and willing to continue to learn on the job. (Staffing information in the *Directory of Child Life Programs in North America* would suggest that this is what most hospitals have done—for the training backgrounds listed are quite broad in their scope.) All of the above criteria apply equally to staff in outpatient clinics. Ability to relate well with parents is particularly important in the outpatient department; so is a flair for providing short-term, age-appropriate activities for the steady stream of patients.

Ideally, in terms of overall inpatient coverage, one should aim to have at least one play staff member for every 15 patients; the ratio should be considerably lower in areas where staff are working with infants and toddlers. If there are very few staff available, first consideration should be given to children under 5 years of age; children with no visitors; children in isolation with infectious diseases or burns; and children undergoing surgery.

Because of financial restrictions, many hospitals set up their play programs by using volunteers to provide and supervise activities, but there are some obvious drawbacks to such an alternative. A principal disadvantage is that volunteers, except in very rare circumstances, do not come on a daily basis. Consequently, unless they are in hospital for a long time, the children fail to develop a significant relationship with the play opportunist and therefore may be less willing to play, talk, or act out upsetting experiences. In turn, the volunteer is unable to observe the children's play and social behavior over consecutive days and to report such observations to medical staff. On balance, however, some volunteer play programs can help. They are, at very least, a step in the right direction, for their existence shows that someone has recognized the need for hospitalized children to play.

Whether volunteers assist or direct a play program, certain conditions will make their involvement more effective. One person should be responsible for volunteer selection, orientation, placement, and supervision. Volunteers should be selected for their maturity, reliability, empathy, discretion, and knowledge of and talent with children. Orientation and training give a volunteer a context in which to work; similarly, supervision and feedback let the volunteer feel his or her time and effort are noticed and valued. When hospitals do not have a coordinated volunteer program under the direction of one person, the level of involvement and effectiveness is not high, and is usually short-lived.

LOCATION AND DESIGN OF PLAY SPACE

In the writer's opinion, it is advantageous to have play spaces located within or close to patients' wards. Some children, particularly young ones, become fretful if they have to go to other parts of the hospital complex—it is a large enough task to adapt to the strange surroundings of a hospital ward without having to take on the entire building! Play spaces far from the children's unit require staff to supervise comings and goings. Moreover, play spaces are much more likely to be used for both formal and informal activities if they are within sight of or easy access to the nursing station. Play space in the outpatient clinic should also be within sight and hearing of the booking desk. Parents want both to see where their children are and to hear when they are called for their appointments. One Canadian hospital has used curved, waist-high plexiglass in its outpatient clinic, which gives children the sense of being set apart but gives parents and clinic staff continuous visual access.

The design of play spaces should incorporate doors wide enough and floor space sufficient to accommodate a number of children in beds and wheelchairs as well as ambulatory patients; storage space for play materials and crafts supplies; movable furniture so that defined play areas can be created and dismantled as needs arise; space to display children's work and to ensure that certain materials are always invitingly evident; and a two-way communication system with the closest nursing station (if the space is not within its visual field). Such a list borders on the obvious, but the important thing to remember is that practically any space—even old, dimly lit ends of corridors—can be transformed into productive play spaces with a clear vision of the needs to be served and a touch of creativity (see Chapter 9 for a fuller discussion of this topic).

Outdoor play spaces are among recent developments in environments for hospitalized children. Hospitals with outdoor playgrounds report that outside play for hospitalized children yields not only enjoyment but also better appetites, continued growth, development of gross motor skills, and improved cooperation with physiotherapy programs. As with interior space, almost any design for an outdoor play space will work. However, certain considerations should be kept in mind:

1. Shade. While fresh air and sunshine are a nice change from the indoors, too much sunshine can be hazardous, so children should be able to retreat to shade. (Sometimes, children cannot be in direct sunlight because of specific medical conditions or treatments.)
2. Terrain. Among the exciting features of outdoor playgrounds are small hills and streams, grass, and sand; however, a hospital playground also needs paved areas for children in beds and wheelchairs.
3. Storage space. Provision for storage of playground equipment in a locked shed right on the playground saves considerable time in getting ready and cleaning up at the end of activity periods.
4. Water. Water has one-hundred-and-one uses on an outdoor playground! Once plumbing has been established, the provision of a bathroom (accessible to children in wheelchairs, too) should be considered; it saves transporting children back and forth to their wards.
5. Communication. "What if the doctor comes and wants to see him?" Two-way communication with the hospital building ensures not only that playground staff can be notified if someone has to return indoors but also that the playground staff can notify the unit staff if any incidents occur.

PROGRAMS

Any good library has extensive resources to help plan activity programs for children. Hospitalized children have the same needs for play and activity as well children, but because of limitations (traction, therapy, isolation, bed rest), play staff have to be particularly inventive. A comprehensive play program for hospitalized children should plan for age-appropriate activity; it should also recognize and accommodate different play needs, ranging from diversion and entertainment to the mastery of new skills and for the therapeutic play that works out upsetting experiences through role play. Activities may include the following:

- music: listening, playing rhythm instruments, singing, making instruments from scrap materials;

- games: board games such as Scrabble and active games such as hide-and-go-seek and pingpong;

- arts and crafts: (It's nice to take something home that was created in the hospital);

- stories: listening, telling, and reading;

- movies: cartoons, often the highlight of a hospital experience; good educational films as well;

- messy materials: . . . sand, water, and clay;

- work activities: helping out in the playroom and on the ward;

- dramatic play: pretend cooking, dressing up in old clothes, puppets and puppet shows, role-playing doctor, nurse, patient, and operations;

- construction: stacking and fitting toys, blocks, puzzles, creations from junk;

- special events: birthdays, holidays, special guests or entertainers; (One hospital has a yearly turtle race and another has a yearly mini-olympics;

- plants, animals, and fish: learning, talking about, and caring for growing, living things;

- field trips: places of interest in the community and also in the hospital.

Such a list could go on and on (especially if all the things particular to a hospital setting that can act as catalysts to activity and learning were to be added.)

Most of the activities mentioned can be part of an activity program in an outpatient clinic as well. The overall aim of providing play activities in a hospital setting is to help children—be they infants or teenagers—to feel comfortable, to express themselves, to explore, to grow and develop, and to optimize what they can do.

Materials. Large amounts of toys and materials need not be purchased for a play program. A few carefully selected, durable materials are preferable to many poorly made toys. Also, starting with a basic inventory allows for orderly additions as needs arise. Activities listed previously assume that certain necessary materials will be on hand, including hospital clothes and equipment for role-playing. In addition, toys for infants should be available, including rattles, mobiles, and toys of tactile interest.

An important point to remember when selecting play materials is that children often see certain play possibilities in materials that adults cannot see. For example, to a little boy a hank of wool to be wound for pompoms and other wool toys becomes a headdress, a lion's mane, and any number of things! Play materials should be selected not only for safety features and durability, but also for complexity; a toy that does only one thing quickly bores a child. Most important: It should be remembered that the best toy in the world is a person who is interested, responsive, and willing to "play back." It is not enough to have great toys and materials for a play program; people are crucial to the stimulation of play. Staff should be selected, then, not only on the basis of training but also on the basis of their ability to be good "players."

Resources for a Play Program

A number of useful books and pamphlets are available to anyone interested in hospital play programs. Readers are especially advised to refer to works by Azarnoff,[1] Azarnoff and Flegal,[2] Bopp,[3] Cleverdon,[6] Glaser,[14] Harvey and Hales-Tooke,[4] Petrillo and Sanger,[21] and Plank.[23] All provide excellent guidelines for setting up play programs in pediatric settings. Also, most of them include good sections on the implications of, and ways to provide for, therapeutic hospital play.

Some organizations have been consistently concerned with the development of quality play programs in pediatric settings. The Association for the Care of Children in Hospitals is an interdisciplinary organization with an international membership, (chiefly from Canada and the United States). The Association has several study sections (groups of professionals with common concerns); one such section is the Child Life Activities study section. For anyone planning a play program in a pediatric setting, this study section can provide guidance and moral support.* The Association has a number of publications in addition to its regular journal which would be of value: *The Hospitalized Child Bibliography,*[10] *The Directory of Child Life Activity Programs in North America,*[8] *Ideas and Activities with Hospitalized Children,*[14] and *Guidelines for*

---

* Association for the Care of Children in Hospitals, P.O. Box H, Union, W. Va.

the Development of Hospital Programs and for the Personnel Conducting Programs of Therapeutic Play for Pediatric Patients.[3]

Comparable organizations exist in Britain and Australia. In Britain: The National Association for the Welfare of Children in Hospital;* in Australia: The Association for the Welfare of Children in Hospital.† The Australian Association has published an excellent annotated bibliography, *Play and the Hospitalized Child.*[19]

Conclusion

For those who say, "Well, what you've said about play is nice, but most hospital experiences are very short; surely, kids can get along without playing for a couple of days," there are two studies that challenge their point of view.

One study looked retrospectively at a very large sample population to see if there were correlations between hospitalization in early life and later problems. In his conclusion to the study, Douglas states:

This study provides strong and unexpected evidence that one admission to hospital of more than one week's duration, or repeated admissions before the age of 5 (in particular between 6 months and 4 years) are associated with an increased risk of behaviour disturbance and poor reading in adolescence. The children who experienced these early admissions are more troublesome out of class, more likely to be belligerent and more likely to show unstable job patterns than those who were not admitted in the first 5 years . . . The children most vulnerable to early admissions to hospital are those who are highly dependent on their mothers, or who are under stress at home at the time of the admission. There is evidence that early admissions to hospital are more frequent today than 25 years ago and that readmissions are more frequent. Length of stay may have been reduced, but the proportion of children who experience long or repeated admissions is no less in 1975 than in 1946 and in fact, may be greater.[11]

In short, Douglas suggests that the hospitalization of children in the late 1940's has had long term morbidity. While he agrees that psychosocial aspects of pediatric care have improved, he fears that incidence of admission and long stays of children under the age of 5 have not changed. A recent study[5] has supported his fears. Of 74 hospitalized children under 6 years of age, 93% were between birth and 4 years of age; 43% were between birth and 12 months; 63½% had been hospitalized before, and 53% had been hospitalized for more than 7 days. Looking at these figures in connection with Douglas's conclusions, it follows that, in terms of age, length of stay, and repeated admissions, a large percentage of this patient population was "at risk." How many children in other hospitals are also "at risk"?

Things are changing in pediatrics: Parental visiting is more extensive; children are being prepared for hospitalization and surgery; play programs are provided—but are things changing everywhere or fast enough?

Although there have been no controlled research studies that have specifically evaluated and analyzed the effects of play programs in pediatric settings, there is strong reason to believe that play is crucial for children's social, emotional, intellectual, and physical growth, as well as overall health. Those who work in play programs in ped-

---

* National Association for the Welfare of Children in Hospital, 7 Exton St., London SE1 8VE, England.

† The Association for the Welfare of Children in Hospital, 5 Union St., New South Wales 2150, Australia.

iatric settings have always believed that such service is important to the children, parents, and medical staff. Anecdotal evidence shows that play in all its forms makes a difference, not only in growth and development but also in children's adjustment to the pediatric setting and thus, ultimately, to rates of rehabilitation and recovery.

Can hospitals afford to have play programs? Azarnoff and Flegal have answered this question. "It is a good idea, it is indispensable, and it is right for children. When deciding whether it deserves maximum support, the question to ask is whether the hospital can afford not to have it.[11]

There is still much to be done. A major challenge in the coming years for those concerned with the quality and effects of total pediatric care is to ensure that children are not denied opportunities for constructive play just because they suffer the experience of hospitalization.

REFERENCES

1. Azarnoff, P. A play program in a pediatric clinic. *Children* 1970, *17*, 218.

2. Azarnoff, P., & Flegal, S. *A pediatric play program.* Springfield, Ill.: Charles C. Thomas, 1975.

3. Bopp, J. (Ed.). *Guidelines for the development of hospital programs; and for the personnel conducting programs of therapeutic play for pediatric patients.* Union, W. Va.: Association for the Care of Children in Hospitals, 1971.

4. Casler, L. The effects of extra tactile stimulation. *Genetic Psychology Monographs*, 1965, *71*, 131–175.

5. Church, B., Kelly, P., McArel, G., et al. To visit or not to visit? That is the question. Unpublished manuscript, Dalhousie University School of Nursing, Halifax, Nova Scotia, 1977.

6. Cleverdon, D. (Ed.). *Play in a hospital.* New York: The Play Schools Association.

7. Crocker, E. *Child life programs in the maritime region: A study of the non-medical needs of and future directions for hospitalized children.* Halifax, Nova Scotia: Atlantic Institute of Education, 1974.

8. Crocker, E. (Ed.). *Directory of child life activity programs in North America.* Union, W. Va.: Association for the Care of Children in Hospitals, 1977.

9. Dennis, W. Causes of retardation among institutionalized children. *Journal of Genetic Psychology*, 1951, *96*, 47–59.

10. Donnelly, M. (Ed.). *The hospitalized child bibliography.* Union, W. Va.: Association for the Care of Children in Hospitals, 1976.

11. Douglas, J. W. B. Early hospital admissions and later disturbances of behavior and learning. *Developmental Medicine and Child Neurology*, 1975, *17*, 456–480.

12. Ellis, M. J. *Why people play.* Englewood Cliffs, N.J.: Prentice-Hall, 1973.

13. Gilmore, J. B. The role of anxiety and cognitive factors in children's play behavior. *Child Development*, 1966, *37*, 397–416.

14. Glaser, H. (Ed.), *Ideas and activities with hospitalized children.* Union, W. Va.: Association for the Care of Children in Hospitals, 1970.

15. Haller, J. A. (Ed.). *The hospitalized child and his family.* (See esp. Appendices A & B.) Baltimore: Johns Hopkins, 1967.

16. Harvey, S., & Hales-Tooke, A. *Play in hospital.* London: Faber & Faber, 1972.

17. Hebb, D. O. *The Organization of Behavior.* New York: Wiley, 1949.

18. Kunzman, L. Some factors influencing a young child's mastery of hospitalization. *The Nursing Clinics of North America*, 1972, *7*, 13–26.

19. Langley, E. (Ed.). *Play and the hospitalized child.* Parramatta (N.S.W.), Australia: Association for the Welfare of Children in Hospital, 1976.

20. Newcombe, P. The effects of maternal interactions on some infant behaviours and implications for infant care workers. Unpublished manuscript, Atlantic Institute of Education, Halifax, Nova Scotia, 1974.

21. Petrillo, M., & Sanger, S. *Emotional care of hospitalized children: An environmental approach.* Philadelphia: Lippincott, 1972.

22. Piaget, J. *Play, dreams, and imitation in childhood.* New York: Norton, 1962.

23. Plank, E. N. *Working with children in hospitals.* Cleveland: Case Western Reserve University Press, 1971.

24. Rheingold, H. L., & Samuels, H. R. Maintaining the positive behavior of infants by increased stimulation. *Developmental Psychology,* 1969, *1,* 520–527.

25. Scarr-Salapatek, S., & Williams, M. L. The effects of early stimulation on low birth weight infants. *Child Development,* 1973, *44,* 94–101.

26. White, R. W. Motivation reconsidered: The concept of competence. *Psychological Review,* 1959, *66,* 297–333.

27. Yarrow, L. J., Rubenstein, J. L., Pederson, F. A., et al. Dimensions of early stimulation and their differential effects on infant development. In L. J. Stone, H. T. Smith, & L. B. Murphy (Eds.), *The competent infant.* New York: Basic Books, 1973.

28. Zubek, J. P. Effects of prolonged sensory and perceptual deprivation. *British Medical Bulletin,* 1965, *20,* 38–42.

ADDITIONAL READING

Axline, V. M. *Play therapy.* Cambridge: Houghton-Mifflin, 1947.

Bloom, B. S. *Stability and change in human characteristics.* New York: Wiley, 1965.

Bowlby, J. *Attachment and loss: I. Attachment.* Jordon, England: Hogarth Press, 1969.

Bronson, W. C. The growth of competence: Issues of conceptualization and measurement. In H. R. Schaffer (Ed.), *The origins of human social relations.* London: Academic Press, 1971.

Brooks, M. Why play in the hospital? *The Nursing Clinics of North America,* 1970, *5,* 431–441.

Caldwell, B. M. What is the optimal learning environment for the young child? *American Journal of Orthopsychiatry,* 1967, *37,* 8–22.

Caldwell, B. M., & Richmond, J. B. Social class level and stimulation potential of the home. In J. Hellmuth (Ed.), *The exceptional infant.* New York: Brunner/Mazel, 1967.

Caplan, F., & Caplan, T. *The power of play.* New York: Doubleday, 1973.

Chodil, J., & Williams, B. The concept of sensory deprivation. *The Nursing Clinics of North America,* 1970, *5,* 353–365.

Crocker, E. Do they really pay you to play? *Nova Scotia Medical Bulletin,* 1973, *51,* 192–193.

Erikson, E. H. *Childhood and society.* New York: Norton, 1950.

Gellert, E. Reducing the emotional stresses of hospitalization for children. *American Journal of Occupational Therapy,* 1958, *12,* 125.

Gregg, E. (Ed.). *What to do when there's nothing to do.* New York: Dell, 1968.

Groos, K. *The play of man.* New York: Appleton, 1901.

Hardgrove, C. B., & Dawson, R. B. *Parents and children in the hospital: The family's role in pediatrics.* Boston: Little, Brown, 1972.

Hartley, R. E., Frank, L. K., & Goldenson, R. M. *Understanding children's play.* New York: Columbia, 1952.

Jolly, H. Play is work: The role of play for sick and healthy children. *Lancet,* 1969, *2,* 487–488.

Maccoby, E., & Masters, J. C. Attachment and dependency. In P. A. Mussen (Ed.), *Carmichael's manual of child psychology* (3rd ed.). New York: Wiley, 1970.

Mason, E. A. The hospitalized child: His emotional needs. *New England Journal of Medicine,* 1965, *272,* 406–414.

Millar, S. *The psychology of play.* Baltimore: Penguin, 1968.

Moustakas, C. *Children in play therapy.* New York: Ballantine, 1972.

Noble, E. *Play and the sick child.* London: Faber & Faber, 1967.

Patrick, G. T. W. *The psychology of relaxation.* Boston: Houghton Mifflin, 1916.

Piers, M. W. (Ed.). *Play and development.* New York: Norton, 1972.

Rheingold, H. L. The effect of a strange environment on the behaviour of infants. In B. M. Foss (Ed.), *Determinants of infant behaviour* (Vol. 4). London: Methuen, 1969.

Robertson, J. *Young children in hospitals.* New York: Basic Books, 1958.

Rubenstein, J. Maternal attentiveness and subsequent exploratory behavior in the infant. *Child Development,* 1967, *38,* 1089–1100.

Rutter, M., & Mittler, P. Environmental influences on language development. In M. Rutter & J. A. M. Martin (Eds.), *Young children with delayed speech.* New York: Heinemann, 1972.

Spencer, *H. Principles of psychology,* Vol. 2, Part 2 (3rd ed.). New York: Appleton, 1873.

Sutton-Smith, B. S. *How to play with your child and when not to.* New York: Hawthorn Books, 1974.

Tisza, V. B., & Angoff, K. A play program and its function in a pediatric hospital. *Pediatrics,* 1959, *19,* 293.

Wolff, S. *Children under stress.* London: Penguin Press, 1969.

Yarrow, L. J., & Goodwin, M. S. The immediate impact of separation: Reactions of infants to a change in mother figures. In L. J. Stone, H. T. Smith & L. B. Murphy (Eds.), *The competent infant.* New York: Basic Books, 1973.

PSYCHOLOGICAL CONSIDERATIONS IN HUMANIZING THE PHYSICAL ENVIRONMENT OF PEDIATRIC OUTPATIENT AND HOSPITAL SETTINGS

Anita R. Olds, Ph.D.

THE ENVIRONMENT IS THE MESSAGE

In our informal interviews with children . . . we find that their memories are seldom of adults, but usually of places and related sensations—the agony of lying still at naptime, not ever being able to get a swing, having one's back rubbed, digging in the sand under the big tree, having lunch outdoors on the grass.[2,p.2]

The physical discomforts of pain, illness, and injury can be upsetting to anyone. For a child, the anxiety of a visit to the doctor is compounded by the threat of unfamiliar people prepared to impose unknown assaults upon his body, and a frightening institutional setting new to his experience. Large buildings, with long, tortuous corridors, strange pieces of equipment, and mazes of rooms, are staffed by a host of intricately related individuals sporting uniforms, titles, and medical instruments, and functioning according to a set of mysterious social norms. Believing that things are the way they appear to be, and confused by part-whole relationships, it is unlikely that children differentiate the success or failure of the pediatrician and his procedures from the uninviting, frightening physical circumstances surrounding examination and treatment. At the very least, pediatric settings should not aggravate existing levels of anxiety and distress; when they are welcoming, comforting, and supportive they may actually be used in the service of prevention, treatment, and recovery.

Experiences in pediatric environments affect three psychological needs of children, parents, and staff: the need to feel comfortable, the need to feel in control of one's self, and the need to be purposefully active.

The Need to Feel Comfortable

Psychologists know that a child who is comfortable in a space will "lose" himself in it, not by being confused and disoriented, but by feeling safe from attack or intrusion and unself-conscious about his performance. Comfortable surroundings foster playful attitudes towards events and materials, attitudes that help to lower anxiety and to make the child a more cooperative subject for examination and treatment. Comfortable surroundings also help parents better attend to instructions and explanations, treat their children with more patience and understanding, and accept distressing diagnoses with greater calm. Staff, too, are less impersonal in dealing with human needs when they feel relaxed in the setting in which they work.

Yet, the response to human suffering and disability has been to strip therapeutic environments bare, rather than to enrich them as at least partial compensation for a patient's loss of well being. Medical facilities are uncomfortable places because their arousal properties are extreme, whereas moderate degrees of environmental variability are necessary for maintaining optimal levels of mental and physical alertness.

The over-arousing aspects of medical settings are obvious: vast, unfamiliar spaces, ambiguous events, long, disorienting corridors, frightening equipment, and a confusion of people and materials rushing through hidden areas, engaging in mysterious and painful activities. Less obvious are the ways in which such settings deaden arousal: cold, shiny tile floors, multiple tables and chairs of identical design and hard finish, dull-colored walls lacking recesses or changes in texture, endless corridors each of which looks like the other, ceilings of uniform height, fluorescent lights which spread a constant, indiscriminate, high-powered glare over all activities—all convey an environmental sterility and uniformity that is boring and distasteful.

Warm, welcoming, friendly spaces are sensorily rich and varied. In fact, the old adage, "Variety is the spice of life," is the best guideline for making pediatric facilities comfortable. Elements used in personalizing homes, such as pillows, plants, soft furniture, are essential for humanizing institutions. So is the intentional variation of physical parameters such as scale (small spaces and furniture for children, larger ones for adults; areas for privacy, semiprivacy, and whole group participation; materials at child eye level and at adult height); floor height (raised and lowered levels, platforms, lofts, pits, climbing structures); ceiling height (canopies, eaves, skylights); boundary height (walls, half-height dividers, low bookcases); lighting (natural, fluorescent, incandescent, local, indirect); visual interest (wall murals, classical art, children's paintings, views to trees and sky); auditory interest (the hum of voices, mechanical gadgets, music, birds chirping, children laughing); olfactory interest (fresh flowers in a vase, plants in warm earth, medicines and antiseptic solutions); textural interest (wood, fur, carpet, fabric, plastic, formica, glass); kinesthetic interest (things to touch with different body parts; things to crawl in, under, and upon; opportunities to see the environment from different spatial vantage points). Moderate variation of each of these elements can transform a stark, stressful institution into a comfortable and pleasant place.

The Need to Feel in Control

Institutional settings are organized by persons other than the client for the shared use of many strangers. As Milgram has demonstrated,[1] those who work and appear to belong in such settings become vested with authority to direct and control outsiders, and to effect changes in the institution's physical or social structure. In fact, the sterile design of medical facilities bespeaks a literal "hands off" policy to those who do not work there—and even sometimes to those who do. (This perception may account for the paucity of attempts on the part of employees and medical personnel to humanize such spaces, despite frequent acknowledgement that the environment is debilitating.)

Authorities demonstrate their status nonverbally by knowing their way around, and by actively utilizing spaces or facilities that are part of the institutional setting. On the other hand, clients experience a sense of required submissiveness and a reduced legitimacy to function autonomously in such environments, since they are unable to behave in customary ways, to stake out territories (other than seat or bed) over which they have jurisdiction, or to control their activities and levels of social interaction. Instead, they must be on the alert for and obedient to institutional expectations for how they should behave. Children, being less adept at deciphering such social rules, provoke parents to compensate for their immaturity by placing unaccustomed demands for proper performance upon them.

To overcome this loss of control and status, the client should be helped to feel that he belongs, that is, that he can make his way easily through the institutional spaces, and that he has activities to perform which grant him some control over territory, materials, and social encounters.

Interpretable physical layouts, reinforced by good orientation devices in entries, lobbies, corridors, elevators, waiting and treatment rooms, will enable clients to perform the simplest of human activities—getting where they want to go. Good orientation requires simple, visible signs or cues that occur with regularity and at critical turning points to keep people on route. A survey of the number of times personnel are interrupted to give directions can reveal the difficulty with which strangers orient themselves in a building, the strain on staff to be traffic cops, and the major loci of confusion. Since children do not attend to cues utilized by adults, pediatric facilities must provide orientation devices at child level. Objects to spin; buttons to push; something to touch, poke or peer into; a sequence of photographs of children or animals at work or play—all are ways to welcome and orient young patients, as well as to designate pediatric areas, especially when they are located in mixed-use facilities.

Any material or posture which respects the capacity of child and parent to understand and contribute to medical matters is a reinstatement of their status and self-respect. The provision of educational materials on prevention and treatment acknowledges the client's right, need, and capacity to care for his own body.

Facilities specifically intended for parents and children (coat racks, coffee machines, water fountains, reading lights, diaper-changing tables, and conveniently located lavatories), which enable them to fulfill basic personal needs and to be helpful to themselves or others without assistance, are all proof that they belong. Parent lounges, children's playrooms, and waiting spaces, which through their design and provisioning genuinely support play, a choice of private and semiprivate conditions, and the rearrangement of some furnishings to suit individual preferences, legitimate the client's right to entertain and occupy himself while on institutional territory.

The Need to Be Purposefully Active

Frightened, submissive, and subjected to extremes of over or underarousal, the well being of patients and parents is further violated by the opportunity to engage in but one activity: waiting. There is waiting to be scheduled, registered or admitted; waiting to be examined; waiting for laboratory tests and treatment; waiting for results; waiting for meals; waiting for visitors and play leaders; waiting for recovery; and waiting (finally and hopefully) for release from the confinement of the institution. Although chairs and beds are provided to support the body while it waits, rarely is enough provided to sustain the eyes, ears, hands, brain, and muscles that grow limp, useless, and restless with the interminable waiting.

To offset the waiting, parents and children must be given genuine options for activity, engagement, and interaction. There must be things for adults alone, children alone, and adults and children together to touch, look at, and work upon, and there must be spaces and facilities which support maximal use of and engagement with materials. A box of crayons, locked in a closet except when the nurse is around, is not, from a child's standpoint, having "something to do." Nor are a few materials placed haphazardly around a room suffice as entertainment, and usually, for lack of appropriate storage, work surfaces, and play space, they end up being destroyed or stolen in short order.

Pediatric facilities must provide parents with entertainment such as magazines, newspapers, and educational pamphlets, and they must provide children with physically identifiable, protected play areas where materials are visibly displayed and can be actively used. Where space is limited, some small area still must be carved out for play. A platform 4–12 inches off the floor can often suffice. On it might be a low table (at which children kneel), a rack to hold books, a storage unit with a few craft materials, stuffed animals, construction toys, and games. Two sides of the platform might form a puppet theatre or peekaboo space across which children can communicate with nearby adults and peers (see Fig. 1).

The design of any pediatric space must also support positive social interactions among family members, and also between unfamiliar parents and children. The parent who is pleased with his child's behavior will be less self-conscious about his own public image, more sympathetic to the child's reactions while undergoing examination and treatment, and will provide a positive link in relationships between child and pediatrician. Encounters between unfamiliar parents and children are usually entertaining and distracting. They provide orientation for newcomers, and create a small mutual support-information-exchange network which helps attenuate the loneliness, depression, and embarrassment frequently accompanying illness and disability.

Subsequent pages will present planning and design strategies for creating environments which are welcoming, orienting, comfortable, and rich in possibilities for productive activity and social exchange. To ignore the context in which medical practice occurs by focusing primarily on illnesses and therapy, is to evade the substantive support which environmental design can give to prevention, treatment, and recovery.

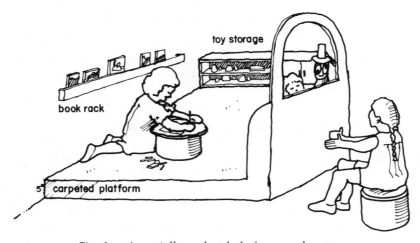

Fig. 1. *A partially enclosed platform as play area.*

114

DESIGNING WAITING SPACES

Despite their differences, general strategies for the successful design of all types of outpatient and inpatient waiting spaces will be discussed: clinics, emergency and outpatient departments, specialized treatment services (cast/brace, preoperative, x-ray), lounges, and private offices.

Preliminary Design Considerations

The design of any waiting space should proceed from identification of the functional requirements of its users. Such requirements are reflected in the three needs previously discussed (comfort, control, and activity), and in the customary movements and actions of the room's occupants (removing coats, sitting, tending children, filing, telephoning). Pediatric waiting areas are challenging to design because of the variety of needs usually present. Populations are transient, of differing cultural and economic backgrounds, varying in age from infant to adult, and varying in extent of illness, anxiety, and vigor. Some patients wait for 5 minutes, others for 5 hours. Inevitable variances in scheduling and human punctuality lead to periods of overcrowding, equipment clutter, and poor supervision, as well as to times of depressing emptiness. The inherent complexity of such settings generates a long list of functional requirements, the most important of which will be considered as strategies for planning are presented.

The three primary factors to consider in organizing any waiting area are (a) the position of major transit zones, (b) the arrangement of seats, and (c) the location of the play space.

Begin by emptying the room (psychologically if not physically) of all movable elements, so only the fixed features remain. Then, based on the location of doorways, identify the major zones of transit as people move between entries, as well as those corners and protected areas which remain. Wherever possible, a single path, entry-to-reception-to-exit, should be created, so as to maximize the territory available for sitting and play. If transit zones are multiple or confused, relocation or elimination (or both) of some doorways should be attempted. The most protected area of the room must be devoted to play, while seats and reception may occupy spaces around the transit areas. In this way, children's activities can proceed with a minimum of interference, and with minimum need for solid barriers around the play space, which might cut off visibility and communication between this area and the sitting zone (see Fig. 2).

Windows, walls of glass, or an open door allowing visibility into the waiting space from the corridor, psychologically prepare both client and receptionist for entry, orient them to major channels of commerce through the building, prevent a child on the wrong side of the door from getting hurt, and even provide visual relief for a small space. For purposes of orientation and control, it is usually most efficient to place the receptionist near the entrance. However, being asked to give one's name and identification before actually entering a space is a formal, institutional mode of welcome, not appropriate to all situations (psychiatry, for example) or to small, intimate rooms where the welcome might better be made by the space itself, with the receptionist seated somewhere in the interior. As the hub of the communication network, the receptionist needs to be located near clients, physicians' offices, files, and the like, but she must have sufficient distance to efficiently carry out her tasks without imposing them on clients. Both parties should feel they can rely on, yet not be forced into communication with, one another.

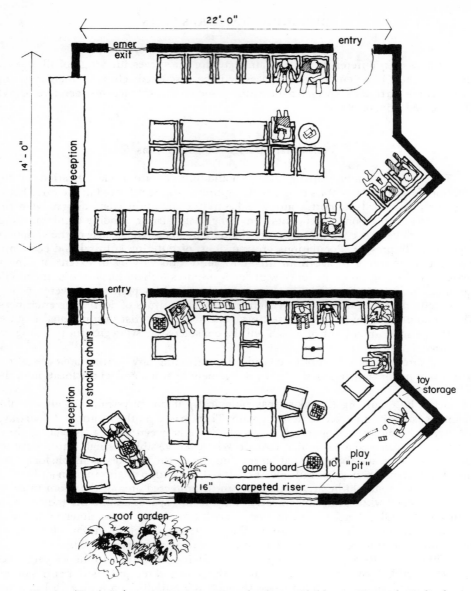

Fig. 2. *(Top.) Before renovations, Dental Clinic, Children's Hospital Medical Center, Boston, Mass. (Bottom.) Proposed renovations for Clinic, featuring seating clusters, a play area, game tables, and a relocated entry.*

Moreover, the receptionist has another duty to perform (perhaps to be added to the job description), which must be reflected in the position of the reception desk, if the success of a pediatric waiting space is to be assured: surveillance of the play area and materials. A well planned play area is essential for controlling activity and use, but no design can replace the power of supervision to constrain negative behaviors. Placement of the reception area within good visual and auditory range of the play space can, without hiring additional personnel or taxing the receptionist, reduce vandalism and pilferage, and so guarantee the purposeful activity of patients and parents.

Arranging the Sitting Area

Typically, waiting room furniture is pushed against the walls of the room, creating an airport "line-up" effect that precludes either privacy or social exchange. The result, in spaces with more than half a dozen seats, is deadly. Each individual is in full view of the multitude, with no place to look, no place to hide, no place to perform even simple actions without being subject to critical public appraisal. Small wonder that people sit immobile and withdrawn, staring blankly into space, or seemingly engrossed in the printed page.

The first requirement for humanizing the sitting area is the elimination of most of this line-up by creating seating clusters, of at least two chairs and a table, placed in an L-shaped configuration (see Fig. 3). Oddly enough, this arrangement makes available more area for sitting or other uses because less space is required in access to and from seats. It also makes the room appear less congested and more interesting. The L-shaped arrangement does require seats with fairly solid backs, however, since most people feel uncomfortable with their backs exposed.

In arranging seating clusters throughout the waiting space, an easy flow (rather than a sharp separation) between sitting and play zones should be attempted. Waiting adults are often relieved of their boredom when given the chance to watch children at play or to interact with them. Young children are prone to vacillate between mother's seat and the play area, and to feel uncomfortable unless mother is in view. In support of

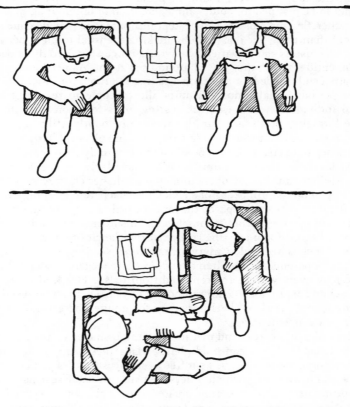

Fig. 3. *(Top.) Wrong: Seats arranged in a "lineup." (Bottom.) Correct: Two seats and a table in an L-shaped arrangement.*

these needs, and for provision for simultaneous stimulation and supervision, some seating clusters should be made to face the play area, while elements of other clusters can be oriented indirectly towards the play. Privacy can be achieved (for teenagers, or in lounges where parents need to express grief, compose themselves, discuss personal matters) by turning a few seats away from the play space, or by retaining some of the line-up.

Seating clusters act as separate areas (see discussion which follows), diversifying the waiting room and permitting clients to engage in different activities simultaneously. Teens find ways to be alone and aloof from younger children, solitary adults can retreat from the crowd, a child in a hospital "johnny" does not feel so exposed, and groups of related individuals may gather together, minimally interfering with or being intruded upon by strangers. Casual conversation occurs most readily when people are oriented at right angles to one another and can easily engage or disengage eye contact. Furthermore, the improved orientation and decreased physical separation of interlocutors reduces the need to raise one's voice to be heard, lowers the overall noise level of the room, and supports conversational intimacy. Thus, a comfortable balance of community and privacy is achieved.

Furnishings and Activities

To meet the range of needs found in pediatric waiting spaces, furnishings and activities should be planned for adults alone, children of different ages, and adults and children together. Seating clusters can be kept intimate if any single couch or unit does not hold more than three persons (thereby making the total number per cluster about six). The size of clusters can be varied by having a range of one- to three-person units as well as some child-sized chairs, placed around the room. As need and census dictate, stacking chairs can be added, or subtracted to free the room for other functions during nonoverflow periods. Small, modular units allow people to rearrange the furniture according to individual needs, whereas seating units for more than three not only increase the formality of a space but also tend to be poorly utilized, since unrelated individuals prefer not to sit side by side without some physical barrier between them. Couches with separate cushions will be filled more quickly than those designed as one long mat. At least one three-seat unit should be available for a sick or tired child to stretch out; Mother can then be unencumbered while her child rests. Newer modular seating units open up to form beds (for a sick child or a parent sleeping overnight); they thus added flexibility to small spaces that must fulfill a range of functions. A basket, carriage, or small canvas satchel for infants can also conserve seating space.

Banquettes built into an existing corner, at right angles to a wall, at floor level, or on a platform 7 inches high, add variety to traditional seating units. They provide soft, inviting places for parents and children to cuddle, for teenagers to socialize, or for adults to supervise play even while being removed from it (see Fig. 4, also Fig. 8).

Rocking chairs are invaluable for promoting physical contact between a parent and child, for comforting tired or ill children, or for giving energetic ones constructive opportunities for movement.

The vital links in creating and maintaining the L-shaped configurations are small tables and end-stands. These can hold plants, magazines, pamphlets, lamps, and the like. However, some tables must be kept free as surfaces for personal belongings, coffee cups, snacks, and baby bottles which otherwise usurp valuable seating space and make the room appear cluttered. Most seating clusters should also have a centrally-positioned low table that acts as a game surface and promotes social cohesion. Indeed, a checkerboard can be permanently glued and varnished to it (note the tables in Figs. 2, 4). A

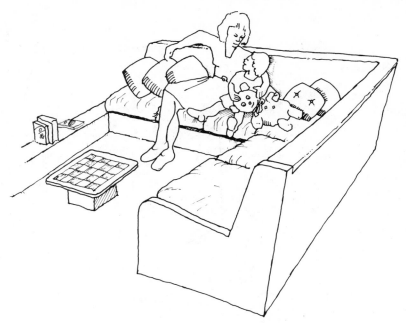

Fig. 4. *Banquette seating.*

shelf under the table, holding inexpensive checker or chess pieces, cards, or other games, will provide immediate sources of entertainment and interaction.

A flap/game table, developed by the author, fulfills a variety of waiting room needs. When the flaps are closed, the surface can be an end table, a low seat, or a footstool (especially for legs in casts). When the flaps are open and lie at the sides of the table completely out of the way, they reveal an internal trough holding a game board and pieces. The trough and flap covers reduce the chances of game pieces being lost or strewn about, and provide for the resumption of play that is interrupted for an exam (see Fig. 5).

Some parents, however devoted, like a few moments to read, rest, or be free not to interact with their children. Also, some pediatric procedures, such as x-ray, require the adult to wait without his child. Therefore, in addition to games, conversation, and casual surveillance of play, some activities must be provided for adults to do alone. Magazines, newspapers, books, and educational pamphlets are essential. These can be placed directly on the tables forming seating clusters, or be displayed on slanted shelves and wall-mounted bookracks in and around the sitting area (see Fig. 6). Pilferage and loss are reduced by placing magazines in binders, and on racks that clearly signal where reading material belongs. Good display units also aid the receptionist to tidy up.

Probably the most friendly, calming support a waiting adult can receive is a cup of coffee or tea. Parents who anticipate a long wait often bring such provisions along, since the coffee shop is hard to visit once parent and child have settled in. A coffee machine, even a small refrigerator for cold drinks, in or near the waiting area, properly located away from transit and play zones and supplemented by adequate numbers of end tables (perhaps with lips around them to minimize the dangers of cups of hot liquids near young children), provides the adult with some much appreciated refreshment.

Contrary to current belief and practice, television, when viewed by a group of waiting people in a public setting, is rarely a source of genuine involvement. As a moving, rapidly changing stimulus, it forces constant visual orientation but receives

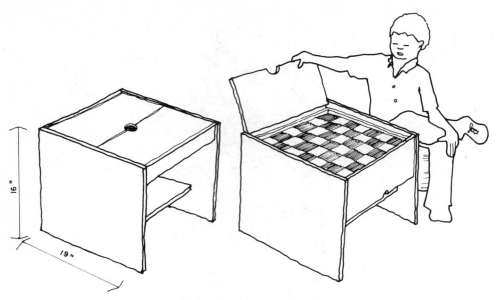

Fig. 5.   *The flap/game table.*

little sustained attention. Most people stare blankly at the set, unable to disengage. Any single viewer is reluctant to select a program of personal choice, and since the volume must be kept low to prevent interference with other activities, viewers at any distance cannot hear. If a set is retained in the waiting area, it should be placed low on a wall or table, accessible to only one or two seating clusters, so that genuine options for watching or not watching are available. Television reduces the parental supervision and stimulation of children, both of which help control discord and vandalism. As a mechanical device, it is a poor substitute for the potential of a well-designed and

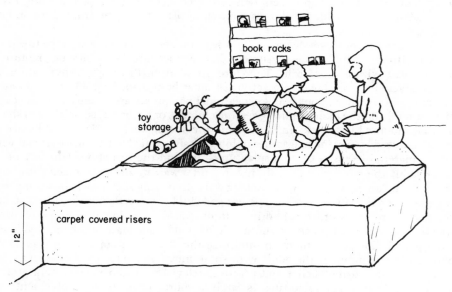

Fig. 6.   *Low carpeted risers, forming an enclosed play "pit."*

well-provisioned waiting space to bring people together in meaningful and socially enjoyable ways.

Additional facilities supporting the basic functional needs of most waiting areas are a clock within easy view, a water fountain with a stepstool for child use, a telephone in a semiprivate contiguous zone, a changing table for infants in the room or nearby lavatory, and racks or hooks for coats and the paraphernalia that invariably accompany pediatric patients. (Such belongings need to be reasonably close to their owners for security, but otherwise usurp seating space.) Stretchers, wheelchairs, and other equipment used near the waiting space should be clearly segregated from sitting and play areas, so the room does not appear devoted to utility storage. Plants, mobiles, mirrors, wall hangings, manipulable puzzles, and trick devices add color, excitement, and visual interest to a bland environment, and are valuable resources for encouraging both passive involvement and social interaction.

Once a comfortable, well-functioning arrangement of furnishings has been achieved, care must be taken to maintain it. This usually requires providing custodians with clearly labeled floorplans, and explanations for the diversified arrangement, so their support may be enlisted, for instance, not to put all the chairs back against the walls by force of habit.

Creating a Play Area

Because productive use of materials occurs best when play is assigned to a geographical area uninvaded by movement, a territory must be set aside or "carved out" of the overall waiting space, in its most untrafficked zone, to be a play area* (see Fig. 2). Despite common practice, a table and chairs put out in a space or corner do not suffice to make a play area, but only to make a work surface and seats. An *area* has five defining attributes: (a) a physical location with (b) visible boundaries indicating where it begins and ends, within which are placed (c) work and sitting surfaces as well as the (d) storage and display of materials to be used on the surfaces to create the activities for which the area is intended; in addition an area, like a room, ideally should have (e) a mood all its own, which distinguishes it from contiguous spaces.

The play area, more than any other facility in the pediatric setting, must visually entice children to explore and use materials. In achieving this goal, the two variables most often neglected are physically visible boundaries and materials displayed for use.

Boundaries

Most children under 10 years of age prefer the floor to tables and chairs as a sitting and work surface. Use of the floor reduces clutter of the play space by furniture, makes distracting actions less perceptible, keeps children from moving underfoot or wandering off and becoming separated from parents. Most importantly, it lowers the energy of the play to levels appropriate to subdued waiting. The result is a more tranquil and productive waiting and play space, but only if the floor surface is protected by physical boundaries which structure its limits, prevent transit across it, and allow visibility and communication to contiguous zones, on at least one side. Since barriers as solid as four walls or as fluid as taped lines are inappropriate, low dividers, storage units, or changes in level must be employed to protect and signal where an area begins and ends. A "pit"

---

* If seating clusters and stacking chairs still preclude a space for play, reduce the size of some seats from 30 to 24 (or 18) inches square.

made from 12-inch-high carpeted risers placed in a U-shaped or rectangular configuration can serve this purpose, as can a platform 4–12 inches off the floor (see Fig. 1), which even makes a small room appear more spacious. (See Fig. 6.)

Storage and Display of Play Materials

A child's invitation to play really is not communicated by Lilliputian furniture and play platforms, but by the visual presence of play materials. The message conveyed by locked cabinets and empty shelves is "Hands off; these materials are too precious for you to use." On the other hand, the message of well-stocked shelves at child height, is "Look, children, at my beautiful wares. Come touch them, come learn and play." In addition to mere presence, however, the way in which materials are stored and displayed affects their perceptibility, accessibility, and use. Too few materials can make a place seem drab and uninteresting, as if there is nothing to do; but too many can make it appear chaotic, so it is impossible to know where to begin. A puzzle invitingly placed on a wide counter may be irresistible, but a puzzle haphazardly piled on a shelf, pieces disarrayed and missing, generates little interest.

Good display also communicates desired patterns of use. If storage shelves and bins are clearly labeled, if they fit the items they will hold and display them attractively and distinctly; if containers are light enough to carry, yet small enough not to usurp all the work surface, then people will be encouraged to care for and put things away because there are cues by which to do so. Transport, loss, and confusion can be further minimized by placing the storage units next to the work surfaces appropriate for the specific materials used (see Fig. 7). Well-organized play areas that distinctively store and display materials beside work surfaces appropriate to the function of the area regulate the use of materials by giving everything a place, and by providing places where things can be found, used, and returned within clear physical limits.

By failing to store and display play materials appropriately, most institutional

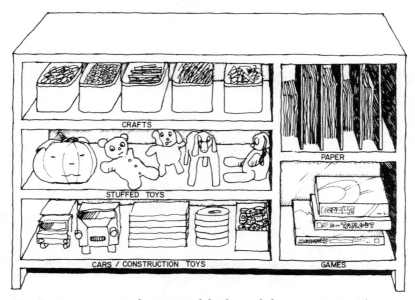

Fig. 7. *A storage unit, showing good display and clear organization of materials.*

122

settings suffer from either chaotic profusion or dire emptiness, both of which foster undesirable behaviors. Donated, cheap, plastic toys with little play value often glut a play space; they encourage chaos rather than manipulation, since it is difficult to see what is available or where things belong. Such toys should be judiciously replaced by a smaller stock of well-designed and well-displayed materials with inherent capacity to sustain involvement.

The public nature of institutions obviously invites depletion of playthings. However, misuse also arises from the frustration of only partial or insufficient support for the full constructive execution of an activity—crayons without paper will be used on walls. But the way to prevent vandalism is not to deplete, or allow depletion of, usable items in a play area. The absence of playthings only frustrates the need to have something to do, and thereby encourages the use, and probable misuse, of available but inappropriate materials such as furniture, walls, and floors.

In the interests of supporting human needs for productive activity, and of preventing general destruction, some money must be set aside for expendable play materials, and some depletion must be assumed. There are many simple and ingenious uses for inexpensive and "scrounge" materials to makes games, collages, dolls, and puppets, with which children can be well occupied. However, someone must take the time to organize materials, to replenish bins, and to prepare activity cards suggesting ideas for use. A notice that sympathizes with the client's need to be occupied, indicates what things there are to do, and requests support for preservation of play items, will often encourage cooperation. A balanced stock of materials, well-displayed in protected play areas that are tacitly supervised by the reception and seating zones, may not eliminate but will certainly reduce undesirable behaviors by giving patients a satisfying waiting experience.

Types of Materials

As many as four different age groups may be present in a pediatric setting: infant, toddler, preschool, school age, and adolescent. The materials purchased to equip a waiting area will depend upon the ages and energy level of patients, the intimacy of the setting, and the intensity of tacit supervision provided by contiguous reception and sitting areas. Catalogs and toy stores can guide the selection of specific age-related items. Materials should be sturdily constructed, have some inherent complexity and, if possible, be usable by more than one child at a time. Unless supervision is direct, toys with small, easily lost, or swallowable pieces should be avoided, as should messy activities such as painting and water play.

Aside from providing some activities for each age group, it is important that the materials represent all or most of eight different categories of play experience. These categories, which include both active and passive play, apply equally to all age groups (except, in a few cases, infants).

1. Quiet activities (reading, manipulatives, busy boards, blocks, construction toys, puzzle and maze books);
2. Crafts (blackboards, crayons, pens, clay, collage materials, weaving);
3. Games (card, lotto, pen and pencil, board, table, and electronic games for 1–6 players; TV tennis, air hockey, bumper pool);
4. Listening activities (music, stories, educational materials);
5. Dramatic play activities (puppets, store play, medical play, masks, dress-up, kitchen play, dolls, miniatures, fantasy toys);

6. Large motor activities (velcro and magnetic darts, ring toss, nerf basketball; games of skill; climbing, sliding, crawling; rocking horse, infant swing, jolly jumper; large blocks, punching clown);
7. Viewing activities (slides, films, television, educational media);
8. Educational and therapeutic activities (casts and braces, x-rays, models of teeth, models of organs; informative films, slides, tapes, and pamphlets; inflatable and foam equipment, water bed, air mattress for sensorily and physically disabled patients).

Ideally, there should be a range of eight different types of play experience at each age level, so as to match the mood, energy, and personal interests of each child present. All ages enjoy a large blackboard or wall mural for sketching, plants, and animals (fish, reptiles, birds where not medically contraindicated), books, music, movies, peer and parent interaction, and the opportunity to examine and test out medical procedures or equipment related to their waiting. Special consideration should be given to ways of educating parents and children about examination procedures to be experienced. Such information reduces anxiety, furthers understanding and cooperation during treatment, and respects the intelligence of patient and parent. A rear-screen projection booth, although initially expensive, can regularly present educational slides and tapes—even a case study of treatment—without supervision.

DESIGNING PLAYROOMS

The Playroom as an Environment

Commercial playthings are designed for healthy children playing in familiar surroundings, where toys act as a diversion and a complement to accustomed activities. Studies of children and animals reveal, in fact, that genuinely playful activity occurs only when young creatures feel comfortable and secure in their surroundings. In hospitals, therefore, where many things are unfamiliar and frightening to children, toys must be supplemented by a total play environment or playroom that is a comfortable, secure retreat from the scary aspects of medical treatment and the loneliness of bedrooms.

Preliminary Design Considerations

The first function of a playroom, whether organized according to medical condition or by age, is to bring children together socially, in a child-oriented context. The ability of children to play cooperatively and productively there is then affected by (a) the amount and variety of things there are to do, (b) the variety of places there are in which to do them, and (c) the organization and accessibility of those things and places within the play space.

Playrooms must be subdivided into activity areas or multiple play spaces, which each support a different function, in order to support a range of activities, from passive to active, for children of all ages. Facilities that encourage family interaction should also be emphasized, since parents need to participate positively in the child's recuperation (see Fig. 8).

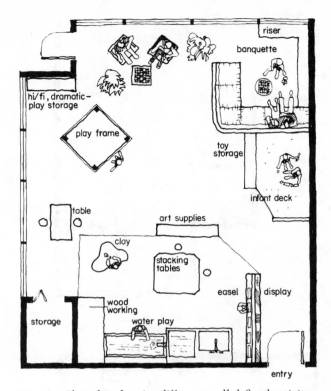

Fig. 8. *Floorplan showing different, well-defined activity areas in a playroom for cardiology patients (infant through adolescent). Children's Hospital National Medical Center, Washington, D.C.*

Well-designed activity areas, intended to support particular functions, can be compared to the rooms of a house. Just as a living room, bedroom, and kitchen vary in function, size, organization, activity level, and the postures they engender, so too should playroom activity areas vary in the things done in them (read, play a dart game, draw a picture), the number of persons they accommodate (1, 3–6, 10–15), the postures they enable occupants to assume (lying, sitting, standing), the work surfaces they provide (tables, floors, counters, walls), their storage and display (open shelves, wall racks, cabinets, surface mounts, and suspension), their modes of boundary (upward and downward changes in level, high and low storage units, free-standing partitions, sliding panels), and the activity levels they support (resting, drawing, climbing).

The functional requirements and basic strategies for design and maintenance of waiting spaces, previously discussed, apply equally to the design of playrooms. Activities involving use of the floor (quiet play, manipulatives, infant activities) should go in protected zones, while those involving work at tables (crafts, games, dramatic play) can be located in more open areas. When noisy and quiet, messy and clean, expansive and contained activities are kept apart, many different functions can be supported at one time (see Fig. 9).

External graphics in corridors are important for helping children to locate the playroom. The view at the entry should suggest comfort, security, and playfulness; it should also give a glimpse of facilities for different ages—an important consideration,

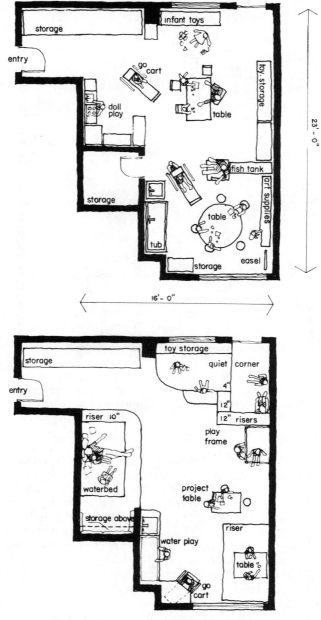

Fig. 9. (Top.) Before: Floorplan of a playroom prior to renovation, showing clutter and congestion. Division 27 Playroom, Children's Hospital Medical Center, Boston, Mass. (Bottom.) After: Improved definition of play areas in the renovated room, increasing the room's usefulness while providing more cleared floor space.

126

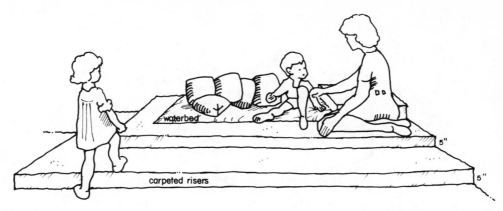

Fig. 10. *A waterbed, an excellent place for children and parents to relax together, also providing soothing stimulation for patients with burns or developmental delays. Low carpeted risers bordering the waterbed can provide additional surfaces for sitting, reclining, play, and physical therapy.*

since teens, especially, will not come to a playroom that looks designed for young children.

Activities and Furnishings

Since commercially available children's furnishings are intended for schools and homes, and not for complex therapeutic settings, versatile facilities for playrooms are still rare. Some custom-designed facilities, developed by the author as especially suited to the needs of hospitalized children, are included here (Figures 10–15) to stimulate new approaches to the creation of exciting, functional playrooms.

The eight categories of play experience discussed for waiting spaces are equally desirable for playrooms, and can be used as the basis for creating different activity areas.

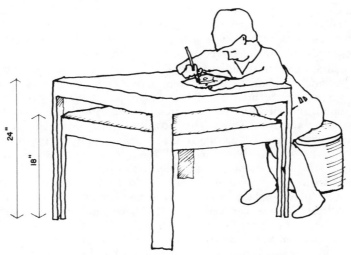

Fig. 11. *Stacking tables conserving floor space and helping to keep table sizes small overall.*

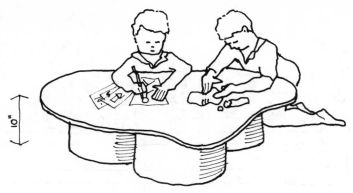

Fig. 12. *A low table, extremely popular, at which children kneel or sit on the floor.*

In playrooms, however, a broader range of craft materials (paint, ceramics, leather, beading, woodworking) and of dramatic play props (kitchen furniture and supplies, dolls, crib, clothing) is usually desired, as is provision for cooking activities (popcorn, blender, cocoa, toaster oven, for teens to use and for all for snacks), and water and sand play. Compared with waiting spaces, playrooms require more display surfaces and more storage units (some of which should be locked to remove from use materials harmful to unsupervised children), more supports for resting (waterbed, hammock, banquette, play pit), a private space (for a child alone or to share with another child or parent), and a space to hold all the children in the room (for parties and communal dining) (see Fig. 10).

To conserve space, to encourage dispersion to all areas of the room, and to make furnishings more versatile, chairs and tables should be kept to a minimum, and boundary-creating units should be designed to serve as sitting and work surfaces for adults and children (see Figs. 6, 10). Tables for more than six children reduce tranquil social interaction, while those that stack keep unit sizes and numbers low, except at times, such as meals, when additional spaces are required (see Fig. 11).

The height of work surfaces, tables, and sinks needs to vary in order to support use by children of different ages, as well as by weak or physically constrained children in wheelchairs, go-carts, or stretchers (see Figs. 13, 14). Tables can be at least at two heights: normal chair height and 10 inches off the ground. Those at which children kneel are extremely popular, because they allow the child greater visual command, and freedom to get the full force of his body into his work (Fig. 12).

A customed-designed unit called a Play Frame is an extraordinarily versatile work surface that provides as many as 20 different activities in as little as a 4-foot-square space: easel, puppet theatre, busy board, house, dart games, play kitchen, and the like. Play panels supporting the different activities may be interchangeably suspended on any of the four sides and at varying heights, so as to accommodate children in go-carts, beds, and wheelchairs. Panels and other items can be stored in the upper portion of the frame. Where space is extremely limited, wall-mounted supports for the panels, rather than the entire frame, can enable comparable versatility* (see Fig. 13).

Messy play with water and sand is a superb activity for a young hospitalized child since it encourages individual expression, is calm, and is slow-paced. Built-in water play tables, with lockable faucets, can keep the activity within bounds of safety and easy maintenance. Covers for the table troughs provide additional work surfaces for unsupervised periods when there can be no water play (see Fig. 14).

Instead of obstructing a playroom with playpens and other infant equipment, a

---

* Credit is due Fred Todd for the initial conception and prototype of this ingenious structure.

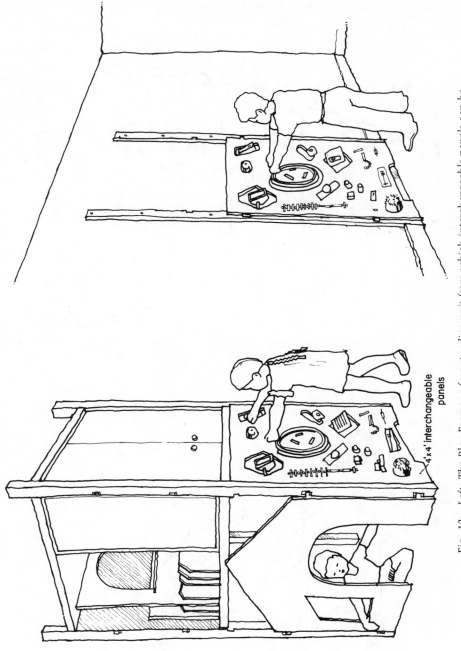

Fig. 13. *Left:* The Play Frame, a free-standing unit from which interchangeable panels can be hung at varying heights to provide a wide variety of activities in a small area. Panels are stored in upper portion of unit. *Right:* Wall-mounted uprights, supports for the play panels when space is too limited for a free-standing unit.

4'x4' interchangeable panels

129

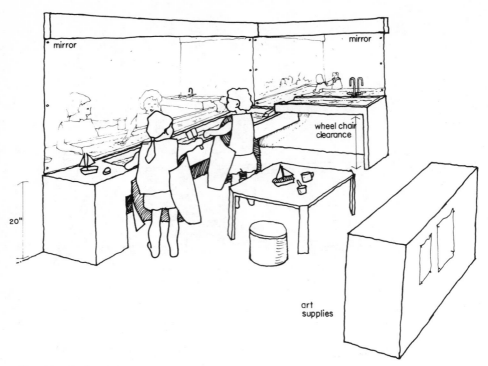

Fig. 14. *Built-in water play troughs, including one to accommodate a child in a wheel-chair, forming part of a messy play area that includes a table and open storage for crafts activities. Water troughs have covers and lockable faucets for unsupervised periods.*

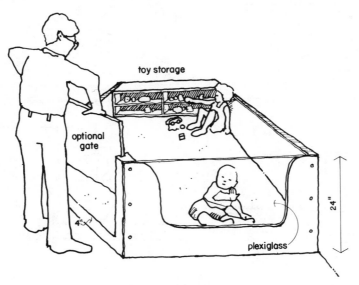

Fig. 15. *A play deck, or platform, enclosed on all sides but the one used for entry. To contain infants and toddlers, a panel or optional gate can be dropped into the entry space.*

semienclosed space such as a deck or "pit" (see Fig. 6) with an optional gate, can contain babies when necessary, but may also be used by adults and older children (see Fig. 15).

In addition to these furnishings, a well-equipped playroom might have wheelchair trays; a telephone; storage for the personal effects and records of staff; a changing table; and ample vertical and horizontal display surfaces for posters, art work, crafts projects, and communications. Mobiles, plants, interactive devices, pillows, wall hangings, fish tanks, and other decorations need to be added to make the space comfortable, interesting, and inviting.

Maintenance of the Playroom

Most playrooms are supervised by trained childlife staff for 8 hours a day, 40 hours a week, while the child and his parents are in the hospital 24 hours a day, 168 hours a week. Long hours of waiting, pain, fear, and boredom connect the brief interludes of supervised play in the playroom. Locked playrooms, or locked cabinets beside empty storage units, are an open invitation to breakins since they so strongly say, "We trust you with nothing and have hidden all the good toys away." A primary goal of the design of any playroom should be to create a secure, safe, and interesting environment that can remain accessible to patients even when the room is not professionally supervised.

REFERENCES

1. Milgram, S. *Obedience to authority.* New York: Harper & Row, 1974.
2. Prescott, E., & David, T. G. The effects of the physical environment on day care. Pacific Oaks College, Pasadena, California, 1976. (Paper commissioned by the Office of the Assistant Secretary for Planning and Evaluation, Department of Health, Education and Welfare.)

ADDITIONAL READING

Fiske, D. W., & Maddi, S. R. *Functions of varied experience.* Homewood, Ill.: Dorsey, 1961.

Lindheim, R., Glaser, H. H., & Coffin, C. *Changing hospital environments for children.* Cambridge, Mass.: Harvard, 1972.

Mehrabian, A. *Public places and private spaces: The psychology of work, play, and living environments.* New York: Basic Books, 1976.

Piaget, J., & Inhelder, B. *The psychology of the child.* New York: Basic Books, 1969.

PSYCHOLOGICAL TESTING
OF CHILDREN

Betty C. Buchsbaum, Ph.D.

The appropriate use of a psychological evaluation can be of critical importance in both preventive and therapeutic work with children. Early identification of children with developmental difficulties or emotional disturbances can often determine whether a child will cope with his life or will be defeated by it. The consequences of an accurate assessment of a child's strengths and weaknesses are extensive. The choice and application of such tools as education, school planning, remediation, family counseling, and psychotherapy depend for their choice and effectiveness on a clear and accurate statement of a child's cognitive and emotional status. Without the required evaluation a child many be left to grow up in a world he cannot understand and in a world that fails to understand him.

In this chapter I shall explore the indications for testing, the nature and application of information obtained, and the limitations of the evaluation process. Knowledge of testing and its implications facilitates appropriate referrals; it also aids in preparing the child and family for the examination procedure.

The three obvious components of a psychological examination are the subject or child being evaluated, the psychologist, and the tests administered. Let us first consider the role of the child and how his characteristics shape the testing process.

THE CHILD

Development and change are among the most predictable characteristics of childhood. At each stage of growth quite different aspects of behavior become prominent. Thus at various periods in a child's life both the reasons for testing and the methods and validity of an examination will differ.

During the first two years of life, the infant's major task is physical growth and, concomitantly, the development of sensorimotor, perceptual, cognitive, and social functions. In addition, a homeostatic equilibrium is expected to be established which becomes stronger and more reliable with age. The disruption or lag in the development of expected capacities (given an "average, expectable environment")[16] alerts the pediatrician to the need for further inquiry. Knowledge of birth history and environmental factors, such as maternal health, attention available to the baby, or neonatal illnesses, provides a medical and social context for understanding developmental deviations. An infant who becomes lethargic during his mother's absence is quite different from one who, under average circumstances, fails to respond to people or does not grasp and manipulate objects. The main purpose of testing at this early age is to explore the question of retardation, organic brain damage, or excessive vulnerability. The last feature characterizes high risk babies who are unable to sustain a more or less adequate state of inner comfort. Hyper– or hyposensitivity to external stimuli, prolonged periods of stress, and the lack of a reliable "stimulus-barrier"[8] that modulates the impact of outer stimuli characterize these infants. Sequential observations and followup over time is indicated for such children, who have a propensity to develop psychiatric disorders later in life.[4]

The day-to-day variability of an infant's physical and psychological status as well as the unpredictability of his responses to an adult contribute to his unreliability as a subject for psychological evaluation. Even using such carefully constructed scales as the Gesell or Bayley scales, reliability correlations tend to be low.[4] Also, results of infant scales do not show a significant relationship with intelligence test results at a later age.[23] Only after language develops and can be tested does predictability from early to later tests improve. As Bayley and others suggest, "At each stage of infant development, intelligence comprises a set of relatively discrete abilities . . . During the early period of development these clusters of abilities are relatively age– or stage–specific; therefore, there is no necessary continuity between intelligence as defined at one stage of development and as defined at another."[23] It has been found, however, that "infant tests may have value in detecting neuromotor abnormalities"[20] and extremely low scores appear to be predictive of retardation in the future.

As growth continues through the toddler stage to five years of age, the child's responses become more accessible and trustworthy. New functions emerge, such as organized speech and grapho-motor skills which are more like the abilities present in older children and adults. Though attention span is still brief, compliance with test demands somewhat variable, and sustained use of a given ability still vacillating, preschoolers nonetheless function more reliably than they did when younger. Thus test data tend to be more consistent upon repetition. With regard to the predictive ability of test findings, a study by McCall, Hogarty, and Hurlburt[23] indicated that after eighteen months, correlations of early childhood scales with performance of school age children was moderate and stable.

As the child grows more complex, the possibilities for deviant behavior become greater and more varied. The preschoolers' speech and play patterns, their reactions to bladder and bowel control, their capacity to socialize with peers, their ability to and strategies for coping with anxiety can reflect either smooth development or areas of difficulty. Ego functioning now encompasses diverse emotional and social components with increased sources of disturbance possible. Hence, in addition to neurological impairment or retardation, features related to personality development become more meaningful. The exaggerated quality of phase-specific issues often deserve scrutiny. Intense temper tantrums, delays in toilet training, excessive stubbornness at two or three years of age, excessive fears at three or four years of age—all are examples of such age-specific behaviors. Moreover, regressions that persist or lack of progress in such functions as speech or motor functioning suggest the need for further study.

Parent interviews, observation of the child, exploration of family and more general environmental issues may be sufficient to understand and to handle a given problem. When diagnostic questions still remain or etiology is uncertain, testing can be most valuable. Generally, however, when cognitive functions do not develop at an appropriate rate or infantile behavior persists, testing should be considered early in the evaluation process. Testing is also of value in determining a young child's strengths. It can assist in establishing whether a parent's difficulties with a child stem from the parent's problems in coping with the child's quite healthy responses or whether the child is indeed showing deviant behavior.

Between two and three years of age, severe pathology may begin to emerge. Early manifestations of emotional and social withdrawal, severe disturbances in relationships with adults, and uncontrollable aggressive outbursts are among the behaviors that require further study. Not infrequently the high risk infant shows aberrant behavior in the preschool years. In such a situation, tests are useful to clarify questions of differential diagnosis; the same behavior, for example, may be caused by mental retardation, organic brain damage, affective deprivation, or inadequate coping resources. Psychological testing can serve to pinpoint the most pertinent aspects of the problem. It also helps to identify children who will not "outgrow" the disturbances that are presented, but who require rapid therapeutic intervention.

During the school-age years, a child's intellectual functioning becomes increasingly stable and predictable. Perception, motor skills, and cognition are less vulnerable to emotional and environmental pressures. Personality organization develops into increasingly differentiated and complex patterns. These factors account, in part, for the greater reliability and predictive value of psychological tests from six years of age forward. Whereas infant intelligence is not a unitary trait, verbal comprehension and reasoning are significant organizers of experience at six years of age. The dominance of verbal skills appears to be related to the more valid and consistent reactions obtained from intelligence tests.

The reasons for testing children of school age are, again, dependent on the expectations of the age. Learning disabilities based on school performance become a prominent issue for referral. In the face of school failures, a psychological evaluation can be critical in distinguishing an emotionally disturbed, inhibited child from one with neurological impairment. Timely use of testing in conjunction with a medical and psychosocial history is often essential in identifying the specific etiology associated with a learning deficit.

Hyperactivity is another prominent symptom resulting from a variety of causes. Depression, organic brain damage, minimal brain dysfunction, as well as childhood psychosis—all can be associated with hyperactive behavior. For example: Ritalin was recommended for two children because of hyperactivity, but only one child responded positively. On testing, the child who improved showed evidence of an organic brain syndrome that was further validated by an abnormal EEG. The second child, with an IQ of 126, showed no evidence of neurological impairment when tested; he was found to be generally anxious, and fearful of separating from his mother. The tendency to label and treat disorders in terms of an ambiguous symptom can be avoided through judicious use of testing.

The pediatrician, especially, is confronted by a variety of somatic symptoms, some of which have no organic basis. Often phobic, hypochondriacal, or hysterical reactions are expressed through somatic pathways. The persistence of physical symptoms, for example, headaches or stomach pains, after physical causes have been excluded can also be better understood through a psychological examination. As with younger children evidence of severe pathology in the form of extremely aggressive or withdrawn behavior in children of school age is a matter for concern. Testing is especially helpful in the understanding of such children since both their age and, often, the nature of their emotional difficulties limit the ability to describe (or even admit to) their problems.

The early adolescent patient is well known for the perplexing and provocative nature of his adjustment efforts. With puberty, physical and psychological events occur which may interfere with school performance, social adaptation, and emotional stability. At best, the adolescent is an unpredictable individual; during the teenage years, it is often critical to understand quickly the nature of disturbances in his ongoing development. Tests may be required to explore the basis for academic failures, for antisocial or self-destructive behavior and reactions of a bizarre nature. The classical symptoms of schizophrenia emerge at adolescence, the suicide rate rises, and drug abuse and promiscuity become sources of concern. Questions relating to the need for hospitalization, school counseling, individual or family treatments take on added urgency during adolescence, because of the patient's predilection for acting out his problems. Testing plays a significant role in rapidly assessing the severity and range of pathological behavior as well as in illuminating the strengths of the patient.

THE PSYCHOLOGIST

In the previous section the developmental stage of the child was emphasized as a determinant in the role of psychological testing. The validity and usefulness of testing instruments depends also on the clinician using them.

Psychologists regarded as qualified for independent practice are those who (a) have been awarded a diploma by the American Board of Professional Psychology, or (b) have been licensed or certified by state examining boards, or (c) have been certified by voluntary boards established by state psychological associations. Psychologists who do not yet meet these qualifications are expected to work under qualified supervision. In the United States, all but seven states require a Ph.D. degree in order to meet certification or licensing requirements for independent practice.[2]

It is probably not necessary to remind pediatricians that eliciting a child's responses as well as interpreting test data constitute a dynamic process linked to the experience and skill of the examiner. The degree to which a child can cooperate and function appropriately in a testing situation is frequently a function of the ingenuity and understanding of the psychologist. The younger the child, the more adept one must be in obtaining test responses; with older subjects, the test situation is relatively predictable but the organization of test results is more complex. The basic goal of an evaluation is to obtain as much relevant information as one needs in order to judge a child's capacities, weaknesses, feelings about himself, focal conflicts, adaptive mechanisms, and potential for healthy development.

In addition to test findings, parent interviews, medical and social histories, and patient observation are utilized. Although diagnostic "hunches" based on limited bits of data may occasionally be accurate, only an evaluation derived from various levels of functioning can yield the depth of understanding that is required. One wants to know not simply whether a child is anxious or inhibited, but rather, what the nature of the inhibition is, with what it is associated, what situations facilitate spontaneity. Moreover, the psychologist seeks to determine the child's available intellectual and emotional resources and to utilize environmental support or treatment.

In addition to knowledge of personality organization, the psychologist must possess a background in child development, and a familiarity with the problems typical for each age as well as with the ways in which these problems are usually met. Pertinent socioeconomic and cultural variables must also be understood as they affect test procedures and results. With reference to minority groups, test findings should be evaluated in terms of the conditions of a child's subculture. Failure on specific test questions may reflect economic and environmental deprivation more than intellectual status. Even so, tests can be used to provide a sample of problem-solving strategies, modes of dealing with adult demands, and attitudes toward school-related work. Furthermore, qualitative aspects of a test point up a patient's style of functioning. Often the projective material and drawings indicate intellectual resources which are not picked up by the structured intelligence test.

Whatever the background of the child, it is the psychologist's responsibility to understand and convey the information revealed by the examinations. Such an understanding includes an appreciation of the limits imposed by a less than good match between test and patient. Ideally, the particular test selected is appropriate both to the problem under investigation and to the background of the child involved, but even so-called culture-fair tests have been found less successful in representing the abilities of underprivileged children than had been hoped.[4] It thus becomes the task of the psychologist to evaluate a test protocol with full awareness of the unavoidable restrictions imposed by a given test.

After completing an evaluation, the psychologist attempts to provide a meaningful and helpful statement about the patient. Usually an interview with parents is advisable in order to present and interpret test findings. Older children and adolescents also profit from a sensitive review of their performance. The psychologist's use of interpretive sessions is therapeutic inasmuch as it clarifies the meaning of the testing process, thus reducing its mystery and implementing the patient's understanding and acceptance of recommendations derived from the clinical procedures.

THE PSYCHOLOGICAL EXAMINATION

The following section will present the major psychological tests and their uses. Only techniques requiring individual administration by a psychologist—as opposed to group-oriented achievement or intelligence tests—will be discussed. The general function of tests is to provide a representative sample of behavior in response to a standardized stimulus situation. A uniform set of tasks is presented to all subjects in a prescribed manner and scored in the same way. The test's efficiency is based on one's ability to generalize from it to nontest behaviors.

The confidence placed in test findings, i.e., the degree to which data can be generalized, depends on the validity and reliability measures of that test. Reliability addresses the following questions: 1. How consistent will test results be upon immediate repetition? 2. How much will scores change over time? 3. How much agreement is there among the scores of different examiners? Validity addresses the questions: Does the test accomplish its purpose? Does it measure what it was designed to measure?

Standardization constitutes a third issue for test evaluation. A standardized test refers to one that is capable of uniform administration and scoring. In addition, the test must initially be administered to a large, representative sample of subjects so that a set of norms or typical performance levels for a given population can be established. The information derived from norms enables a subject to be evaluated in terms of group expectations. A basic criticism of most intelligence tests refers to the lack of normative data for minority groups. The attempt to measure an individual from a particular subculture against norms based on the culture of the majority can be misleading.

General Characteristics of Psychological Tests

In the following review, various tests will be evaluated in terms of their reliability, validity, and quality of standardization procedures. Usually, the structured tests, such as measures of intelligence, reach higher criteria levels than do the unstructured or projective tests. The latter rely more heavily on the interpretive skills of the examiner. The confidence in projective test data is enhanced by the use of a test battery rather than a single test. The broader the sample of behaviors available, the more reliably hypotheses about an individual can be tested. When different sets of data point to the same phenomenon, one can be relatively certain that the patient, not test artifacts, is responsible for the results.

An unavoidable limitation in the application of test findings is the unpredictable nature of life events. When extreme environmental stress is encountered or gross changes in life patterns occur, test findings may not apply. However, to the extent that external conditions can be anticipated, clinical evaluations continue to reflect rather consistent response patterns.

STRUCTURED TESTS

Let us now turn to the structured tests which most often deal with assessing cognition, perceptual-motor functions, and attention. Shortly after Galton's use of measures to investigate individual differences in sensory discrimination and reaction times, more complex functions were explored by Alfred Binet. In 1905, he and Theodore Simon were commissioned by the French government to develop an objective means of identifying retarded children. Their efforts resulted in the first intelligence test constructed. Terman revised the test and adapted it for use in this country. The last revision of the Stanford-Binet Intelligence Scales occurred in 1960[27] and the most recent standardization was completed in 1972.[28]

In presenting a variety of tasks to a population ranging from two years of age to the superior adult level, the Stanford-Binet has served as a standard against which newer tests have been evaluated. Organized as an age scale, it offers many verbal and nonverbal stimuli, such as copying geometric figures, repeating digits, defining vocabulary items, and dealing with abstract concepts. Placement of an item on the scale was based on the number of children passing the item at any given age; therefore, test content as well as item difficulty varies from age to age: for example, more nonverbal tasks appear below the six-year-level than above it. Qualitative examination of test performance reveals areas of strength and weakness. However, quantitative comparisons between verbal and nonverbal behaviors is not possible. The total score, expressed as an intelligence quotient (IQ) represents the deviation of an individual score from the average scores of the subject's age group.

As Lourie and Rieger point out,[21] the Stanford-Binet is particularly useful with respect to the wide age range it covers. The behaviors of young retarded children and older children of above average intelligence can both find adequate representation on the same instrument. The reliability of the Stanford-Binet has been high, and validity studies using school performance as a criterion have been good. However, since the test is highly verbal at the upper levels, children weak in language but stronger in visual-motor ability may be underestimated.

Following the development of two intelligence tests for adults, (the Wechsler-Bellevue, later replaced by the Wechsler Adult Intelligence Scale), in 1950, Wechsler proceeded to construct a similar scale for children. Revised in 1974, the Wechsler Intelligence Scale for Children (WISC-R)[31] differs in a number of ways from the Stanford-Binet. It is applicable to a narrower age range, one that includes children from six years to sixteen years, eleven months of age. Rather than organizing items into an age scale, it divides them into a Verbal and Performance Scale providing separate scores as well as a composite full scale IQ. The subtest items are arranged in increasing order of difficulty and all subtests may be administered. The Verbal subtests include Information,

Comprehension, Arithmetic, Vocabulary, Similarities; Digit Span can be added if desired. The Performance scale contains Block Design, Picture Completion, Picture Arrangement, Object Assembly, Coding, and an optional Maze task. The separate subtest scores permit a more direct analysis of different abilities than is possible on the Stanford-Binet. The obtained IQ represents the degree to which a child deviates from the norms for his age.

One of the purposes of the 1974 revision of the WISC was to include a proportional representation of nonwhites in the standardization procedure. A stratified sample of the population was used, based on 1970 U.S. census reports. Thus for each range tested, subjects included the same proportion of whites and nonwhites as was found in the 1970 census. As Wechsler indicates, the term "nonwhites" included blacks as well as other groups such as American Indians and Orientals.[31] The Puerto Rican and Chicano children tested were classified as white or nonwhite in accordance with visible physical characteristics. In addition to race, other population variables used in the sampling plan were age, sex, geographic region, occupation of head of household and urban/rural residence. In terms of statistical procedures, the WISC-R has taken racial as well as environmental factors into account in establishing norms. However, any individual who may have suffered extreme deprivation, whether nutritional, emotional or cultural, will require special understanding when test findings are interpreted.

In evaluating the Wechsler scales, Anastasi notes their high levels of reliability and their good standardization procedures.[4] Validity studies are rather limited, however. Studies correlating WISC-R and the Wechsler Preschool and Primary Scale of Intelligence (WPPSI)[31] scores with the Stanford-Binet show a significantly strong relationship, with the Verbal scale achieving higher correlations than the Performance scale.

Most space has been devoted to the Stanford-Binet and Wechsler scales because they have been the most frequently used and most researched tests for children. The WISC-R has been an aid in the diagnosis of brain damage. According to Black,[9] a difference of 15 points or more between the Verbal and Performance scales does appear to identify some children with neurological dysfunction. The large number of visual-motor tasks is particularly helpful in detecting evidence of organic impairment.

A more recently developed measure is the McCarthy Scales of Children's Abilities (MSCA),[24] serving an age range from two and one-half to eight and one-half years of age. It is organized into six scales: Verbal, Perceptual-Performance, General Cognitive, Quantitative, Memory, and Motor. A General Cognitive Index is obtained which describes the child's performance in terms of his age group. This index is based on the same statistical concept as is the IQ.

Infant and Preschool Measures. Let us now consider measures used for infants and preschoolers. As was noted earlier, the infant scales are helpful in a restricted sense; that is, they identify clinical groups, mainly organically impaired or severely retarded infants. For a systematic sampling of a baby's current pattern of behavior, several instruments have been developed.

The Infant Schedule of the Gesell Developmental Scales elicits and rates motor, adaptive, language, and personal-social behaviors.[14] Most of the items depend on observation rather than on testlike situations. The schedule can be applied from four weeks to six years of age, but is most frequently used at the lower age levels. The Cattell Infant Scale provides another similar procedure for infant observation.

A more recently constructed instrument is the Bayley Scale of Infant Development, for children two months to two and one-half years of age.[5] In terms of test construction and standardization, the Bayley Scale is the best infant scale available. Areas evaluated include perception, memory, learning, problem-solving, vocalization, the beginnings of abstract thinking, and motor functioning. An Infant Behavior Record contains information about emotional and social behavior, attention span, persistence, and goal directedness.

A relatively new measure of infant functioning is Brazelton's Neonatal Behavioral Assessment Scale.[10] This examination assesses the dimensions of reflex behavior; interactive processes, i.e., the infant's capacity to respond to social stimuli; motor reactions, i.e., the infant's ability to maintain adequate tone, to control motor behavior, and to perform integrated motor actions; organizational processes, i.e., physiological stability in response to stress. The measure has been successfully used in a study differentiating underweight from full-weight newborns where significant differences were found on measures of motor behavior and interactive processes.[1] The development of such a refined assessment of neonatal status should be most helpful in predictive research and clinical studies in identifying the more vulnerable infant. (It should be noted that special training in infant testing is required for valid results from this scale.)

The findings of Piaget have been incorporated into an Ordinal Scale of Psychological Development devised by Uzgiris and Hunt in 1975.[29] It evaluates sensorimotor performance in terms of different levels of organization. Other Piaget–oriented methods of evaluation are being developed for older children; one of these, designed by Laurendeau and Pinard, examines modes of thought in children from two to twelve years of age.[19,29] However, these promising approaches have not yet been sufficiently standardized to become part of a regular test battery.

Moving from the evaluation of infants to the study of preschoolers, an increasing number of tools is available. In addition to the Stanford-Binet, WPPSI, and McCarthy Scales, the Merrill-Palmer Scale of Mental Tests for children from two to five years of age and the Minnesota Preschool Scale for one and one-half to six-year-old children evaluate preschool children.[21] When formal testing is not possible or supplementary information is desired, the Vineland Social Maturity Scale, through a parent interview, provides scorable data about social competence.[11]

A number of tests designed for physically handicapped children can also add to an understanding of the physically normal children. The Columbia Mental Maturity Scale applies to children from three and one-half to nine years of age and yields information about abstract reasoning. This is a reliable and well standardized test which is also available for Spanish-speaking subjects. The Peabody Picture Vocabulary Test (PPVT)[12] is helpful in working with children (two and one-half to eighteen years of age) who have expressive difficulties. A nonlanguage test, the Progressive Matrices developed by Raven, can be used to obtain nonverbal intelligence; it also provides specific information about visual discrimination.[26] A test designed to reduce the impact of cultural factors is the Leiter International Performance Test with tests arranged in age levels ranging from two to eighteen years of age. The Arthur adaptation of this scale, for children from three to eight years of age, was standardized on a middle-class population so that more data from low socioeconomic groups are needed before the effects of cultural factors can be ruled out.[4]

A number of tests have been designed to assess specific deficits. For example, the Illinois Test of Psycholinguistic Abilities (ITPA) focuses on various areas of language development.[17] Used with children from two to ten years of age, it is valuable in identifying early language disorders and providing information for remedial work. Its main drawback is the restricted nature of its normative sample, a largely middle-class population.

A frequently used technique aimed at assessing visual-motor and perceptual functioning is the Bender Visual-Motor Gestalt Test.[7] It requires subjects to copy geometric designs of varying complexity, thus revealing neurological maturity and the management of motility. Koppitz[18] has provided a scoring system for children (five to eleven years of age) so that an age scale with reference to errors is available. Other visual-motor tests include the Graham-Kendall Memory for Designs and the Benton Visual Retention Test. A more elaborate study of visual-motor functions is the Marianne Frostig Developmental Test of Visual Perception.[13] An associated remedial program is used in conjunction with the test and is geared to work with children susceptible to learning difficulties.

A study of motility patterns can be obtained from the Lincoln-Oseretsky Motor Development Scale for children (six to fourteen years of age). It is helpful in exploring issues of minimal brain dysfunction and learning disabilities by examining a wide range of motor behaviors.[4]

PROJECTIVE TESTS

After evaluating a child's intellectual resources, a diagnostic picture is not complete. For most children beyond the age of three years, projective or unstructured methods of studying personality are also included. The relatively undefined projective test permits the child to perceive and organize stimuli in a way uniquely his own. His responses provide insight into his style of thinking and emotional organization not otherwise available.

One of the most frequently used projective methods is the Rorschach Test. This test consists of a series of ten cards made up of inkblots and presented in a uniform manner. In the process of reporting his perceptions, the subject reveals the nature of his feelings, sources of anxiety, and modes of dealing with his emotional responses. Cognitive as well as affective dimensions are reflected. Available developmental studies provide a framework for judging children's responses.[3] An understanding of the protocol is not derived from discrete scores, but rather from the patterning and relationships among those scores. This fact, among others, contributes to the difficulty in establishing high validity and reliability correlations for the Rorschach Test.

While the Rorschach is unique in yielding information about personality structure, other methods offer insight into the quality of interpersonal relationships. Murray's Thematic Apperception Test (TAT)[25] presents pictures about which the subject is asked to tell a story. Though norms and scoring procedures are available, the TAT is most often interpreted qualitatively. Among the dimensions explored are the story themes, quality of personal relationships, the direction of outcomes, and the nature of story organization. Since the TAT is most suitable for older children, Bellak has devised the Children's Apperception Test (CAT) for children from three to ten years of age. In this version, animals are presented in situations with which a child can readily identify. (A later modification replaced the animals with people, but maintained the original scenes.) The thematic tests suggest how the child views himself in relation to others, his way of responding to parental figures and siblings, and his feelings about sexual and aggressive impulses. Each protocol emphasizes different issues, depending on what themes most concern the child.

Other tests which also focus on content and use pictures as stimuli include the Make-A-Picture-Story Test in which children select given figures in order to compose their stories.[4] The Michigan Picture Test and the Cartoonlike Blacky Pictures Test are also available but less frequently used tools for eliciting fantasy.

For young children whose verbal responses to the CAT and Rorschach are often limited, structured play sessions provide additional insight. Doll families, furniture, and household equipment permit the child to dramatize his own relationships to significant people in his life as well as to express inner needs and drives. The Bolgar-Fischer World Test is another form of a play interview used as a projective technique with children.

For use with older children, sentence-completion tests help to focus on specific lines of inquiry. Questions directed at eliciting the content of fears, ambitions, and other attitudes are formulated as open-ended sentences. The Rotter Incomplete Sentence Blank is an example of this type of test.[4]

Drawings provide a fruitful medium for evaluating expressive behavior. The Goodenough Draw-A-Man test, for example, can be used as a vehicle both for assessing intelligence and for interpreting aspects of personality. When used formally, features of the drawings are scored and evaluated in relation to age; Harris has provided age norms for children from kindergarten through ninth grade.[15] When used as a projective device, aspects of the drawing such as line quality, size, and placement on the page are examined; the subject is also asked to tell a story about the figure. Although Machover[22] first used drawings for projective purposes, subsequent validity studies have not supported her interpretations. As supplementary information, however, they have proved useful in clarifying diagnostic questions. Illustrative is the suggestion of neurological dysfunction when figures are rotated or are grossly asymmetrical.

Dynamic material also can emerge, particularly when the drawings and associations are combined. Buck's House-Tree-Person Test is another grapho-motor technique used for personality evaluation. The addition of nonverbal tasks to the test battery contributes an expressive mode that complements the heavily verbal orientation of the other instruments.

It is noteworthy that each test, although designed to focus on specific behavior, can be used in a variety of ways. Thus, cognitive measures reveal a patient's style of responding and manner of relating to another person, while projective tests reflect vocabulary, thought organization, and cultural background. Although each technique is a rich source of data, no one test can be used alone (except when very limited information, e.g., IQ, is required). It is the search for intertest consistencies as well as the awareness of unexpected contradictions that characterize the clinical process. The combination of intelligence and personality tests provides stimuli sufficiently varied so that different levels of functioning can be explored. Thus an intelligent child who fails in school, or a child whose aggressive outbursts have developed because of frustrations related to a perceptual disability can be understood and helped.

Special Features of the Psychological Examination

One may question the choice of a psychological examination over a clinical interview. Let us dissect the testing experience and view the elements that are unique to testing. Behavioral observation reveals the patient's ability to comply with the examiner's requests and to deal with the failures that inevitably occur on items of the intelligence test. Comparing the adequacy of reactions to the structured and unstructured tests is also informative. For example: A child may feel comfortable when asked intelligence test questions wherein he knows what is expected; in contrast, anxious or evasive responses may occur on the projective tests. Analysis of test data permits the delineation of specific strengths and deficits in cognitive and perceptual-motor performance; difficulty in concentration and attention is also revealed. The capacity to perceive reality as others do (or the nature of distortions that may occur), central areas of anxiety, and available coping mechanisms are among the insights revealed by the projective material. Clearly, not only diagnostic questions are answered; rather, a picture of the child emerges that calls for specific educational and therapeutic procedures. The objectivity and specificity of test data result in a gradual accumulation of facts that clarify and delimit more impressionistic findings.

Administering a full test battery is a rather lengthy undertaking, lasting four or more hours. Among the factors affecting testing time is a child's age and ability to cooperate, the number of tests required, and the types of tests used. One would not refer a patient for an evaluation routinely. Where severe pathology, learning disability, neurological impairment, retardation, or neurotic inhibitions are suspected, testing should be considered. Periodic examinations are also useful for children known to be vulnerable or who have experienced severe trauma; for such children, the tests can provide a monitoring function of significant preventive value. The pediatrician's knowledge of a patient's family background and medical history offers an excellent base from which to judge the need for referral.

In this chapter, not every test has been mentioned nor every testable aspect of behavior noted. I have attempted, however, to review the kinds of problems which require testing and to report on the measures most frequently used. It should be added that the testing process, from the initial referral through the examination and the formulation of a treatment plan, is a dynamic one. Its effectiveness does not depend on the mechanical application of tools. The ultimate success of a clinical study is based on the definition of a child's needs and an investment in determining how those needs can be met.

REFERENCES

1. Als, H., Tronick, E., Adamson, L., & Brazelton, T. B. The behavior of the full-term but underweight newborn infant. *Developmental Medicine and Child Neurology*, 1976, *18*, 590–602.

2. American Psychological Association. *Biographical directory of the APA, 1975*. Washington, D.C.: 1975.

3. Ames, L. B., Learned, J., Metraux, R., & Walker, R. *Child Rorschach responses*. New York: Hoeber, 1952.

4. Anastasi, A. *Psychological testing* (4th Ed.). New York: Macmillan, 1976.

5. Bayley, N. *The Bayley scales of mental and motor development*. New York: Psychological Corp., 1969.

6. Bellak, L., & Bellak, S. S. *Children's apperception test*. Larchmont, N.Y.: C. P. S., 1949.

7. Bender, L. A visual motor gestalt test and its clinical use. *American Orthopsychiatry Research Monographs*, 1938 (No. 3).

8. Bergman, P., & Escalona, S. K. Unusual sensitivities in very young children. *The Psychoanalytic Study of the Child*, 1949, *3–4*, 333–352.

9. Black, F. W. WISC verbal-performance discrepancies as indicators of neurological dysfunction in pediatric patients. *Journal of Clinical Psychology*, 1974, *30*, 165–167.

10. Brazelton, T. B. *Neonatal Behavioral Assessment Scale. Clinics in Developmental Medicine* (No. 50). Philadelphia: Lippincott, 1973.

11. Doll, E. A. *Vineland Social Maturity Scale: Manual* (Rev. Ed.). Minneapolis: American Guidance Service, 1965.

12. Dunn, L. M. *Peabody Picture Vocabulary Test*. Minneapolis: American Guidance Service, 1965.

13. Frostig, M. *The Marianne Frostig Developmental Test of Visual Perception*. Palo Alto, Cal.: Consulting Psychologists, 1964.

14. Gesell, A., & Amatruda, C. *Developmental diagnosis*. New York: Hoeber-Harper, 1949.

15. Harris, D. B. *Children's drawings as measures of intellectual maturity: A revision and extension of the Goodenough Draw-A-Man Test*. New York: Harcourt, Brace, & World, 1963.

16. Hartmann, H. *Ego psychology and the problem of adaptation.* Transl. by D. Rapaport. New York: International Universities Press, 1958.

17. Kirk, S., McCarthy, J. J., & Kirk, W. D. *Examiner's manual, Illinois Test of Psycholinguistic Abilities* (Rev. ed.). Urbana: University of Illinois Press, 1968.

18. Koppitz, E. M. *The Bender Gestalt Test for Young Children.* New York: Grune & Stratton, 1964.

19. Levine, M. Psychological testing of children. In L. Hoffman & M. Hoffman (Eds.), *Review of Child Development Research* (Vol. 2). New York: Russell Sage Foundation, 1966.

20. Lewis, M., & McGurk, H. Evaluation of infant intelligence. *Science*, 1972, *178*, 1174–1177.

21. Lourie, R. S., & Rieger, R. Psychiatric and psychological examination of children. In S. Arieti, (Ed.), *American Handbook of Psychiatry.* 1974, 2, 15–36.

22. Machover, K. *Personality projection in the drawing of the human figure: A method of personality investigation.* Springfield, Ill.: Charles C. Thomas, 1949.

23. McCall, R. B., Hogarty, P. S., & Hurlburt, N. Transitions in sensorimotor development and the prediction of childhood IQ. *American Journal of Psychology*, 1972, 27, 728–748.

24. McCarthy, D. *McCarthy Scales of Children's Abilities.* New York: Psychological Corp., 1972.

24a. McGuire, J. M. Current psychological assessment practices. *Professional Psychology*, 1976, 7, 475–484.

25. Murray, H. A. *Thematic Apperception Test Manual.* Cambridge, Mass.: Harvard, 1943.

26. Raven, J. C. *Progressive Matrices.* New York: Psychological Corp., 1956.

27. Terman, L. M., & Merrill, M. A. *Stanford-Binet Intelligence Scale: Manual for the Third Revision, Form L-M.* Boston: Houghton Mifflin, 1960.

28. Terman, L. M., & Merrill, M. A. *Stanford-Binet Intelligence Scale: 1972 Norms Edition.* Boston: Houghton-Mifflin, 1973.

29. Uzgiris, I. C., & Hunt, J. McV. *Assessment in infancy: Ordinal scales of psychological development.* Urbana: University of Illinois Press, 1975.

30. Wechsler, D. *Wechsler Preschool and Primary Scale of Intelligence.* New York: Psychological Corp., 1967.

31. Wechsler, D. *Manual: Wechsler Intelligence Scale for Children—Revised.* New York: Psychological Corp., 1974.

THE PROCESSES OF CONSULTATION AND REFERRAL

Richard M. Sarles, M.D.
Stanford B. Friedman, M.D.

In the primary health care of children and adolescents, recent years have seen a greater emphasis upon issues related to their psychological, social, and emotional needs. Such emphasis has been especially evident within the field of pediatrics, whether under the label of child development, behavioral pediatrics, or comprehensive care to adolescents. The advantages of treating the total child and his family has been championed by pioneers in the field of pediatrics for decades, and is consistent with the historic emphasis on disease prevention by those most concerned with the health of children.[5] A number of factors, however, have recently contributed to increased interest in integrating psychosocial factors into the health care of children and youth: a decreased morbidity and mortality of many "physical" childhood diseases, a longer life expectancy of individuals suffering from wide range of chronic diseases and a concomitant concern for their care, a greater focus on multidisciplinary research and delivery services within pediatrics, and a growing general interest in improving the quality of life in society. Ultimately, the achievement of a more comprehensive care of children will rest on the willingness and ability of pediatric training centers to support such an approach in the education of future pediatricians.[2]

Nevertheless, even the ideally trained pediatrician (or family medicine practitioner) will at times identify psychosocial and learning problems that exceed his expertise. Further, it must be acknowledged that, as with other aspects of pediatric care, not all physicians will have an equal interest in or inclination toward the psychological and social aspects of health care. Thus, for the *optimal* health management of children and adolescents, consultation or referral is often indicated.

GENERAL INDICATIONS FOR CONSULTATION OR
REFERRAL

Physicians providing the primary care to children and adolescents are potentially in the most opportune position to diagnose and manage most of the common, less severe psychological, social, and learning problems present in their practices.[4] The longitudinal collection of health-related data, as well as "knowing the family" are of enormous importance; they give such a physician an advantage over any mental health professional who becomes involved only after a problem has been identified. Long-term contact with children and their families often can give significant insight into the genesis of a problem, and contribute to the type of intervention suggested to the family. Family strengths as well as family problems are frequently well known to the family's pediatrician or family practitioner. Further, his rapport with the family may take the consultant some time to duplicate. In short, the mental health specialist is not always best, even for the child with an emotional or learning problem. Recognition of this fact can help to differentiate between "dumping" a problem case on a professional colleague and requesting consultation or referral.

Obviously, physicians in pediatrics or family medicine are not the providers of primary care in all instances; new patients continually enter into their practices or may be seen—especially in the hospital setting—for some special purpose. In such cases, although lacking a previous contact with the family, the practitioners may believe a mental health consultation or referral is indicated.

In the course of eliciting information from the patient or parents, or from nursing or house staff during a hospitalization, it often becomes clear that the child is exhibiting signs of emotional or developmental difficulties completely different from the chief complaint or stated purpose of the office visit. A long-standing history of behavioral or academic problems in school, poor peer relationships, excessive sibling rivalry, and various other behavioral disturbances at home or in the community should be reason for the physician to consider the need for a behavioral consultation.

In some cases it will be learned that the child having significant emotional or learning difficulties has been receiving counseling or medication (or both), but has shown no response to these treatment interventions. It would be appropriate in some instances to suggest a further behavioral consultation and evaluation to the parents. It is important and professionally courteous to contact the person who has been treating the child in order to explain the reasons for the current consultation, and to assure him that a full report of the consultation will be sent to him to insure continuity of care for the child and the family.

Parents occasionally will request another opinion concerning their child's behavior problem; this right to further consultation should never be denied. Only the insecure professional has fears of consultation from professional colleagues. In isolated cases, however, the parents' desire for an additional consultation may be a form of denial of their child's difficulty; in other words, their request may represent a form of "doctor-shopping" through which they are hoping to find a dissenting opinion. It is important in such instances to schedule a conference with the parents, the referring physician, and the consultant to clearly delineate the diagnosis and the recommended treatment plan.

Referral also is indicated on those occasions when the physician may feel uncomfortable working with certain cases. For example, cases of juvenile delinquency or homosexuality may create feelings in the physician which can interfere with evaluation or treatment. It is important for the physician to recognize and accept such feelings, and to refer these cases to other professionals. No professional should be expected to be able to work efficiently with all types of problems or all families. While not always necessary, it may be advantageous in some instances for the physician himself to seek professional help in order to unravel some of his own feelings engendered by certain kinds of problems. Insistence on management of such cases in order to settle one's own problems is unwise as well as unfair, both to the patient and the physician.

Certainly, if the child (or family) is a close relative or in the physician's own family, referral is always indicated. When the patient (or the family) is well known socially to the physician, referral also is indicated. The necessity to explore personal material, such as sexual behavior and family relationships, moves beyond the boundaries of normal social interaction. The necessity to delve into such material can place the physician, the patient, and his family, in such an embarrassing position that further social relationships may be altered.

Suicidal behavior should always be viewed as a sign of a weakening of the adolescent's coping mechanism. Suicidal behavior usually represents a last plea for help when all other mechanisms have failed. It is a serious symptom and should not be ignored. Generally, it is here advisable to seek consultation to investigate the presence of serious psychopathology that might pose a threat of a repeat, possibly fatal, attempt. Consultation also emphasizes the concern of the physician, and underlines the serious nature of any problem which necessitated the adolescent's need to resort to suicidal behavior. Suicidal behavior in any child before puberty is extremely uncommon and usually represents a seriously troubled child. Consultation should always be obtained in these cases.

If a history of repeated drug or alcohol *abuse* is obtained, consultation should be strongly considered. Such behavior generally indicates the adolescent's attempt to seek relief from feelings of excessive anxiety or depression using alcohol or drugs as self-medication. To dismiss or minimize this behavior as normal teenage experimentation is to do an injustice to the patient by not providing proper medical opinion and treatment recommendation. Such denial by the physician may reflect his own personal discomfort, based on an individual or family problem with alcohol or drug abuse.

Psychosomatic conversion reactions represent a significant percentage of cases seen in pediatric practice.[3] Most physicians develop the ability to begin to think of this diagnostic possibility even while taking the initial history from the patient or the parents. With experience, an intuitive differentiation of organic from functional illness develops. Obviously, a reasonable, diagnostic, organic workup should be initiated, but investigation of psychosocial and intellectual factors should be explored concomitantly. The diagnosis of conversion reaction should never be made simply by the exclusion of organic disease, but rather by the inclusion of positive findings, such as the illness' fulfilling an unconscious conflict, or serving secondary gain.

It is often true that the child with a problem such as conversion symptoms, for instance, can be best cared for by the primary care physician, but not all professionals are adequately trained or even interested in such cases. Although many pediatric residency programs recognize the need for training in child development and behavioral disturbances, such training is often overshadowed by the more traditional subspecialty disciplines, such as cardiology, infectious diseases, neonatology, and hematology. Too, in actual practice, the primary care physician often feels pressured to comply with current medical trends that "treat the total patient" when he may have received less than adequate training in the behavioral areas. In such cases, it is usually preferable for the physician to recognize his limitations and interest and recommend appropriate consultation. Parents generally acknowledge the physician's honesty in admitting his own limitations, and appreciate the concern and interest he shows when consultation is suggested for their child.

THE HOSPITALIZED CHILD

In general, behaviors that are disruptive to the hospital routine and are upsetting to the physician and nursing staff generate the greatest number of referrals for consultation with specialists in psychiatry, psychology, or behavioral pediatrics. The most disturbing behaviors are overt aggression toward staff or patients, suicidal behavior, psychosis, inappropriate sexual behavior, and refusal to comply with medical treatment. Many of these behaviors demand immediate consultation to protect the patient, the staff, and other patients on the ward.

The child who creates no behavior disturbances but is withdrawn and silent is often viewed as a "good patient," and no thought is given to the need for a behavioral consultation. For example, the child who cries the first day or night following hospital admission and then "settles down" is seldom defined as a problem. A characteristic reaction of some children to hospitalization is an initial phase of active protest followed by a period of depression that is manifested by withdrawal and silence.[1] In reality then, the "good patient" in many cases may actually be a depressed child who is equally in need of psychological consultation as the more overt problem child. Hospitalization may also lead to regressive behavior in some children. Manifestations may include bed-wetting, fecal or urinary incontinency, aggressive behavior, immature behavior, and clinging behavior. Although most pediatric centers recognize this phenomenon as a normal occurrence, the behaviors are often so disturbing to the staff and parents that a behavioral consultation may be useful.

Staff Relationship with the Problem Patient

Modern pediatric inpatient facilities must necessarily be efficient and orderly. Coordination of time schedules is necessary to insure a smooth functioning unit. House staff rounds, nursing medication times, dietary serving times, consultation rounds, blood-drawing, playtime, change of shift conferences, and admission and discharge procedures all need to fit together somehow. Patients with medical illnesses generally do not create undue anxiety or tension for the ward staff. Standardized medical treatment methods, with relatively predictable responses, provide structure and support for the staff.

The emotionally disturbed child, however, touches upon uncleared diagnostic categories, unstandardized treatment modalities, and unpredictable outcomes. In addition, despite professional and public education, mental illness is still far less acceptable and understandable to patients and staff than physical disease. Thus, the general attitudes toward the emotionally disturbed child in most pediatric wards is one of discomfort. When a child (or children) demands special attention because of any one of the many types of behavior problems, the carefully tuned workings of the pediatric unit can be disrupted. When this disruption occurs, the daily work schedule may not be completed; certain tasks may then have to be transferred to a later time—perhaps to the next shift. In such instances, the staff's inability to finish the work deprives them of certain satisfactions and rewards associated with the completion of these tasks, and feelings of anger and frustration may result. In addition, the staff may experience feelings of guilt about leaving their own incompleted work for the oncoming staff. Naturally, the oncoming staff, faced with additional work, may also experience feelings of anger and frustration. If this cycle is repeated too often, poor staff morale results.

The resultant anger experienced by the staff is often manifested in covert hostility between house staff and nursing staff. Occasionally, this anger will be displaced onto dietary services, other ancillary services, or surgical subspecialty personnel. Nevertheless, the anger of the staff is seldom consciously directed toward the physically ill problem child. This may stem from the feeling among health care professionals that physical illness is beyond the control of the child. It may also be fostered by the erroneous belief that to be a caring professional, one must like or accept every patient as he is. In almost every instance, however, such anxiety results in a poorly functioning unit with increased absenteeism in the nursing staff and avoidance of the ward by the pediatric house staff. Ultimately, this behavior leads to a decrease in the level of patient care.

Management of the Problem Patient

Specific management of behavior disorders such as aggressive behavior, inappropriate sexual behavior, suicidal behavior, depression, or psychosis is quite different for each group of disorders, and in addition, generally needs to be individualized for each patient. Although a detailed outline of management principles for each behavior disorder is beyond the scope of this chapter, a general outline of principles that may be applicable to the management of many behavioral disorders can be offered. Preventive medicine is a basic principle of pediatric practice. Certain steps may be taken early by the hospital staff to prevent or minimize behavior problems, and to maximize the management of these patients who do present as problems.

In the case of the young child, it is frequently advisable to allow the parents to sleep in the child's room, in order to provide security and parenting. If, for any reason, it is impossible for the parents to stay, they should be encouraged to spend as much time as possible with the child, and to provide the child with reminders of home. Personal pajamas and slippers, a teddy bear, and a "security blanket" can help to make the transition to the hospital less frightening and lonely. For the older child or adolescent, a telephone is supportive in maintaining ties with friends. Visitors are generally helpful and should be encouraged. (In cases of drug abuse and suicidal behavior, an exception to the unlimited visitor rule should usually be enforced. Until a thorough evaluation of such cases is completed, the risk of "street drugs" entering the ward may be substantial and, naturally, needs to be prevented.)

In those hospitals where there is a special adolescent unit, an admission "hand out," naming key ward personnel and time schedule, rules, and regulations on the ward, often helps to establish behavioral limits. A ward meeting of patients and two or three staff members is another method of practicing preventive problem management. By discussing issues before they become manifest or by using positive peer pressure to regulate ward behavior, individual patient problems can often be more easily managed. These meetings can be held as often as each day, but, to be effective, should never be less than once each week. A task orientation should be maintained; issues such as food selection, game room privileges, and behavior of visitors are usually topics to discuss of common concern.

Of equal or greater importance than the weekly ward meeting for teenagers is the need for a regularly scheduled ward staff meeting. The pressures of a busy pediatric unit make it imperative for all professionals associated with the ward to have the opportunity to meet as a group at least once a week. Representatives from nursing, social work, dietary, psychology, child life, and housekeeping should all be encouraged to attend, as well as residents, fellows, and faculty from pediatrics and child psychiatry. Responsibility for these meetings should be shared, and each discipline should assure their staff's attendance. One member, with experience in group dynamics and group processes, should be designated as the leader or facilitator of these meetings. A balance of task and process orientation should be maintained, allowing time not only for imparting necessary information, but also for discussing interpersonal and patient-staff issues. It should be made clear that these meetings are *not* group therapy sessions, but are sessions designed to enhance communication among the many professionals and staff working on the ward, to share common concerns, and to collectively seek solutions to problems. Such interaction should ultimately provide higher quality care to patients.

Even with the most ideal preventive preparations and weekly staff meetings, patient problems still occur. Individual behavioral consultations with a liaison service should be available—and utilized. Liaison services are generally provided by child psychiatry, child psychology, or behavioral pediatrics. In addition, nursing liaison and pediatric social work often provide consultative assistance to the ward staff.

The behavioral consultation often can clarify the underlying reasons for the child's behavior. Understanding the predisposing factors generally makes the staff more comfortable and willing to work with the problem child. For example, the knowledge that the child's "unreasonable" fear of hospital procedures is caused by his experience of the death of a friend or sibling may help the staff to be more empathetic and tolerant towards him. The consultant also may be able to provide suggestions concerning psychotropic medications or methods of behavioral modifications as indicated. Lastly, the consultant can offer crisis intervention or brief therapy for the child and family; he may also suggest an alternative placement or treatment facility for the severely disturbed child.

PREPARING PARENTS FOR CONSULTATION

When a psychosocial or learning problem is initially suspected, the primary care physician begins the preparation of the parents for consultation with a specialist in behavioral disorders during the first discussion of the differential diagnosis, and both physical and emotional factors as potential causes of the symptoms are included in this discussion. If the need for behvioral consultation is discussed only after all organic factors are excluded, parents often feel the referral is being made only because of the lack of positive physical feelings. A negative bias may be cast on the behavioral specialist by both the physician and the parents when the feeling is conveyed that "since all else has failed, let's try a psychiatrist."

In some cases, however, even when the primary care physician carefully and correctly introduces this possibility early in the diagnostic workup, the parents may resent and resist exploration of emotional factors. It may be helpful in such cases to address the parents' concern for their child's health and welfare; in explaining the need for a behavioral consultation, the physician suggests that this consultation is an additional service to the complete and comprehensive care of their child. It should be emphasized that such consultation does not imply the child is "crazy," or emotionally disturbed, but that it suggests emotional factors may, totally or in part, account for their child's difficulty. A useful example most parents can understand is the feeling of "butterflies in the stomach" before an examination, when speaking in public, during a marriage ceremony, or at other times of stress. A tension headache is another common symptom which can be used to demonstrate that a person can experience physical distress or pain without actual structural or physical disease being present.

When overt behavioral disorders occur during hospitalization, in school, or in the community, parents are generally more willing for behavioral consultation. Psychosocial components also are generally more obvious to parents in cases of suicidal behavior, drug or alcohol abuse, and sexual promiscuity. Psychotic behavior is usually so frightening and upsetting to parents that it usually leaves little question for the need for consultation.

In some cases, however, parents unconsciously foster aberrant behavior in their children, often projecting the blame onto school or peers; in other cases, parents deny any problems with their child. Such a denial may represent the parents' need to avoid consultation so as not to reveal their own interpersonal or marital difficulties, or a problem such as alcoholism. Nevertheless, the physician should present his honest appraisal of the situation with appropriate recommendations for a behavioral consultation, and without trying to please or appease the parents by avoiding a discussion of his true assessment of the clinical situation.

If the parents agree to consultation, it is important for the primary care physician to inform the parents of the consultant's name and the reasons he was selected to consult. Parents should know what credentials the consultant possesses, how closely the physician works with the consultant, and the physician's own professional opinion of the consultant. The referring physician should always make the initial call to the consultant, discuss the reasons for consultation, and, if the child is hospitalized, arrange for a time at which he can introduce the consultant to the patient and his parents.

Parents should be informed that the consultant will probably want to see both parents together to collect important data concerning the child's development as well as a detailed family history. The number of visits generally required for a consultation and its approximate cost also should be discussed with the parents. Following the consultation, the primary care physician should meet with the parents to discuss the findings and recommendations of the consultant. If psychotherapy is advised and the parents display reluctance to follow this recommendation, the primary care physician should be careful not to support the parents' hesitation. Such a stance engenders lack of faith in the consultant who was recommended by the physician himself. In addition, such a position suggests expertise by the primary care physician in a field where he has just recently recommended consultation. If, however, both parents and physician drastically disagree with the findings and recommendations of the consultant, a second independent consultation should be suggested.

PREPARING THE CHILD FOR CONSULTATION

The young child should be informed that a doctor who is known by the primary care physician will be visiting him. As has been mentioned, if the child is hospitalized, it is desirable that the primary care physician introduce the child to the consultant. The child should be told that his parents and the physician himself are concerned about some aspects of the child's behavior: his inability to get along with friends, his anger, his nightmares, or his ability to cope with his physical illness (to cite some examples). In the case of a psychosomatic symptom, the child needs to be informed that pain or illness is often caused by emotional feelings or worries. The child should be informed that a doctor who is an expert in these kinds of problems will see him to try to find out what the worries are and how to make them go away. It should be emphasized to the young child that the consultant is the kind of doctor who plays with children and talks with them about their feelings and about any thoughts that may worry them.

In the case of an older child or adolescent, the physician begins to prepare the patient for consultation even while obtaining a physical and psychosocial history. As the need for a behavioral consultation becomes more obvious, the physician should focus increasingly on social and emotional aspects of the child's or adolescent's life. Often the teenager will become indignant and confront the physician concerning the personal nature of his questions. The physician should not retreat or become defensive, but should reemphasize the need for such probing personal questions in order to fully understand the symptoms or illness with which the patient is troubled.

It is often helpful in such instances to acknowledge that the adolescent's sexual thoughts and behavior, his (possible) drug usage, and his relationships with parents, peers, and siblings are important to know about and understand. Explaining the close interrelationship of the mind and body to the older child or adolescent may help him better to understand the connection between emotional and personal life and physical well being. As with parents, most teenagers can understand, for example, how nervous excitement before an exam can cause an increased number of trips to the lavatory or can cause "butterflies."

As the child approaches adolescence, he begins to struggle with developmental tasks common to this period. Problems of body image, the striving for individual and sexual identity, the striving for independence from the family, and the search for an intimate relationship outside of the home often results in confusion and wide swings of mood. Because of these changes, it is common for many teenagers to wonder about the state of their own mental health. When the primary care physician touches on psychosocial areas of their life or suggests a consultation with a psychotherapist, many teenagers react with active or passive protest. This protest is often a response to their own worst fear about themselves: that they really are "crazy." In most cases, the physician can reassure the teenage patients that they indeed are not.

The physician should explain, however, that the teenager's behavior—whether it be suicidal behavior, drug or alcohol abuse, aggressive behavior, depression, or social isolation—does signal a departure from normal. His symptoms do indicate that some excessive stress is causing such aberrant behavior. Nonargumentative firmness on the part of the physician concerning the need for consultation is essential. Although the physician may acknowledge the adolescent's anger or dismay, he needs to assert his professional responsibility to render his best medical opinion even if it is not to the liking of the patient. It is seemingly paradoxical that a sturdy posture in this regard is often reassuring to the patient, for it conveys the idea that someone is listening and hearing his troubles, and is concerned about his behavior.

In cases of overt psychosis wherein reality testing is seriously impaired, psychological preparation of the patient may be impossible. The physician should not assume, however, that the patient is totally oblivious to his surroundings and, therefore, fail to display human concern and dignity. In fact, the physician can act as a stabilizing, reliable, and predictable influence for the patient. The physician should introduce the consultant as a doctor trained to help patients whose thoughts are confused or jumbled. (It may even be helpful for the primary care physician to offer to remain during the first consultative session as a source of security for the patient.)

In most instances, the child or adolescent should be informed of the number of visits usually required for a consultation and the length of each visit. If psychological testing is to be part of the consultation, this procedure also should be explained. If the patient inquires about the cost of the consultation and evidences concern, the physician can assure the patient that this decision can be only made by his parents. He can emphasize that the patient's parents are concerned enough, and care enough, to be willing to spend whatever it may cost to receive proper help.

SELECTION OF A CONSULTANT

The selection of the proper mental health professional or agency is critical to optimal patient care, and may represent the most important role the primary care physician can assume in caring for a child or adolescent with a psychological, social, or learning problem. The common practice of suggesting a list of competent specialists protects the physician from any accusation of favoritism, but in actual practice is not particularly helpful to parents wishing the very best care for their child. A specific referral to a mental health professional or agency is usually to be preferred; it also relieves the family of wondering later if they made the best choice.

The referring physician should select the mental health professional with the same care that he customarily would use in seeking a surgeon, for instance. A child or teenager with an emotional problem often needs a careful evaluation that may demand a high level of professional competence. Psychotherapy and counseling are expensive, and should not be undertaken without proper indication and defined therapeutic goals. On the other hand, the failure to intervene also can be costly to a family, and later intervention can be literally, too late. The fact that the results of psychotherapy are frequently unpredictable, and certainly not always successful, only increases the responsibility of the primary care physician to make a thoughtful referral.

It is of prime importance that the physician know the mental health resources that exist in his community. This knowledge should include the therapeutic approaches utilized, the level of professional competency, and the fee structure. To obtain such information may take a deliberate effort on the part of the physician—perhaps by having lunch with an experienced and respected mental health professional. This type of contact is undoubtedly time-consuming, but it helps to assure meaningful referrals and, ultimately, saves future time.

It is highly desirable for the physician to have ongoing personal contact with a specific individual in any mental health agency he uses, particularly if the agency is large or bureaucratic. Such a contact person should be someone to whom the physician can relate repeatedly regarding his patients and their families. Failure to allow such a relationship to exist is the physician's first clue that the agency may be inflexible and not organized to work in a collaborative fashion with providers of primary health care.

In many communities, the physician may have little choice, because mental health services may be limited. He must then weigh using what is available locally against using more adequate services that may necessitate significant travel for the family. In other communities, the physician may have to select from a wide array of services. This situation may be confusing for the physician; he has to make some assessment of numerous mental health workers in private practice and in multiple agencies, and even within an agency or mental health center, there may be a variety of services available. Moreover, mental health services may be available through sources not normally considered, such as a medical school's department of pediatrics, a department of social services, or public health nursing.

What kind of mental health professional is best suited to treat children and adolescents with psychosocial problems? Should the physician turn to a child psychiatrist, a social worker, a psychologist, or a counselor? Is private care to be preferred over clinic care? These questions cannot be addressed in a general way, and they are dependent upon multiple factors. It must be realized that no single mental health profession has sole claim on competency; all fields include individuals that are professionally inadequate. This unevenness of professional skill increases the importance of the physician's systematic evaluation of the mental health resources he wishes to utilize in his community.

Each community is different in terms of its mental health resources and its maintenance of standards of care. Where there is a medical school, a faculty appointment may offer some assurance of competency, as may affiliation with a reputable agency. The writers are often asked, very appropriately, by practitioners for advice regarding a potential consultation or referral, and there is usually a professional colleague in every community who can serve this function. If not, information can be obtained from the local or state mental health association, the chairman or chief resident of a nearby department of psychiatry or pediatrics, or the local medical social work or psychology organization. Lastly, the potential consultant's educational and training credentials may be helpful.

Most physicians formally engaged in psychotherapy have been trained in psychiatry. Three years of training are generally needed to be board-eligible in psychiatry and neurology. Two years of general psychiatry and two years of child psychiatry training are needed for board eligibility in child psychiatry. Certification in child psychiatry is allowed only after certification in general psychiatry.

The major accreditation procedure in social work is membership in the National Association of Social Work, and only those with a master's degree in social work (or the equivalent) are eligible. Psychologists vary greatly in their educational background, and may have a degree at the master's or doctoral level. Most are listed in the directory of the American Psychology Association. Many states have licensing procedures for psychologists and social workers engaged in psychotherapy, and the physician should be hesitant to utilize an individual lacking such certification in those states where such laws exist.

It should be emphasized that accreditation and organizational affiliations indicate, at best, minimal standards of professional competence. The physician must seek specific advice regarding the competence of individuals in his particular locality.

It is well beyond the scope of this chapter to discuss treatment modalities. However, the referring physician should be knowledgeable about major psychotherapeutic approaches so as to explain them to his patients and their parents. Thus, he should be reasonably familiar with the orientation of individual and group therapy, behavior modification techniques, family therapy, and the psychoanalytic approach to therapy.

The role of the primary care physician does not cease once the referral has been made. He should contact the family and the mental health professional or agency to see that an appointment has been made. With the appropriate permission, he should provide a written summary of the pertinent information to the agency, and expect from them a written evaluation and treatment plan. These form the nucleus of an ongoing communication that allows the primary care physician to maintain an integrative role in providing total care to his patients.

REFERENCES

1. Bowlby, J. Childhood mourning and its implication for psychiatry. *American Journal of Psychiatry*, 1961, *118*, 481–498.
2. Friedman, S. B. The challenge of behavioral pediatrics. *Journal of Pediatrics*, 1970, *77*, 172.
3. Friedman, S. B. Conversion symptoms in adolescence. *Pediatric Clinics of North America*, 1973, *20*, 873.
4. Friedman, S. B. Behavioral pediatrics. *Pediatric Clinics of North America*, 1975, *22*, 3.
5. Richmond, J. An idea whose time has arrived. *Pediatric Clinics of North America*, 1975, *22*, 517.

═══PSYCHOSOMATIC DISORDERS═══

Jules R. Bemporad, M.D.
Charles Wuhl, M.D.

Introduction

Psychosomatic diseases may be defined as specific disorders in which problems of psychological adjustment are associated with biological processes in such a manner so as to produce an organic illness. It may be argued that according to this definition all diseases are psychosomatic since emotional or adaptational factors may influence the course of any illness. Such a unitary concept of disease may indeed be valid, and the degree of influence exerted by psychological factors may be the defining factor in disease. In psychosomatic diseases, these psychological factors appear to have an extremely significant influence in the maintenance, amelioration, or cure of the disorder. This does not mean that the cause of these diseases is psychological, but rather, that, granting a genetic or constitutional predisposition, the disease process is inordinately responsive to the vicissitudes of psychic experience.

Psychosomatic diseases also have to be differentiated from so-called conversion symptoms which appear to be purely psychological in origin. Conversion symptoms (for example, paralyses) appear to be solutions to psychological problems which may express an underlying conflict in a symbolic manner. The actual physical disability does not follow the anatomical distribution of sensory-motor innervation. In addition, the autonomic nervous system is not involved, there is no primary tissue damage, and there is no metabolic predisposing factor. These disorders respond to direct psychiatric intervention, and the manner through which the body is affected is still unknown.

Psychosomatic disorders, in contrast, are mediated by the autonomic nervous system, resulting in tissue damage such as ulcerations of the bowel. There is usually (but not always) some metabolic predisposition, such as high pepsinogen levels in ulcers, or allergy in asthma. Finally, the actual symptom appears to be dictated by a biological rather than a psychological diathesis. The individual automatically reacts to certain emotions or stresses in a characteristic physiological manner. Therefore while conversion reactions appear to be mediated by the higher centers and culminate in highly evolved defensive operations to threatening situations, psychosomatic diseases are more affected by the vegetative parts of the nervous system and result in bodily changes that appear to lack both a defensive purpose or a symbolic significance in the service of intrapsychic needs.

Historical Review

The modern history of psychosomatic medicine may be divided into two periods: 1940–1960, and 1955 to the present. In the former period, the emphasis was on specificity; importance was placed on the discovery of which factors determined a person's susceptibility to a particular disease. Also studied were intrapsychic mechanisms and specific psychological factors that determined the choice of organ system and disease. In the latter period, as more sophisticated research techniques and broader perspectives developed, other factors have been taken into account. Among these are genetic transmission of possible predisposing agents, the social matrix in which illness occurs, and the concept of nonspecific stress. Other research has focused on the actual neurophysiological mechanisms that link cognitive or emotional experience with organic illness.[31]

Early Contributions

Of historical importance in the study of psychosomatic medicine are the works of Flanders Dunbar and Franz Alexander. Dunbar's work[7] was based upon an extensive review of the literature, and the examination of 1600 hospital admissions. For each of a variety of illnesses, she delineated one or more features in several areas of the individual's psychosocial life and formulated personality profiles of illnesses including arrhythmias, coronary occlusion, and hypertensive cardiovascular disease. For example: An individual with hypertensive disease demonstrated a lifelong pattern of anxiety, perfectionism, compulsivity, and difficulties with authority figures. However, later studies showed that there was no consistent correlation between a certain personality profile and a type of psychosomatic illness.

Franz Alexander[3,4,5] also attempted to determine psychological factors that accompany, or possibly cause, psychosomatic illness. He focused on unconscious unresolved neurotic conflicts rather than on manifest personality traits in determining specific psychological factors associated with any particular illnesses. His work postulated that the affective component of the neurotic conflict, as it is denied external expression, discharged excessively into internal and vegetative pathways. The eventual result is somatic disturbances or organic lesions. Alexander felt that some constitutional organ vulnerability is a necessary, though not a sufficient, cause of psychosomatic illness. Two clinical examples which may illustrate Alexander's formulations are peptic ulcer and ulcerative colitis.

Alexander reported that patients with peptic ulcers have severe conflicts with the expression of oral dependent strivings, which are inconsistent with their ego ideals. He felt that these strivings, when denied gratification and external expression, are discharged through the hypothalamus along autonomic pathways to the stomach. The stomach then reacts as if continually hungry for mother's milk, and this results in excessive acid secretion and eventual ulceration.

Alexander felt that ulcerative colitis is caused by disappointment in, resentment toward, and sense of loss of the loved one. As these feelings are not expressed, the patient tries to please the loved one in an archaic way learned during toilet training:

producing a bowel movement. This eventually leads to explosive diarrhea and eventual ulceration. Various other illnesses such as rheumatoid arthritis, bronchial asthma, neurodermatitis, Grave's disease, and essential hypertension were explained in similar ways.

Alexander also made a clear distinction between conversion hysteria and the *visceral neuroses*, a term he used to refer to the psychosomatic disorders. In conversion hysteria, according to Alexander, symptom formation acts to resolve unconscious conflicts, while in visceral neurosis the basic conflict is not resolved. This unresolved conflict leads to the formation of a chronic affect that is accompanied by its appropriate physiological concomitants, even though the affect remains repressed or suppressed. The physiological changes that accompany the chronic emotional state associated with unresolved conflict are those changes that give rise to altered functions within the specific organ system. If these changes are sustained for long enough periods of time, alterations in structure and eventually disease occur.

Alexander also postulated that in each instance there is a specific, related "onset situation." He felt that some current situation in the patient's life affects him emotionally, and in such a way that the old conflicts are reactivated, together with the affective counterpart. These affects can not be expressed openly and so are discharged internally, leading to metabolic abnormalities. In a similar formulation, Ruesch[31a] believed that the core problem in psychosomatic illness is the persistence of infantile conflicts in the adult personality.

This approach to psychosomatic illness stressed the individual in isolation; it searched for causes of illness in aberrant personality factors or in the persistence of childhood conflicts. While giving a tacit acknowledgment to constitutional factors, these early investigators relied heavily on the individual's psychological makeup in accounting for the specificity of disease.

In the late 1940's and early 1950's, another model of disease began to find application in the study of psychosomatic disease. This model centered on Hans Selye's[36] brilliant work on the body's hormonal response to stress. Selye's work introduced the concept of nonspecific stress as a precipitant of metabolic changes which are adaptive for a short time but may result in disease if chronically employed. Selye termed this reaction to stress the *general adaptation syndrome* and delineated three successive stages.

The first stage is an "alarm reaction" which results from the stress or noxious stimulus which the animal initially experiences. This stage is itself divided into two parts. The first, or shock stage, consists of various physiological reactions, among which are hemoconcentration and tachicardia. The pituitary gland is then stimulated to produce ACTH, which in turn stimulates the adrenal cortex to produce corticosteroid hormones, thus maintaining body fluid balance and building up sugar stores. In the latter, or countershock phase, the adrenal cortex is enlarged because of great activity during the shock stage; one now finds a reversal of the tissue changes seen earlier.

In the second stage, or "stage of resistance," the hormonal reaction is at a minimum, and the organism is adapting to the continuing stress. The lesions of the shock phase disappear completely because of these adaptive mechanisms.

The third stage of the general adaptation syndrome is the "stage of exhaustion"; the adaptive mechanisms break down from prolonged or severe stress. The hormonal needs of the organism are excessive. The symptoms of the alarm reaction intensify, the adrenal glands enlarge, depletion of adrenal cortical hormones now takes place, and exhaustion and death result.

In England during World War II, under the stress of bombing raids, individuals were known to develop acute gastric hemorrhages and ulcers. Under experimental conditions, prolonged nonspecific noxious stimuli have produced psychosomatic diseases, e.g., arthritis and hypertension, in white rats. Selye felt that any noxious stimulus, including psychic stress, might cause the general adaptation syndrome to commence. It recently has been felt that the hypothalamus is the initiator of the adaptation syndrome.

Recent Contributions

In the past two decades, research on psychosomatic illness has broadened so that social factors, such as crowding or recurrent life changes, have been considered as possibly causative. At the same time, investigation of constitutional factors, such as congenitally high pepsinogen levels, has attempted to identify those at risk for a specific illness. Much of current thought is less concerned with an individual's psychological makeup than with the presence of some biological predisposition that can be actualized by any environmental stress. The development of an actual definition of *stress* has occasioned much recent work. Of more importance, perhaps, has been the evolution of a multifactorial view of psychosomatic illness which considers a certain interaction of constitutional, predispositional, psychological variables, which results from childhood experience, and social stress, which may precipitate the actual illness.[27] Therefore, psychosomatic disease is currently conceptualized as a result of a complex combination of diverse factors, each necessary but not sufficient in its own right to determine pathology.

This multifactorial approach is well exemplified in the work on peptic ulcer by Mirsky and others.[27,37] They delineated a group of individuals with genetic hypersecretion of pepsinogen. This inborn trait made these individuals at risk for peptic ulcer. However, additional determinants, such as specific childhood experiences, were needed in order to cause a vulnerability to stress in adult life that resulted in the formation of an ulcer.

There are other illnesses where risk studies could find an appropriate application, since there are diseases known to possess biological markers: Gout, using hyperuricemia as a marker, could identify subjects at risk;[16] in rheumatoid arthritis certain immune proteins are indicators. In coronary heart disease, multiple factors are present: obesity, cigarette smoking, exercise habits, heredity, hypertension, blood lipids, and the like.

Another area recently studied is the effects of psychological stress on endocrine function, in work carried out on experimental animals.[1,21,25] The resistance of the host to a variety of pathogenic organisms, as well as the viability and rate of growth of implanted neoplastic tissue have been shown to be influenced by psychological stress.[19]

Research on the roles of early life experiences, conditioning, and genetic endowment, has been carried forward. Infantile and childhood experiences have been shown to influence subsequent adult susceptibility or resistance to illness. Adar and Friedman[1,2,10] have studied solitary versus crowded conditions of raising animals, and have found these to influence adult susceptibility to a number of microorganisms and viruses. Levine[22] has studied the effects of subtle early manipulations (handling), on eventual adult behavior (excitability). He has also studied the relationships of these early experiences to adult physiological responses, such as the responsiveness of the pituitary-adrenal system.

Henry[11] studied the susceptibility of mice to the development of hypertension and associated adrenal changes. He correlated the effects of psychological stress, and studied differences in early rearing and experiences with the later development of hypertension. Biological, psychological, and social aspects were also studied, and their interrelationships taken into account. With increased crowding, social disorganization, and confrontation, the mice developed hypertension with pathological consequences.

In the human neonate, research has focused on the identification of some inborn constitutional differences between infants in their psychophysiological reactivity.[6,23] The differences people experience in their susceptibility to certain illnesses may be partially accounted for by these variations.

Studies have been made of variations in physiological activity during the various stages of sleep, as well as activity that occurs between the waking and sleeping states. Profound physiological activity has been shown to occur during rapid eye movement (REM) sleep. Kales and Tan[14] showed that the bulk of nighttime acid in peptic ulcer patients is secreted during REM periods. Nocturnal angina was studied by Nowlin and his associates[28] who found that these episodes were experienced almost exclusively during REM periods.

In the 1970's, personality constellations have been studied as a means of identifying individuals at greater risk for particular illnesses. As initially suggested by Dunbar, certain personality constellations have been identified by Friedman and Roseman[9] as related to the proneness to coronary artery disease. They termed this personality the "Type A" individual: upward striving, a perfectionist, with a tendency toward impatience.

As already noted, several factors play key roles in the etiology of psychosomatic disorders; one factor that has been studied in depth is stress. Psychological stress interacts with other factors in precipitating psychosomatic diseases. Stressful factors often found to be of importance involve loss of love, separation, or stimulation of aggression.[38]

In attempting to better define what stress means, Lazarus[21] noted that certain conditions must be present for a particular stimulus to evoke a stress reaction. The stimulus must signify harm to the individual, it must be communicated symbolically, and he must regard it as dangerous to his psychological well-being. When a stimulus is felt to be threatening to the individual, various processes are activated that aim to reduce or eliminate the anticipated harm. Some of these coping devices are accompanied by physiological changes which can result in organic damage.

Several investigators have felt that the various stresses and changes in one's life greatly increase the likelihood that one may fall ill of virtually any disease. This conclusion has followed from observations that individuals having recently undergone a major stress or change in their lifestyles are more prone to illness. Rahe[12,30] has developed a life events inventory in which individuals are asked to check off the various changes that have occurred in their lives over a period of time, ranging, possibly, from death of a spouse to a change in one's employment. The emotional significance of each event had previously been determined. Based upon its emotional significance (previously determined), each item is assigned a score. The individual's readjustment to the events is also taken into account; he is asked to judge the intensity of the various life occurrences and the length of time necessary to adjust to them.

In following such patients, there has been seen a significant correlation between a high score and greater susceptibility to a variety of illnesses—heart attacks, cancer, influenza. Retrospective studies have shown that subjects with tuberculosis experienced higher scores on their life events inventory for the ten years prior to the onset of illness than did a control group.

Mortality, and morbidity of bereavement is another area in which physical health highly correlates with nonspecific effects of psychological stress. Rees and Lutkins[31] studied a community in Wales in which the experimental subjects were all those individuals who experienced the death of a close family member. Control subjects were matched for age, sex, and marital status. The two groups were followed for a period of one year, during which time it was noted that the death rate of bereaved subjects was seven times that of controls.

Engel[8] and Schmale[34,35] demonstrated that real, threatened, or symbolic object loss highly correlates with the development of illness of any type. They felt that the psychological state of the individual contributes to the timing of the onset of disease. The "giving up–given up" complex describes the setting in which illness occurs. The characteristics of this complex include a feeling of not being able to function to full capacity, a consideration of one's future as bleak and unrewarding, and an impression of relationships as less secure or no longer gratifying.

CURRENT CONCEPTS OF PSYCHOSOMATIC
ILLNESS

From this brief historical survey, it becomes apparent that the investigation of psychosomatic disorders has expanded in two major directions. Early studies focused on the psychological problems of the individual in isolation; more recent approaches have investigated the interaction of predisposing biochemical factors with precipitating psychological events, and another line of research has grown to consider the environmental context in which the disease originated. There has been less reliance upon the nature of unconscious conflicts or personality variables as explanatory hypotheses, together with, on the one hand, a greater effort to discover genetic or constitutional prerequisites for illness, and on the other, an equally rigorous search for the social or familial interactions that may influence the course of illness. As Minuchen, Baker, Rosman, et al.[26] have indicated, the open system model of psychosomatic illness has replaced the former linear model. The newer model attempts to integrate multiple factors, such as specific types of family organization, involvement of the patient in familial conflicts, and the role of some physiological vulnerability. This newer view of psychosomatic illness is more suited to the complexities involved in these diseases, discarding as it does, facile unidimensional explanations.

This broader view has resulted from the failure of previous theoretical models to fit clinical findings. For example, when large numbers of patients were studied, no specific personality profile has been demonstrated. Knapp and Nemetz,[18] on the basis of intensive psychological investigations of forty asthmatics, were unable to find any single personality type or single significant conflict. Their only generalization ventured was that those individuals with more severe asthmatic problems seemed to be more emotionally disturbed. However, this finding might indicate that the degree of personality disturbance might be secondary to the degree of physical impairment.

Other alleged personality characteristics of patients with certain psychosomatic diseases either have been discounted or have been explained on a nonpsychodynamic basis. As an illustration of the latter, Purcell[29] has made some astute observations on the asthmatic child's tendency to cry softly (or not at all) rather than to weep openly as nonasthmatic children do. Such a finding led Alexander (partially) to postulate that the asthmatic wheeze is a substitute for the suppressed cry for the mother. Actually, Purcell comments, loud crying may initiate an asthmatic attack, so the child may learn to express his displeasure quietly or in nonemotional ways, rather than risk a full-blown asthmatic episode.

Such criticisms in no way deny the importance of psychological factors. They are very significant, but they are specific for each individual, and they defy generalization. One patient may become threatened by separation, another may not tolerate intimacy—there is no specificity in terms of psychological conflict or personality profile for each disease. What does appear specific, however, is the innate physiological organ response.

The question of psychological precipitant becomes a separate one for each patient. States that constitute stress consist of the arousal of emotions which the individual cannot adequately handle. This, in turn, leads to an overwhelming or flooding of the self and, in predisposed individuals, an automatic arousal of metabolic reactions resulting in an organic symptom. It is this lack of ability to master certain emotions that renders the individual vulnerable to exacerbations of illness whenever environmental changes arouse such emotions within him. Quite often, the physiological changes occur so rapidly that these symptoms mask the precipitating affective state; at other times, the emotions may be so painful that the individual immediately suppresses his feelings. Hence, these precipitating affective states are often difficult to detect. (This difficulty is all the more troublesome in the study of children with psychosomatic disorders, since they often have difficulty in verbalizing emotional states.) When these triggering emotions can be discovered eventually, however, psychotherapy is greatly advantaged. Psychotherapeutic intervention cannot be directed at the organic symptom of illness, but is aimed, rather, at helping the individual achieve mastery over precipitating emotions: recognizing them, expressing them, and eventually ceasing to be threatened by them. In children, therapy is also directed at eliminating the excessive occurrence of situations which evoke these emotions within the family unit.

The variability of these threatening emotions may be illustrated by the development of asthmatic children. The writers feel that most asthmatic children who are seen in latency age can be divided into three categories. The first group are those children who are dependent, passive, and almost totally restricted to the family group; these children seem to respond to any threat of separation from the maternal figure with an asthmatic attack. The second group are those children, overly independent, who strive toward mastery especially in the intellectual sphere; these children consistently deny dependency strivings and their asthmatic attacks are often precipitated by frustration in their drive toward mastery. The third group are those children in whom there is little emotional or psychiatric disease concomitant with their asthmatic problems. This last group (possibly the bulk of asthmatic patients) is rarely seen by child psychiatrists, and is normally treated by pediatricians and allergists.

For most asthmatics, regardless of their later personality structure, the first asthmatic attack seems to occur in late infancy, around 2 or 3 years of age. Most have shown prior manifestations of allergic diseases such as eczema, hives, or milk allergy. Usually the asthmatic attack is precipitated by an infectious disease such as bronchitis or pneumonia. The initial attack, understandably, provokes anxiety in the family and the child. Repeated attacks elicit from the mother an over-concern for the child and a continuous anxiety over the occurrence of a repeated attack. Moreover, the asthmatic attack is not only precipitated by allergic factors but may result from a state of psychological stress to the organism, and in this sense asthma is often a reaction to a feeling of anxiety within the child. Since, at this age, anxiety is connected with separation from the mother, a pattern emerges in which the asthmatic attack occurs upon separation from the mother and is often ameliorated by being reunited with her. Thus, the mother and child form a dyadic relationship in which each becomes reluctant to separate from the other for fear of provoking an asthmatic attack. Asthmatic attacks are not seen here as manipulative or as an attempt to be reunited with the mother but, rather, as a physiological counterpart of separation anxiety. The child does not talk himself into having an anxiety attack; instead, he automatically experiences one when separated from the mother, since this leaves him in a state of anxiety and stress. Although the asthmatic child may use the threat of an asthmatic attack manipulatively, it is doubtful that the child can experience an asthmatic attack except as a result of an allergic or emotional tiggering mechanism.

Depending upon the mother's needs, each of the three types of asthmatic children can evolve. In the first type (in which the child remains dependent upon the mother), the mother usually has a great fear of the child's asthmatic attacks. Therefore, she does everything she can to lessen the frequency of these attacks—usually, spending an inordinate time with the patient and becoming overprotective. She discourages activity which she feels might result in asthmatic attacks, such as sports or situations wherein the child might be exposed to an infectious disease. The mother feels comfortable only when she is with the child, for she fears that the child may experience an asthmatic attack in her absence and may not be helped.

Actually, the mother is infantilizing the child and sabotaging attempts at autonomy and independence. Again, it is not that the mother uses the asthma to fulfill her own needs for a dependent child (although this may occur in a few cases); the situation is such that the mother has to reassure herself, because of her own anxiety over the child's illness. Thus, a relationship evolves that robs the child of normal confrontation with his environment. The child is discouraged from assertive or exploratory behavior; he is restricted and kept at home.

As this dependency is reinforced, the effect on the child is often disastrous. He becomes less and less able to form adequate defenses against normal anxiety and he comes to rely exclusively on the mother for protection and comfort. In turn, he becomes ever more vulnerable to anxiety and stress, since he has little experience with mastery or self expression. When, later on, he tries to break away from the mother, he is met with situations which provoke anxiety and again lead to an asthmatic attack. Repeated attacks may cause a further binding to the mother, a deepening of the dependency and more liability to future asthmatic attacks.

An 11-year-old Hispanic female asthmatic had missed a considerable amount of school as a result of her illness. On evaluation, she appeared socially immature and seemed content to let her mother speak for her. History revealed that the child stayed at home with her mother excessively because of a mutual fear of an asthmatic attack. Therapy consisted of initially explaining the psychological factors that played a role in the child's asthmatic condition. The child was gradually encouraged to venture out on her own, being told that she might experience some wheezing but that she could always obtain help, even when away from the mother. It was suggested that the child begin to carry medication with her and to decide when she should take it. This helped to give the child a sense of mastery over her illness and to have her appreciate that her illness was to be her responsibility. At the same time, the mother was seen and allowed to express her anxieties about the child's asthma. These feelings were respected by the therapist but it was made clear to the mother that she had to deal with her own anxiety if her child was to develop normally. While overprotection worked in the short run to protect the child from asthma or from anxiety, it was explained that, in the long run, these well-meaning efforts would be counterproductive. Eventually, the girl was able to be with friends, or in an afternoon activity group without anxiety and with a minimum of respiratory difficulty. Once along the path of individuation, she enjoyed age-appropriate activities without the mother. While she still continued to have some asthmatic attacks, she was able to lead a fairly satisfying life despite her illness.

The second type of asthmatic patient has a similar mode of onset. Rather than giving in to dependency needs, however, this type of patient actively fights against a dependent way of life. This patient see his asthma as a burden rather than as a face-saving escape from the responsibilities of life, but he similarly responds to situations of conflict and anxiety with asthmatic attacks. He generally feels betrayed by his asthmatic attacks and most often experiences them when his drives toward mastery are frustrated.

For example: A patient who was supposed to be in a school play for which he had prepared, experienced an asthmatic attack on the evening of the play. As a result, he could not be in the play, and he felt angry about not being able to perform and resentful of the asthmatic attack. Actually, the asthmatic attack may be seen as a result of this patient's ambivalence over being in the school play. Such a state of conflict, which in others might have produced a sense of nervousness or "butterflies," produced a severe asthmatic attack in this patient. Here again, the asthmatic attack was a direct response to a feeling of anxiety—anxiety centered on fear of failure or of making a fool of himself in front of an audience rather than on separation from mother or frustration of dependency needs.

The genesis of the asthmatic dyad between mother and child in these patients seems somewhat similar to that seen in the dependent patient type. However (perhaps because of less need on the part of the mother), this type of child is not always overprotected or pampered. The mother is concerned, and reacts with anxiety to the asthmatic attack but stresses competitive goals and achievement as well. Often an overly competitive relationship exists with a sibling or with a parental figure. As a result, this type of asthmatic is often in conflict as he attempts to make up for what he feels is a genetic inferiority. Because of the enforced limitations in sports or physical activity, this child often attempts to excel in scholastics or other nonphysical modes of achievement such as music or art. Too, this child often sees his mother as a threat to his quest for super-adequacy in that the mother, out of her own anxiety, cautions him against assertion and independence.

Often, this type of child is reported in psychoanalytic literature. Markedly conflicted about the maternal figure, on the one hand, he strongly desires independence and achievement while on the other hand, he is not sure of his ability to fulfill these desires and, on occasion, will tend to revert to a more dependent and passive mode of relating. In brief, this type of child overcompensates for his illness, denies dependency needs at any cost, and becomes a pseudomature, overreliant, adultlike child. An extreme example of this type of asthmatic follows.

Subject was a 13-year-old boy who strenuously fought against the idea that he had a physical illness. This child insisted on going out for varsity sports even though he often experienced an asthmatic attack after practice (a fact he concealed from his coach and his parents). He prided himself on hunting with a bow and arrow in the most severe weather. In addition to feats of physical prowess, he felt compelled to make outstanding grades and to participate in extracurricular activities. His parents described him as in a constant state of tension over the accomplishment of the numerous tasks he set for himself. He became angry when he experienced an asthmatic attack and complained that it was holding him back from what he wanted to achieve. Unfortunately, his state of anxiety combined with his disregard for limits on his activity made his asthmatic condition worse rather than better.

This child was seen in fairly intensive psychotherapy as he presented with complex psychological problems that had been internalized and were relatively independent of the environment. Initially he resisted therapy, viewing it as a further confirmation of his alleged weakness and inferiority. In time, however, he was able to form a good working relationship with his therapist and to drop his facade of a superachieving, independent individualist. He was able to reveal his sense of inferiority about having asthma as well as his overcompensating defenses against it. He was able to understand that his reaction to his asthma, although intended to allow him to see himself as physically healthy, was actually increasing the severity of his illness. A pattern of repressed sibling rivalry emerged in which the patient felt he had to maintain superiority over his younger brothers in order to feel adequate. His parents had unconsciously given him the role of the serious, achieving, and (in his mind) favored child, and he was still following their commands. He projected his parents onto his teachers and his brothers onto fellow students, so that he carried his childhood family situation over into teenage activities outside his home.

While this boy might have had problems even without asthma, the illness greatly impeded his needed sense of superiority and made him strive all the more. As he became aware of his behavior patterns and realized that others would accept and respect him without superior achievement, his asthma greatly diminished.

The third type of asthmatic, probably the most frequent type, is the child who has some emotional problems but not of a gross or incapacitating sort. This child also first experiences his onset of asthma in late infancy but because of different family dynamics does not develop into an asthmatic personality type. This type of child seems fortunate in having parents who do not over-respond to the asthma and who can bear their own anxiety over the child's illness. At the same time, the child is not made to feel weak or incapacitated because of the disease. Such asthma is treated as a physical illness and the reciprocal dependency between child and mother is not established.

The Open Systems Model

So far we have focused primarily on the child's problems in isolation; we have also considered the family unit only as it is appreciated by the child patient. A systems approach to psychosomatic problems in children advocates a consideration of the child's illness in the context of a larger family disturbance. It is believed that the course of illness becomes much more understandable when seen in this broader framework. The basic postulate of the systems approach is that the child's symptoms are triggered and maintained by the family with the result that the illness becomes necessary for sustaining the family's pathological equilibrium. In a broader context, it may be said that the family, as a unit, requires the child to remain sick and prevents cure. Such a view is supported by the frequent finding that the removal of a child from the family atmosphere produces an abrupt amelioration in symptoms. The staff of the Children's Asthma Research Institute and Hospital in Denver report that about 40% of the children lose their asthma soon after admission.[24] The dramatic effects of this "parentectomy" in most psychosomatic conditions certainly implicates familial interactions in symptom maintenance.

Some preliminary studies using this approach were conducted by Jackson and Yalom[13] in their investigation of eight families with a child with ulcerative colitis. These families demonstrated some consistent characteristics that could be related to the maintenance of the child's condition. The families were described as extremely restricted in terms of social or extrafamilial activities; venturesome behavior was discouraged by phobic warnings about the dangers of the world. A deadly quiet atmosphere existed, with no tolerance for the expression of feelings, especially negative ones. Overall, an air of hopelessness and unhappiness pervaded the families, together with a tacit agreement that this gloomy outlook would not be mentioned in front of other family members. It becomes apparent how such a family style would increase the dependency of a sick child, stifle the expression of his emotion (or leave him unprepared to deal with the arousal of feelings), and generally add to his sense of ineffectiveness in coping with his illness. A final significant finding was a preoccupation with physical health and a tendency of the family to use the child's illness as an excuse to further restrict its activities. Jackson and Yalom are careful to state that this family pattern does not cause ulcerative colitis, but that it may limit the child's ability to deal with the disease.

Further pathological interrelationship patterns have been documented in detail by Minuchin and his coworkers.[26] From the study of families which contained children with hyperlabile diabetes, asthma, anorexia nervosa, and other psychosomatic illnesses, this group was able to characterize a psychosomatogenic family. They found that these families manifested four major types of pathological transactions: enmeshment, over-protectiveness, rigidity, and lack of conflict resolution. Enmeshment describes a certain interdependence of relationships, an intrusion of personal boundaries, and poor differentiation of each individual in the family. Overprotectiveness implies a constant eliciting of nurturing and protective responses, with an excess of queries about fatigue or discomfort. This overconcern with health (or the lack of it) deflates any attempt at criticism in that complaints of not feeling well are utilized to ward off possible confrontation.

Rigidity refers to the family's heavy commitment to maintain the status quo, a lack of flexibility that causes problems when events occur that require change. As a result, the family seeks out "detours" or "avoidance circuits" to prevent change, and a "symptom bearer" becomes a particularly useful device in the face-saving maneuvers that maintain the family system's equilibrium. A sick child allows the family to resist threatened change, to deny the conflict that change may bring, and to detour from the true conflictual area by focusing on the child's illness. In this sense, the child's illness becomes a ready defense for the family to employ whenever external events threaten its precarious equilibrium. Lack of conflict resolution results from the three characteristics already mentioned. Enmeshment, overprotectiveness, and rigidity make these families unable clearly to face or resolve problems in a definitive manner. Unresolved conflicts, therefore, threaten the family again and again, and continue to activate the family system's avoidance mechanism, including the precipitation of illness in the child.

These pathological characteristics of the family transactions encourage the use of illness as a communication, as a way of fending off criticism, and as a way of avoiding change and conflict. The sick child becomes the focus of all attention, and thereby relieves other family members of the necessity of confronting their own problems. Whenever these problems can no longer be denied, the child is believed to be subtly encouraged to once again have a "flare-up," thus allowing the family to continue to function in its own manner and to avoid the impending problem. The child, sensing the stress within the family unit, responds with the needed symptom that will be employed as a detouring mechanism. The family then responds to the child's symptom with concern and protection, thus rewarding and maintaining the illness.

Minuchin's group claims a high rate of success, in terms of symptom reduction, with the use of family therapy. The amelioration of illness is indeed impressive and their treatment method is undoubtedly sound in selected families. However, their model of pathological family transactions should not be taken as typical of all families with a child who suffers from a psychosomatic illness. Their sample consists of children whose symptoms have been refractory to adequate medical treatment and whose families are obviously disturbed. The valuable descriptions and treatment programs described by this group appear applicable only when the child's illness synergistically meets the needs of a pathological family. This is not the case for the majority of children with psychosomatic disorders.

Approaches to Treatment

The major thrust of this chapter has been to stress that any attempt to treat psychosomatic disorders must consider physiological, psychological, and sociological factors. The child therapist, therefore, must work closely with a pediatrician to assess the biological contributions to the illness. Kaplan[15] has aptly called the biological contribution to psychosomatic illness the *somatic barrier,* stressing the point that these aspects of the disorder are not amenable to psychotherapy. Psychiatric treatment cannot lower blood pepsinogen levels or the production of antibodies to certain allergens; these aspects of the disorder must remain in the pediatrician's or the internist's domain. The psychotherapist can treat only the emotional aspects of the illness and these are often considerable, as has been discussed. The aim of therapy is not directed at the actual physical symptom but at the psychological antecedents of the symptom. In some cases, wherein the genetic predisposition is exceptionally high, major symptomatic improvement cannot be achieved, but at least the patient may learn to cope with his illness in a more satisfactory manner. Thus Langford,[20] in reviewing the effects of psychotherapy on 63 of 109 children with ulcerative colitis, concluded that while psychotherapy did not affect the basic disease process, it did enable the child to adapt better both to physical and emotional stress, and thereby to function more successfully in life situations.

Once the assessment of physical contribution to illness has been completed, the therapeutic investigation should center on detecting those psychological or environmental stresses that cause flare-ups.

The therapist must define the internalized processes that cause the child to be flooded with unpleasant emotions which, in turn, produce somatic symptoms. The child should be taught how to identify these affective states, to verbalize their effect, and eventually to master them. Many children believe that a show of anger will alienate or hurt others; this inhibition can be worked through in the therapy process. Other children, whose individuation has been blocked, believe that they cannot cope without the help of parental figures; the thought of separation is so frightening that it results in an exacerbation of the illness. Often the parents have communicated this sense of anxiety to the child, for example, in cases of school phobia. Such children require therapeutic intervention that encourages their sense of adequacy and decreases their fear of the world. Some children have learned to use their illness to elicit desired parental behaviors; here, the adoption of a more direct form of mediation is needed. Obviously, the parents of these children must be involved in the therapeutic efforts. If the stresses are produced by the family, as elucidated by Minuchin's group, then a family approach to therapy is indicated. The parents must be made to appreciate how the child reacts to their tensions, and how the illness is unconsciously used by the family to avoid confrontation with problems. In extreme instances the child's illness may be holding the parents together or may be serving to give meaning to their lives.

Sometimes the pathological interactions are so entrenched that the child must be physically separated from the family. The approaches taken to the inpatient treatment of such children have been outlined by Kluger[17] of the National Jewish Hospital in Denver, which has an active program for chronic asthmatic children. In brief: The experience at the hospital deflates the power of the child's symptom. An asthma attack no longer has the disruptive social consequences that it did at home. The physical symptom is not followed by a frantic trip to the emergency room, or absence from school the next day. Likewise, in this setting the child is encouraged to communicate his wishes verbally, not to utilize the symptom as a social mediator. The child is told to carry on despite his illness. Gradually, the somatic illness is conceptually separated from communication of emotional needs; it thus loses much of its reason to exist. As the child begins to assert himself through appropriate channels, the frequency of asthma decreases. The adults in his surroundings respond to direct verbal, rather than indirect somatic, communication. With this treatment, Kluger believes, the child slowly develops a new identity, that of a person who, despite some illness, can cope with life and function independently.

Most of these inpatient studies have dealt with asthma, so we do not as yet know the effect of milieu therapy on other psychosomatic diseases. One of the writers (J.R.B.) has had experience with a 2-year inpatient treatment of an 11-year-old girl with severe ulcerative colitis.

> The disease responded fairly rapidly once the child had psychologically separated herself from her family and had formed close attachments to staff and patients. During her hospital stay, the parents were seen regularly for conjoint therapy (with the girl later joining the sessions).
>
> This family was highly self-restricting, with a chronic undercurrent of hostility and tension beneath a bland facade. The parents had surreptitiously used the patient as a go-between to mediate communications that each parent did not wish openly to acknowledge to each other. Both parents were chronically depressed, exuding an aura of helplessness and despair. They had forced the girl to take on an adult role in the family and to care for them. While the child was angry over having to sacrifice her own gratification for that of her parents, her own guilt prevented any expression or even any prolonged awareness of her own anger. The girl appeared trapped in a suffocating situation where an attempt to gain independent satisfaction was sensed as a betrayal. She acquiesced to her parents' covert demands, but was plagued with troublesome dreams and later with the onset of rectal bleeding.
>
> Away from the parents, in the safety of a hospital situation, she was able to recognize her own anger and to express it to her therapist. She also felt free to enjoy herself without guilt or fear. The girl did not return home until extensive changes were evident in the family as well as in her own personality. As of this writing (ten years past discharge), there has been no recurrence of the disease process.

While it is impossible to generalize from one case, the establishment of specific inpatient treatment centers for children suffering from psychosomatic diseases other than asthma may be indicated.

Summary

Following the initial and heuristic contributions of Alexander[5] and Dunbar,[7] the field of psychosomatic medicine has grown in scope and sophistication so as currently to present a comprehensive concept of illness. Through the efforts of workers in this field, an appreciation for the complexities of all diseases has developed to include genetic, psychological, and sociological factors. Most recently, concepts of general systems theory have been utilized so that health and illness are seen as states of relative equilibrium and adaptation. Romano[32,34] has succinctly formulated this view, regarding health and disease as phases of life which depend at any time on an organism's reciprocal relationship with its environment. The degree to which any organism can successfully master internal or external stresses so as to maintain a successful equilibrium depends on genetic, experiential, and environmental determinants. The so-called psychosomatic disorders are considered to be those greatly but not exclusively affected by psychological factors.

REFERENCES

1. Ader, R. The influences of psychological factors on disease susceptibility in animals. In M. L. Conalty (Ed.), *Husbandry of Laboratory Animals.* London: Academic, 1967.

2. Ader, R., & Plant, S. M. Effects of prenatal maternal handling and differential housing in offspring emotionality, plasma corticosterone levels and susceptibility to gastric erosions. *Psychosomatic Medicine,* 1969, *30,* 227–286.

3. Alexander, F. *Psychosomatic medicine.* New York: Norton, 1950.

4. Alexander, F. *The scope of psychoanalysis.* New York: Basic Books, 1961.

5. Alexander, F., & French, T. M. *Studies in psychosomatic medicine.* New York: Ronald Press, 1943.

6. Bridger, W., Birns, B., & Blank, M. A comparison of behavioral ratings and heart rate measurements in human neonates. *Psychosomatic Medicine,* 1965, *27,* 123.

7. Dunbar, H. F. Emotions and bodily changes: A survey of literature on psychosomatic interrelationships. *Psychosomatic Medicine,* 1948, *10,* 134–144.

8. Engel, G. L. A psychological setting for somatic disease: The giving up–given up complex. *Proceedings of the Royal Society of Medicine,* 1969, *60,* 553–555.

9. Friedman, M., & Roseman, R. H. Type A Behavior Pattern: Its Association with Coronary Heart Disease. *Annals of Clinical Research,* 1971, *3,* 300–312.

10. Friedman, S., Glasgow, L. B., & Ader, R. Psychosocial factors modifying host resistance to experimental infection. *Annals of New York Academy of Science,* 1969, *164,* 381–393.

11. Henry, J. P., Meechan, J. P., & Stephen, P. The use of psychosocial stimulation to induce prolonged systolic hypertension in mice. *Psychosomatic Medicine,* 1967, *29,* 408–432.

12. Holmes, T. H., & Rahe, R. H. The social readjustment scale. *Journal of Psychosomatic Research,* 1967, *11,* 213–218.

13. Jackson, D. D., & Yalom, I. Family research on the problem of ulcerative colitis. *Archives of General Psychiatry,* 1966, *15,* 410–418.

14. Kales, A., & Tan, T. Sleep alternatives and medical illness. In A. Kale (Ed.), *Sleep physiology and pathology.* Philadelphia: Lippincott, 1969.

15. Kaplan, R. H. Considerations in the psychotherapy of psychosomatic disorders. Paper presented at a meeting of the Society of Medical Psychoanalysts, New York, 1977.

16. Katz, J. L., & Weiner, H. Psychosomatic considerations in hyperuricemia and gout. *Psychosomatic Medicine,* 1972, *34,* 165–179.

17. Kluger, J. M. Childhood asthma and the social milieu. *American Journal of Psychiatry,* 1969, *8,* 353–366.

18. Knapp, P., & Nemetz, S. J. Personality variations in bronchial asthma. *Psychosomatic Medicine,* 1957, *19,* 443–465.

19. La Barba, R. C. Experimental and environmental factors in cancer: A review of research with animals. *Psychosomatic Medicine,* 1970, *32,* 259–274.

20. Langford, W. S. The psychological aspects of ulcerative colitis. *Clinical Proceedings of the Children's Hospital.* Washington, D.C., Children's Hospital, 1964.

21. Lazarus, R. S. *Psychological stress and the coping process.* New York: McGraw-Hill, 1966.

22. Levine, S., & Denenbero, V. H. Early stimulation effects and mechanisms: Stimulation in early infancy. In A. Ambrose (Ed.), *Stimulation in Early Infancy.* Proceedings of: The Study Group of Functions of Stimulation in Early Post Natal Development, London, 1967, pp. 3–72.

23. Lipton, E. L., Stenschneider, A., & Richmond, J. B. Autonomic function in the neonate. VII: Maturational changes in cardiac control. *Child Development,* 1966, *31,* 1.

24. Maurer, E. The child with asthma. *Journal of Asthma Research,* 1965, *3,* 25–79.

25. Miller, N. E. Learning of visceral and glandular response. *Science,* 1969, *163,* 434.

26. Minuchin, S., Baker, L., Rosman, B. L., Leibman, R., Milman, L., & Todd, T. C. A conceptual model of psychosomatic illness in children. *Archives of General Psychiatry,* 1975, *32,* 1031–1038.

27. Mirsky, I. A. Physiologic and social determination of psychosomatic disorders. *Diseases of the Nervous System*, 1960, *21*, 950–956.

28. Nowlin, J. B., Troyen, W. G., Jr., Collins, W. S., et al. Association of nocturnal angina pectoris with dreaming. *Annals of Internal Medicine*, 1965, *63*, 1040.

29. Purcell, K., Weiss, J., & Mahn, W. Certain psychosomatic disorders. In B. Wolman (Ed.), *Manual of Child Psychopathology*. New York: McGraw-Hill, 1975.

30. Rahe, R. Epidemiological studies of life changes and illness. *International Journal of Psychiatry in Medicine*, 1975, *6½*, 133–146.

31. Rees, W. D., & Lutkins, S. G. Mortality of bereavement. *British Journal of Medicine*, 1967, *4*, 13–16.

31a. Reiser, M. Changing theoretical concepts in psychosomatic medicine. In Arieti, S. (Ed.), *American handbook of psychiatry*, Vol. IV (2nd ed). New York: Basic Books, 1975, pp. 447–501.

32. Romano, J. Basic orientation and education of the medical student. *Journal of the American Medical Association*, 1950, *143*, 409–412.

33. Ruesch, J. The infantile personality. *Psychosomatic Medicine*. New York: Ronald Press, 1943.

34. Schmale, A. H., Jr. A relationship of separation and depression to disease. *Psychosomatic Medicine*, 1958, *20*, 259–270.

35. Schmale, A. J., Jr., & Engel, G. L. Giving up–given up complex illustrated on film. *Archives of General Psychiatry*, 1967, *17*, 135–145.

36. Selye, H. *The physiology and pathology of exposure to stress*. Montreal: Acta Psychiatrica Scandinavica, 1950.

37. Weiner, H., Thaler, M., Reiser, M. F., et al. Etiology of duodenal ulcers. *Psychosomatic Medicine*, 1957, *19*, 1–10.

38. World Health Organization Expert Committee on Mental Health. *Thirteenth Report*. Geneva, Switzerland, 1964.

MENTAL DEFICIENCY AND BRAIN DAMAGE: DIAGNOSIS AND MANAGEMENT

James D. Block, Ph.D.

MENTAL RETARDATION

Within fairly wide limits of environmental conditions, most children develop not only physically similar organs and motor abilities but also a basic repertory of functionally similar behaviors. Mental retardation (MR)—*generally* deficient development of normal cognitive behavior—has been more or less systematically studied since the beginning of the last century. The results of early investigations, beginning with Itard's account of his training of the "wild boy of Aveyron" in 1798, as well as the development of current concepts make an interesting history in themselves.[15,44]

In clinical practice, the pediatrician is concerned principally with the diagnosis of MR. Once the diagnosis is established, the important nonmedical aspects of the case are usually managed by other specialists, particularly the educator. However, since management of any kind is obviously contingent upon detection or identification, the pediatrician's role is a critical one. Moreover, the incidence of MR is far greater than most of the life-threatening or debilitating childhood diseases; recent estimates[78] suggest the static incidence of MR to be about 1% (3% if one includes those individuals who are labeled MR at some point in their lives and then lose the label).

Diagnostic Criteria

Although various diagnostic manuals, such as the *International Classification of Diseases* (ICD)[38] and *The Diagnostic and Statistical Manual of Mental Disorders* of the American Psychiatric Association (APA),[5] outline the diagnostic criteria and classification of MR, probably the most authoritative and rational criteria is the diagnostic manual of the American Association on Mental Deficiency (AAMD).[33] This organization, the largest of its kind in the world, focuses on retardation, and its publications are usually the source for other groups' classifications. Despite its name, the medical diagnostic term employed by the AAMD is *mental retardation*. Other terms, such as *mental deficiency, psychomotor delay* and *developmental delay*, are either of historical interest or are euphemisms.

The term *mental retardation* is correctly applied only to those deficiencies noted during the developmental period, that is, before 18 years of age; thus this diagnosis is explicitly excluded in cases of amentias associated with later-life disease or trauma. Moreover, it is a diagnosis explicitly designating a condition which may or may not be permanent. Thus, despite the general connotation of MR to the layman, the health professional may qualify its permanence in appropriate cases. It is important to note that the AAMD suggests the MR diagnosis be applied only to cases of significant deficiency in both intellectual and adaptive (or self-help) behavior.

Although not generally acknowledged, early workers evolved a rule-of-thumb regarding the significance of the deficiency: adult development of less than 10 years, two-thirds that of the normal maximum of 15 years, was considered sufficiently deficient to require specialized treatment or education.[79] Since the intelligence quotient (IQ) for the adult at that time (early twentieth century) was generated by the ratio of mental age (MA) to chronological age (CA) × 100 (e.g., 10 years/15 years × 100 = 67), the number 67 thus came to represent the cutoff percentage, or IQ, for *all* age groups, both adults and children. For many reasons, this ratio method was found to be of limited validity: mental age does not develop in a linear fashion with chronological age, nor is the amount of variability equal at different age groups, nor does intellectual development plateau at 15 years of age.

In the 1930s and 1940s and more recently as well, Wechsler's tests (The Wechsler Adult Intelligence Scale [WAIS], Wechsler Intelligence Scale for Children–Revised [WISC-R], and the Wechsler Preschool and Primary Scale of Intelligence [WPPSI]) were developed. The tests used a new method of defining the degree of mental deficiency, which most current tests now employ. Similar methods have been generated for a major older test, the Stanford-Binet Intelligence Scale. The definition is based on the number of standard deviations (s) below the average for an age group that a particular child's score falls. Scores more than 2 standard deviations below average are considered deficient. The test average is generally arbitrarily set at 100; $s = 16$ for the Stanford-Binet; $s = 15$ for the Wechsler tests. Thus MR is defined as an IQ below 68 on the Stanford-Binet test, or below 70 on the Wechsler scales. Although other tests may differ in numerical expression of average or of standard deviation, the general rule of $2s$ for significant deficiency still applies.

A very thorny issue arises as regards the measurement of self-help or adaptive behavior, since such behavior, as well as intellectual achievement, must be deficient to establish MR according to the AAMD criteria. At present, the only generally employed scale is the rather dated Vineland Social Maturity Scale,[21] which is based on parents' reports. Other scales, such as the Balthazar Scales of Adaptive Behavior,[8] the British Progress Assessment Charts[34] and the AAMD Adaptive Behavior Scale[4] (which recently has been adapted to school-aged children of all ages living at home),[49] are not generally accepted among clinicians as criterion measures for deficient adaptive behavior. The Vineland is still quite useful if a few allowances are made for changes in living style and for urban dwelling. However, it should be noted that in clinical practice the intelligence scale is the prime indicator for both physicians and psychologists in the diagnosis of MR,[2] and a theoretical case can be made for a definition of MR solely based on IQ.[16] Additionally, in institutionalized populations, the IQ is as highly related to specific adaptive behaviors as is a direct measure of general adaptive behavior.[42] In fact, from theoretical calculations it can be deduced that if the two scales did *not* have a high correlation (.8–.9), there would be an unacceptably *low* incidence of MR.[75] In clinical practice, instances of great discrepancy between IQ and adaptive behavior scales are rare (if cases of clearly inappropriate application or interpretation of intelligence tests as well as extreme parental denial or exaggeration are excluded). An interesting development in this regard—probably a portent of the future—is the Griffiths scale,[32] in which adaptive behavior is included as one of the subtests from which the general intelligence is calculated. (It should be noted that the foregoing is not necessarily true with respect to race differences in IQ and adaptive behavior; although IQ may differ, the adaptive behaviors may be equivalent.[2] The issue of race and intelligence continues to be highly controversial.)[51,43]

Curiously, and quite inconsistently, an addendum to the AAMD diagnostic manual throws all objective criteria to the winds, and states that in the last analysis clinical judgment is the definitive criterion for MR. Superficially, this permits a greater degree of judgment to the clinician, but it creates even greater diagnostic problems than it solves—in fact, it is so regressive that it is best ignored. Even in the most extreme case of a strongly denying parent, the Vineland scale can be adjusted by the clinician to conform to probable reality. Furthermore, the difference between the denying parents' estimate and the clinician's estimate may be utilized as a rough measure of the extent of their denial! Additionally, most experienced clinicians (beware of the inexperienced clinician here!) can generate an "estimated IQ" based on some concrete observations. In such difficult cases, one should arrange for periodic monitoring of the child (at least annually), until satisfactory observations can be obtained. This is usually possible after a year or so of additional maturation or after the young child had had some experience in a nursery school or kindergarten.

Levels of MR

Early classifications of MR distinguished among three categories: idiot, who never developed more than simple receptive and expressive language, if any; imbecile, who could learn to speak but who could never learn more than simple written speech, if any; and moron, or "feebleminded" (in England), who could never learn to employ oral or written language to express complex abstract concepts. Aside from the horribly negative connotation of the terms to the general public, this nomenclature does have the attribute of simplicity, and some of the terms are still employed in Europe.

In this country, a similar tripartite classification is used in educational systems, wherein is distinguished the educable MR, or EMR, with an IQ approximately 50 to 75 (note that the upper limit, 75, is well above the medical AAMD limit of 67 or 69); the trainable MR, or TMR, with an IQ approximately 25 to 49; and the lower-functioning individuals who have no uniform designation, although "low trainable," "conditionable," "custodial," and "vegetative" are terms frequently encountered. Many research studies simply distinguish between MR individuals with IQ's above and below 50, since the incidence of demonstrable organic damage increases markedly in the group below 50.[58]

The standard AAMD terminology, and one with which pediatric specialists should be familiar, distinguishes among four categories of MR: mild, moderate, severe and profound. For many years now, individuals have been classified psychometrically, that is, in terms of the number of standard deviations that their IQ score is below average. The present classification: from 2–3s, mild; 3–4s, moderate; 4–5s, severe; more than 5s, profound MR. It is evident that the conversationally casual use of terms such as "mild" or "severe" MR should be avoided, since their meaning is associated with operationally specific, diagnostic categories.

Of more than historical interest is that an earlier edition of the AAMD diagnostic manual (1961) defined MR in terms of IQ scores more than $1s$ below the mean. This view differed at that time from common precedent, i.e., the two-thirds (IQ 67) criterion, as well as from any conceivable hope of educators to provide remedial education for the approximately 16% of the population which was thus defined as MR. Understandably, educational systems did not take this view seriously, and left their definition of EMR unaltered. The 1973 AAMD diagnostic manual fortunately reverted closer to the traditional definition.

However, it should be noted that IQ's presently falling from $1s$ to $2s$ below the mean are in a kind of diagnostic limbo. From 1961 to 1973 they could justifiably, according to the AAMD manual, be called "borderline mental retardation," and are still referred to and coded as such in the present ICD and APA manuals. However, since the AAMD redefined this group in 1973 as not mentally retarded, an MR label for these individuals serves no purpose; not even educational allowances are generally made for this group, apart from "slow" classes and tutorial help. At the Developmental Center of Maimonides Medical Center, "borderline intelligence" is used for this group, and the APA code is omitted in order to avoid any mislabeling of the child as MR by other agencies. Actually, the use of the borderline IQ range as a diagnostic label is appropriate only for the educator's purposes. It is probably best not employed as a medical, or even quasi-medical, diagnostic category. There is obviously little consensus on the definition of this group: the APA defines it as IQ 68–83; the ICD, as IQ 68–85; the Wechsler and Binet manuals, as IQ 70–79; and the 1961 AAMD manual as IQ 70–80, 75 or 80–90! It is relevant to note that the French provide special school education for children up to IQ 85.[41] There is much to be said concerning the needs of such borderline IQ children for intensive, specialized instruction, now generally unavailable in schools in the United States.

Etiology

Since the brain is the organ of behavior, significantly deficient cognitive abilities, whether general (MR) or delimited (specific learning disabilities), must be a product of deficient brain function. Deficiency, however, is not synonymous with damage. The patient with Down's syndrome, for example, although cognitively deficient, develops an undamaged cerebrum in accord with its genetic code, a primary deficiency. The brain of the congenital hydrocephalic, on the other hand, is developmentally distorted by the unfolding of genetic codes essentially unrelated to cerebral neural development, a secondary deficiency.

Most of the mild MR group are of unknown etiology and, except for a possibly large but as yet unknown factor of sociocultural components,[11] it chiefly comprises individuals with primary deficiency caused by polygenetically determined cerebral deficiency. The majority of individuals with IQ below 50, however, evidence historical, physical, and neurological signs—or all of these,[58] suggesting the MR to be a secondary cerebral deficiency. The frequency distribution of IQ's in the population does not conform to the normal curve of expected distribution, assuming intelligence to be a polygenetically transmitted trait: there is a significant excess of IQ's below 50.[20] This is generally interpreted as representing the effect of the additional inclusion of at least two distinctly different populations in which intelligence has been affected by factors other than by polygenetic transmission.

There are, of course, the familiar cases of perinatal infection, intoxication, trauma, dysplasia, chromosomal abnormalities, and others.[37] In such cases, the nature of the medical diagnosis is clearly indicated, and a differentiation for the degree of mental subnormality is provided within the framework of the major diagnostic codes. It is equally clear in most such cases that the MR is a symptom of the condition.

In those cases in which there is no known physical cause, the MR may either be caused by an as yet unknown physical condition or may be associated with an extreme of normal polygenetic inheritance. In the latter case, the precise nature of the disorder awaits delineation by the geneticist and neurophysiologist; present diagnostic practice is to indicate the MR and its level as the primary condition, suitably decimal-coded for unknown etiology. "Familial MR" is an obsolete designation because nutritional, cultural, and medical care factors may well increase the incidence of MR within certain families.[11]

There has been an interesting recent revival of speculation regarding the role of the X sex chromosome in the genetic transmission of intelligence. This is based upon observations of the excess incidence of males in the highest and lowest intelligence groups and resulting greater variability of IQ among males, the decline in IQ with inbreeding in females but not in males, the greater correlation of the IQ of children with maternal rather than paternal IQ, and other evidence.[50] The hypothesis asserts that alleles on the two X chromosomes in the female interact so as to moderate extreme effects of any one chromosome, whereas this cannot occur in the male with just one X chromosome. Despite criticisms of the theory,[6] it still has considerable explanatory power.

There are, of course, well recognized sex-linked recessive traits associated with MR, in addition to disorders associated with autosomal aberrations. (Down's syndrome is the best known of these.)[55] Abnormal chromosomal patterns are now known to be more common than previously suspected, since only about one-quarter of such infants have distinguishing physical features.[52] It is essential that the pediatrician be familiar with the broad range of inherited disorders associated with MR, including metabolic and neuroectodermal syndromes,[37] not only for appropriate patient care but for counseling of the parents and siblings in regard to their future progeny. Agencies throughout the country associated with the National Foundation for Genetic Disorders can provide important supportive tissue analyses as well as expert genetic counseling services to the pediatrician. A government serial publication, the *Congenital Malformations Surveillance Report*, provides continually revised data on the incidence of various congenital malformations.[14]

Who Makes the Diagnosis?

Diagnosis of cognitive developmental problems in the preschool child is of focal interest to the pediatric specialist. The common belief that early test results are not predictive of later IQ are indeed true, but only within the normal range. Although still somewhat controversial,[35] amassed results now indicate high probability that children—even infants—found to function within the retarded range will continue to function as retarded in later life in the absence of a remediable medical condition.[54,83,84] This gives impetus to the detection of deficiency as early as possible. Remedial services can then be instituted equally early so that the child may better learn to the limits of his intrinsic capacity. In fact, to extrapolate from animal studies,[67,70] there is the possibility that increased early stimulation may facilitate actual neuronal growth and associated cognitive capacity.

Detection of moderate and lower levels of MR presents little diagnostic problem— the mother most frequently notes the first signs. Nor are those syndromes problematic that are easily identifiable at birth (or soon after) that are associated with deficient later development, such as Down's syndrome, microcephaly, and the like. With the increasing use of amniocentesis for prenatal diagnosis, an eventual reduction in the incidence of certain chromosomal and metabolic syndromes can be expected, but there is little immediate hope of their elimination. Such births occur in mothers with negative histories; some religious groups do not favor abortion, even of identified abnormal fetuses. The most difficult problems for the pediatrician in these cases are that of informing the parents of the expected lack of development, and of providing supportive medical care, including referral to appropriate community resources for caretaking, management, and counseling.

Detection of mild retardation in the preschool child presents particular difficulty for the pediatrician. On the one hand, there is the risk of false identification and resultant unnecessary emotional trauma to the family, accompanied by the risk of nuisance malpractice suits. On the other hand, there is the risk of depriving the genuinely needful child early extra stimulation. Pediatricians generally carefully observe important developmental milestones, and some are skilled in the use of sophisticated developmental scales such as the Gesell Developmental Schedules[26] or the Bayley Scales of Infant Development.[9] All are acquainted to some extent with critical-age screening scales, such as the Denver Developmental Screening Test[24] or a similar scale available from the American Academy of Pediatrics.[77] Since most scales have well-defined critical levels based upon adequate standardization, it is good practice to heed their results religiously, just as one would a low blood cell count or any other abnormal laboratory test. If a critical age has been reached without the appearance of a given developmental milestone, in the patient's best interests it is imperative that a complete evaluation be planned in order to establish a definitive diagnosis. Periodic reevaluations, if needed, should also be planned. In the child under 18–24 months of age, the pediatrician may have the appropriate skills for such a thorough examination; but in the older preschool child, the developmental or child psychologist needs to be called upon for his specialized skills in assaying the broad range of cognitive abilities of older children.

Originally a part of the law mandating Medicaid, but only now being implemented, is a provision for developmental evaluation of eligible preschool children. The development of methods for screening these children, a responsibility assigned to the American Orthopsychiatric Association, has been rife with controversy, and no generally accepted criteria have yet been evolved.[82] In medical center practice, screening methods currently range from adequate to abysmal, according to the fiscal wonts of the institution, the time devoted to examination, the skill levels of the examiners, and other bureaucratic complexities.[56] Private patients may be referred for more uniformly thorough and competent examination by specialists who not only assume the ethicolegal responsibility for accurate diagnosis, but also are useful in referring patients to appropriate management facilities.

The detection of mild retardation, unfortunately, has yet to be efficiently accomplished. More than three-quarters of mild retardates are still detected only when they reach school age,[78] and then usually by the school psychologist. Although the medicolegal status of MR diagnosis by the school psychologist is generally cloudy, the legally given label of EMR or TMR by the school has vast repercussions on the quality of the child's schooling, the emotional climate of the child and family, and their expectations for later adult life. The competence of school psychologists varies considerably, as might be expected in any profession, and school systems provide varying amounts of experienced senior staff supervision. Some communities are able to provide a team of specialists for diagnosis, for example, the Evaluation & Placement Unit in New York City. However, the range of services available in the school varies enormously among the states, and even the most comprehensive is usually overloaded by a long waiting list.

Of considerable aid in detecting suspected MR has been the recent, nationwide establishment of community mental retardation (developmental, mental health) centers.[90] These contain variously composed teams of pediatricians, psychologists, language specialists, social workers, and psychiatrists, generally with the extensive backup services of an affiliated medical center. The team approach offers extensive investigation of etiology, associated medical conditions, and the availability of services. However, neither the school's diagnostic services nor the community mental retardation center offers more than do informed, experienced private practitioners in the various specialities. Private examinations are always more rapid, although they are subject to review by the school's agencies, a process that may delay appropriate class placement.

Prognosis and Management

Mild MR constitutes about three-quarters of the patients with MR, and as stated earlier, about three-quarters of mild retardation is detected by the school. Also, approximately the same percentage of individuals lose the label after they finish school.[78] They continue to be just as intellectually limited,[30] but manage with good social competence to find suitable means of living which do not entail an MR identification. "Suitable means of living" may extend from nonidentified status, but full financial support by the community (welfare), to successful competition in the free job market. Most of the remainder of mild retardates live with their family and are increasingly employed in sheltered workshops for the handicapped.

There is a growing movement for the establishment of supervised group-living facilities, or hostels, for the MR. These facilities provide a rich social life as well as a continuing resource when families can no longer provide a home. With appropriate training, the mild MR can be expected to achieve academic skills to about the fourth grade, and social and self-help skills equivalent to about those of the average person 12 years of age. Social skills are obviously of greater importance for successful adult adjustment, equal, actually, to the importance of stable personality development. In well over three-quarters of mild retardates no etiology or associated organic condition is demonstrable, therefore life spans are not significantly below those of the general population.[64] Community resources for this population therefore need to be extensive, extending to geriatric care in suitable facilities (not as yet available to any extent).

Marriage and childbearing are not infrequent in this group. Controversy surrounds the issue of sterilization, but in no state is it legally mandated[48] although the MR may be legally denied other rights, such as voting or driving a car. Most opinion is vociferously opposed to "blanket" sterilization, and many states have acted to prevent indiscriminate sterilization with but casual regard for informed consent.

The moderate retardate, constituting about 15% of the MR group,[78] requires lifetime services not much different in degree from the individual who retains the mild MR identification. This includes sheltered workshops for the most capable, or a social day program for those with less ability. Hostel placement is feasible, with somewhat greater supervision than with mild MR; in many cases, the two categories of individuals are housed together. Although they may speak in complex sentences, the moderate MR cannot be expected to achieve more than the most elementary academic tasks (simple addition; writing a few words or their name; the reading of signs, ads, and perhaps simple prose). Self-help skills may develop to the level of an average nine-year-old person. Such skills include all basic toileting, eating, and, with training, limited independent travel. Although organic dysfunction is more common in this group, life expectancy is not greatly affected, and thus services must also be available for the full life span of these persons.

The severely and profoundly MR which constitute about 10% of the MR population,[78] require intensive lifetime services. During infancy, the community generally has few resources for their home care. When they become older, they represent the only population that large state residential institutions will now most readily accept. State facilities are now encouraging the home care of all degrees of retarded infants (with the support of local community facilities) and attempt to reserve full-care residential facilities only for the older, severe and profound retardates. This shift in policy has stemmed from the generally marginally adequate management facilities found in large institutions[7] and some current right-to-treatment legal actions (such as the widely publicized dismantling of the Willowbrook facility in New York City).[18] Because of better medical practice, life span of this group has been significantly improved over past years but it is still well below that of the general population.[64]

Despite the different diagnostic nomenclature, both severe and profound retardates can be found in the same daycare centers, in which socialization, recreation and the learning of basic self-help skills is the primary focus. Group residence is possible for some, but with considerable supervision (equivalent to that of a custodial institution). The lowest-functioning profound retardates who have only vegetative function are the prime candidates for full-time custodial institutionalization. The profound retardate can be expected to achieve no more than limited expressive speech, (if any) a small vocabulary with simple sentences, and the understanding of simple questions and commands. The severe retardate may use complex sentences, with a larger vocabulary of 300 or more words. Neither group will develop academic skills in reading, writing, or arithmetic, or even in concrete tasks such as handling money. The profound retardate will develop self-help and social skills equivalent to no more than that of the average 2- to 3-year-old child, whereas the severe retardate may develop skills up to about that of a 6-year-old child. As with the higher level retardates, those with better social skills make the better adjustment in day centers, and those with antisocial behavior are more likely to be institutionalized.[63]

Facilities for the MR child of preschool age are scarce. When available, such facilities are generally managed by private agencies with some public funds. These agencies include the Association for Retarded Citizens, Association for Help to Retarded Children, the Guild for Exceptional Children, Catholic Charities, and others; they provide invaluable support to the troubled parent as well as many diagnostic, recreational, camp, home care, and other services.

Formal academic public schooling for the mild and moderate MR, i.e., the EMR and TMR groups, is usually available until 21 years of age. This may include extensive vocational preparation and job-finding in a work-study program or in an occupational training center (OTC). For the handicapped teenager, the federal facilities of the Office of Vocational Rehabilitation (OVR) are readily available. After 21 years of age, workshop and hostel facilities are often managed by private agencies. These same agencies may also provide programs for the low-functioning retardates of all ages, where it is not available through the public school system. As might be expected, educational and vocational resources for the MR throughout the United States are still a hodgepodge, with glaring deficiencies notable in many areas.[28] (Useful government serial publications that detail the latest in programs for the handicapped,[61] as well as current legislation and court decisions are available.)[62]

There are two important issues which cannot be discussed at any length here. One concerns the utility of labeling children with an MR diagnosis. Opponents of diagnostic labels generally voice their objections to labeling the mild MR and learning-disabled groups, while admitting the necessity for special categorization of severe and profoundly impaired individuals.[57] It is certainly true that labeling is useless unless it leads to appropriate remedial services. In this society, however, services definitely are more readily generated if a specific group and its needs can be identified. A related issue is that of mainstreaming, of educating the MR with the average child. Many projects have been devoted to testing the efficacy of several possible ways of educating the MR child. Although definitive results are not yet available, neither segregated nor integrated classes necessarily offer the best approach.[87] Since the high-level MR will, it is hoped, live and work in the community as an adult, there is no reason why his/her childhood education should set them apart in a distinctive fashion. To do so generates a syndrome of failure, differentness, and abnormality in both cognitive and emotional spheres. The experience of integration or segregation affects the normal individual as well, in his view of the retarded person. In Sweden, for example, where integration is widespread, there is a positive, helping attitude towards retardates, and little or none of the fear and avoidance that one commonly encounters in this country. Integrated educational facilities would do much to diminish such prejudice, which—like other prejudices—stems in large part from ignorance. The logistics of implementation, however, pose a formidable task for legislators and educators.[53]

CEREBRAL PALSY

The most notable association between classic neurological signs of brain damage and secondary cognitive deficit is found among individuals with neuromuscular disorders, or cerebral palsy (CP). More than half of the CP group is retarded, about one-third has an IQ below 50,[69] and nearly three-quarters below average.[59] The pediatrician must be particularly alert to incipient signs of neuromuscular disorder in the neonate and infant, and should have consultative services of a pediatric neurologist available. He should be particularly cautious in predicting the ultimate cognitive competency in the CP infant. Unlike the patient with Down's syndrome who may be found to be developmentally average at one year of age, yet intellectually mildly retarded at five years, the CP child may prove to be just the reverse. Although, in general, the IQ is quite stable in the CP after 2 years of age,[60] intellectual estimates of the CP infant must be viewed with caution. This is because of the importance of motor function in assaying the developmental level of the infant, compared with the availability of alternative modes of assaying cognitive competency in the older child. Intellectual evaluation of the CP child requires the skills of the rare psychologist who so specializes. Guesses by other specialists are just that.

Periodic evaluation is particularly important in the CP, because, as his motor and language skills are slowly acquired, the child's repertory of modes of learning and self-expression correspondingly increases. Bioengineering and biofeedback methods are of great value in promoting motor and cognitive learning in the CP, as has been demonstrated in a project instituted at the United Cerebral Palsy Center in Roosevelt, N.Y.[13] Centers sponsored by the United Cerebral Palsy Association often furnish the sole educational resource available for the preschool CP child, as well as the severely affected CP of school age. They also frequently provide workshop facilities for the adult CP as well as other handicapped individuals.

The tragedy of CP is not confined to individuals with MR. Individuals with normal or even superior intelligence who have no limb use and whose only input/output channel is speech are perhaps even more tragic. Now largely restricted to trivial recreational activities, they may soon reap great benefits from modern technology in the form of various devices activated by whatever effector they can control, e.g., a muscle twitch, eye-blink, tongue movements, and the like. The recent example of a man with acquired complete quadriplegia who studied and now practices law may be encouraging in this respect.[65]

SPECIFIC LEARNING DISABILITIES

In contrast to the generally deficient cognitive capacities of the MR, is the child who functions normally (or nearly so) in important cognitive areas such as language or visuomotor expression, but who demonstrates markedly deficient abilities in one or several other related areas. With respect to diagnosis, it is unfortunate that in the interpretation of the results of disparate tests in various cognitive areas, there is yet no agreed-upon mode of expressing the degree of differences among the areas, that is, of defining a *significant* specific learning disability. At the Maimonides Center, we extrapolate the historic criterion of MR (general intellectual development of less than two-thirds normal) to provide a criterion of difference between cognitive areas (one area developed to an age-level less than two-thirds of that of another). To eliminate such approximations, evaluation that rests upon a broad-based, statistically coordinated test battery is definitely needed, particularly in order to reveal cases of mild specific disorders.

CP is defined in categories of frank neurological disorder; specific learning disabilities are not so defined, generally. Especially in the young child (under 10 years of age), "soft" motor signs may be found, such as nonspecific generalized motor awkwardness, delayed development (often lateralized) of hopping and standing on one foot, awkward finger opposition, marked motor overflow, motor impersistence, choreoform eye jerks during tracking, and others. Neurological examination procedures have been described for these signs in children, but unfortunately with poor developmental norms.[81] A colleague and I find a finger-tapping task that we have standardized for ages 4 to 75 years useful in investigating lateralized deficiency.[12] Other types of rapid alternating finger movement tasks are available that also indicate subtle, lateralized motor deficit.[19,31]

Motor development is an important aspect of the psychological evaluation of any age individual. It is of prime importance in the infant. For such measurement the Bayley Motor Scale is very rapid and well standardized.[9] Motor dysfunction in the child, whether or not of sufficient severity to indicate frank neurological disorder, may nevertheless suggest the presence of etiologically associated, specific cognitive deficiency. This is particularly true if the motor signs are unambiguously lateralized. In the presence of any motor signs, soft or hard, it is imperative to rule out definitely the coexistence of a learning disability. A language disability in the presence of right lateralized signs, or a visual/visuomotor disability with left-sided signs must be specifically excluded. In diagnostic workup, the conjunction of soft motor signs and a cognitive deficit suggests the presence of a syndrome of cerebral deficiency. However, there is no generally accepted medical diagnostic code for such observation. (At this Center, we generally code diagnostically the presence of the learning disability (APA 306.1), with remarks describing the soft motor signs. If one or more hard signs are present of a severity not justifying a CP diagnosis, we generally code minimal cerebral dysfunction (APA 309.92) with remarks describing the learning disability.)

A presumption of brain damage in learning disabilities is often unsubstantiated by any unambiguous event in the patient's medical history. It may well be that the majority of these cases are polygenetic in origin, a product of primary cerebral deficiency rather than of secondary damage. Reports that suggest support for this speculation are those of a high incidence of a familial propensity for a given type of specific learning disability,[25] the presence of which should be sought in obtaining the family history in a given case.

Specific language disabilities are usually so obvious that they are rarely undetected by school age. Not so are the visual/visuomotor disabilities which are usually detected in the kindergarten to second grade. In the very bright child who has the ability to compensate, the disability may go undetected until the middle elementary grades, or later. Child care specialists should be responsive to mothers' statements regarding nonspecific clumsiness, poor visual orientation, and poor drawing ability. Significant differences between language and nonverbal (visuomotor) abilities can be unambiguously demonstrated by the skilled psychologist in the child as young as 3 years of age, and suggestive evidence may be adduced as early as 18 months of age.

Special schooling for the specific learning disabled child is usually available in the form of small classes with specially trained teachers. They are generally categorized by the nature of the disability, e.g., language or visual/reading/writing. New York City still employs the term *neurologically impaired* for the visually impaired child, even though the practical requirement of positive neurological signs, hard or soft, for admission to the class has been absent for years. On a political-legal level, educators have been lamentably slow in promoting the use of nomenclature suitable for educational needs and goals, independent of peripherally related or even irrelevant terminology and diagnoses from other disciplines.

BRAIN DAMAGE AND ORGANICITY

Precision in the use of terminology is important. The child specialist often encounters the terms *brain damage* and *organicity* in psychological evaluations, generally used synonymously. These are inferred from tests of drawing ability, usually the Bender-Gestalt test,[47] or from patterns of subtest scores on a Wechsler test. The criteria for such designation are themselves subject to considerable scepticism, since criteria associated with the Bender-Gestalt test cause more than 20% of the population to fall in the suspect category.[46] In addition, recent evidence demonstrates that differences among WISC-R subtests must be much greater than hitherto accepted in order to be statistically significant.[45] These issues, however, are irrelevant to that of the use of a term: brain damage. Brain damage is an explicit neurological designation and should be avoided by other specialists if its presence cannot be specifically demonstrated. It would seem more prudent to employ words such as *deficit* or *delay*, which are noncommittal in respect to etiology, whether damage, genetic makeup, sociocultural deprivation, and the like. Naturally, independent concrete evidence for etiology may indeed indicate damage as the source, but active search for unambiguous independent evidence is not always general practice.

In a strict sense, the general use of the term *organicity* is tautological. Whenever a child draws so poorly or shows such a great subtest scatter as to fall significantly beyond the average, the behavior is almost always related to a function of his brain and is indeed organic in origin. However, the term does connote, if not brain damage at least brain dysfunction as the causal agent, thus excluding possible cultural, educational, and other nonorganismic causes. Again, prudence should dictate the use of more precise terminology by the psychologist, as well as more critical interpretation of psychological reports by other specialists.

MINIMAL BRAIN DAMAGE

The waning fad for diagnosis of *minimal brain damage* (or *dysfunction*) (MBD) merits special attention. It has been implicated in such a variety of behaviors and in such pervasive aspects of children's functioning that it has been suggested the term might better be "major brain dysfunction."[10] An NIH publication[17] lists almost 100 different symptoms of this disorder, some mutually exclusive, such as hypo- and hyperactivity; thousands of publications have appeared on this topic over the past decade. Yet there are still no unambiguous diagnostic signs. Even the presence of hyperactivity, the single symptom commonly viewed as pathognomonic for the syndrome, is frequently, upon investigation, found to be inappropriate rather than excessive activity.[86] And, although frank brain damage may be accompanied by greater risk of psychiatric disorder, it predisposes to no specific type of disorder.[69,73] Additionally, even soft neurological signs are not necessary components of the syndrome.[10]

In clinical practice, this diagnosis seems to be employed in several fashions depending on the nature of the specialists. Neurologists may use it in cases of mild nonspecific motor disorder, as a synonym for minimal neurological impairment or minimal CP. The psychologist and psychiatrist often use it to describe children who are inappropriately active with short attention spans, possibly showing signs of "brain damage" in drawing ability or IQ subtest patterns. The educator may employ it for cases of disordered activity, and for those with signs of poor academic competence, particularly in reading and writing. The pediatrician may use it to describe groups of symptoms that do not fall in any general classification, including disordered activity, poor attention span, and, possibly, nonspecific motor awkwardness. In all cases, however, the brain damage, or disorder, is presumptive and possibly gratuitous, since many of the symptoms can well be a learning product of an unimpaired brain. In fact, since there already exist diagnostic terms for most of the individual symptoms (disorders of activity, mild motor impairment, dyslexia, specific learning disability, . . .), the need for a general term that blankets nearly 100 symptoms and presumes or implies brain damage is highly questionable. Diagnosing by symptom in cases in which the etiology is uncertain seems preferable to the use of an all-encompassing term that may effectively impede focal attention to, and treatment of the major aspect of, the disordered behavior.[85] Growing realization of this view may account for diminishing interest in, and less frequent diagnosis of MBD.

Pharmaceutical interests continue to promote medications for as many MBD children as possible. However, the value of medication is questionable when it discourages the search for accurate diagnosis and for specific, focal, remedial measures. Additional negative consequences may stem from the patient's and family's reaction to a diagnosis of brain damage (as discussed later). Moreover, there is also always the possibility of psychotic-like reactions and a suppression of physical growth with some drugs[7] with possible associated physiological effects not yet elucidated. In sum, the pediatrician may be well advised to describe the symptoms in available diagnostic codes, and to refer the patient for appropriate treatment. Such treatment could range from tutorial help for a reading disability, to psychotherapy for an emotional problem, to behavior (modification) therapy for increasing appropriate activity and attention span. There may be situations where providing no treatment except parental understanding is indicated, for those mild motor conditions that will improve solely with maturation and practice.

DIFFERENTIAL DIAGNOSIS

The troublesome trio of MR, autism and specific learning disability pose major differential diagnostic problems for those working with children. The extent of the difficulties are generally a complex interactive function of the age of the child, the degree of MR, and the nature of the specific deficit. Specifically troublesome distinctions are discussed below.

Sensory Deficit

As a first step, peripheral sensory defects, even mild, should not be overlooked in making a differential diagnosis. Infants with impaired hearing and vision may develop some autistic-like characteristics, and may not intellectually develop normally.[23,36,40] The current availability of sophisticated modalities for hearing evaluation, even in the newborn nursery,[22] leave little reason to postpone testing until an age at which conventional audiometric examination can be carried out. Although the newborn nursery may not be the most ideal place, a reliable estimate can be obtained by 3 months of age.[36] The conscientious clinician should never hesitate to utilize such services as readily as he would a laboratory test as a diagnostic aid. Excepting color vision,[88] visual impairment is generally less likely to be overlooked, but complaints or observations of poor visual acuity should not be dismissed on the basis of expected improvement with age, particularly in view of the recent findings of considerably better acuity in normal 5-year-old children than was previously thought to be the case.[74]

Cultural Factors

Diagnosis of cognitive competence must be particularly thorough and appropriate in cases of non-English speaking children or those from minority, lower socioeconomic "ghetto" backgrounds. Many are aware of a tragic, historic misuse of intelligence testing that at one time led to the proposed exclusion of newly arrived, non-English speaking immigrants, presumably for low intelligence on the basis of tests administered in English![43] California is progressive in this respect; recent legislation there mandates evaluation of the child in his own language.[66] Although most other states do not make specific legal provision, competent evaluation may be carried out by the administration of nonverbal tests. Even in cases of presumed English-speaking children, cultural factors may greatly alter their vocabulary. Cultural impoverishment may drastically modify some elements of standard tests; for example, those assessing the child's fund of "common" information and the grasp of basic arithmetic concepts. Socioeconomic and cultural factors may modify the child's general test-taking attitudes and behavior as well, including motivation to succeed, task focus, amount of verbalization and trial-and-error attempts, the appropriateness of relating to the examiner, and the set for speedy performance in timed tasks.

Although research has tended to support the general conclusion of a minimal effect of race and examiner expectancy in testing children,[39,72,91] the general issue is far from being resolved to everyone's satisfaction.[29,89,3] It should be noted that the incongruity of test and child always occurs in the school child referred for generally poor academic performance who is administered a test battery containing a subtest for arithmetic competence! Again, professional diagnostic acumen must be sought for these children. In the absence of better methods, the skilled worker who is well acquainted with the population he is evaluating assigns clinical weights to various tests and subtests according to specific characteristics of the population and of the given child. It would be fortunate if a completely culture-fair test were available, or even possible to devise. A brief flurry of hope was raised by the finding of a sizeable correlation between characteristics of the cortical-evoked potential and IQ,[67] but the magnitude of the correlation is far more theoretical than practical.

MR versus Specific Visual Deficit

The distinction between mild mental retardation and specific learning disorders, generally visual, has been and is still often overlooked. Anyone currently dealing with the evaluation of adult retardates is distressed by the high incidence of individuals with borderline to normal cognitive competence in language, and marked deficiency in the visual-visuomotor area. This combination of findings is diagnostic of a specific learning disability (see Chapter 14). As children, of course, today's adults had the benefit neither of current awareness of the frequency of specific learning disabilities nor of the available diagnostic tests and criteria that reveal their presence. It is imperative today that skilled diagnostic facilities be sought for such a child as early as possible.

MR versus Expressive Language Deficit

In the low level (below mild) retardate, both receptive and expressive language are markedly delayed in appearance as well as deficient in ultimate proficiency. In such a case, the MR preschooler may appear specifically deficient in language skills unless intensive skilled investigation is made into the corresponding level of his nonverbal skills. Remarkable as it seems, such confusion is frequent, beginning with the parent's complaint that the child is normal but "just does not speak." The nonspecialist in developmental evaluation is generally not discriminating in the judgment of specific nonverbal behaviors, and often accepts extremely deficient behaviors as lying within the normal range. (The proliferation of "tests" with ill-defined norms that are distributed by pharmaceutical firms may only create mistaken pseudoexperts.) Very denying or infantilizing parents frequently attribute complex understanding and motives to infantile intellectual understanding and expression. This can result in confusion and disruption of the family structure. Fortunately, such children may demonstrate well developed superficial social skills. Unfortunately, however, when this is encountered in the older, teenage child, the realistic diagnosis, prognosis, and appropriate management may be accepted with great difficulty by the patient as well as by the family.

Children with specific language impairment with expressive deficit most marked seldom present diagnostic difficulty. They rapidly develop compensatory modes of behavioral expression that readily dispel any doubts as to the essential normality of their cognitive competence in nonverbal functions. The major problem in these cases is to (re)institute or intensify environmental demands for language expression in the home and nursery school. This is an important factor that is frequently overlooked in language therapy programs chiefly concerned with speech articulation. I have found useful a systematic program of speech elicitation employing behavior modification methods. This training is equally well applied to low-level retardates in whom speech ability matures late, well after the parents have become accustomed to nonverbal methods of communication and, accordingly, after their demands for speech have become minimal or absent.

Autism

The low-level preschool retardate frequently develops mannerisms such as rhythmic motor movements, bizarre vocalizations, self-stimulatory behavior, superficially appearing affective flattering, lack of attending to speech, and a general social isolation. These behaviors resemble the characteristics of the autistic child. To the developmental diagnostician, possibly the most cogent difference between these syndromes and their associated prognoses, is the complete lack of higher cognitive function in the child who is probably more appropriately diagnosed MR, rather than autistic. Of course, this is easier to assay in the older child who has an expected greater repertoire of behaviors. (This factor may account, in part, for the large proportion of individuals who shift in primary diagnosis from autism to MR as they reach adulthood.)[27]

The specific-language-impaired child with marked receptive deficit often presents aspects of behavior associated with autism. In fact, some workers presently view autism basically as a severe language processing deficit,[68] but whether a continuum of deficit and symptomatology exists remains to be verified. There are, however, many language-impaired children who evidence considerable desire to interact with people, who are emotionally reactive, who respond to new environments with interested curiosity. They may freely express endogenous needs and desires, despite abysmal understanding of the precise intent of speech directed at them. Sometimes, they will free-associate responses to only fragments of what is heard, and thus their responses appear bizarre. Examination by the diagnostic specialist can readily identify these individuals. (Further discussion of the extreme complexities of differential diagnosis in childhood psychosis can be found in Miller and Galenson's chapter [15] in this volume.)

Uncertain Diagnosis

There are children, most often preschoolers, who are not clearly autistic, nor clearly specific receptive-language impaired nor clearly low-level retardates. They are those who collect a series of different diagnostic labels as their parents go from one specialist to another. The educational deprivation of these children during the years spent in shopping for an acceptably definitive diagnosis may be considerable. Unfortunately, there may remain a few pediatricians on the parents' shopping list who still counsel indefinite waiting until the "late-blooming" child "outgrows" the problem, but a growing majority recognize the need for referral to appropriate specialists. A potential peril in consulting only a single specialist is the possibility, with difficult cases, of a presenting problem beyond the scope of his professional acumen. This happens frequently with the psychologist who is fond of the designation of organicity or brain damage, the neurologist who offers a definitive diagnosis of the level of MR (a psychometric concept), or the psychiatrist who tends to view problems chiefly as emotional, sometimes ignoring cognitive and medical aspects of the patient's condition. The best service the pediatrician can offer his patient in a difficult diagnostic case is either to refer the patient to a center where all specialities are represented, or to retain strict case control and data collation, with ultimate interpretations to the parents based on his review of the results of examinations by all relevant specialists.

With respect to early schooling in those cases of uncertain diagnosis, it appears that these children, at least initially, are equally well educated in a language facility, MR facility, or psychiatric facility. Any type of fairly suitable early intervention is certainly better than nothing! Frequent periodic reevaluation by specialists, however, should be diligently scheduled until the nature of the disorder is clarified. This usually happens after a year or so in a preschool program.

THE INFORMING INTERVIEW

When diagnosis of the condition is clear, the often painful (to all parties) facts must be conveyed to the parents. In important conditions, such as major CP or MR, there is the temptation to not tell it all, to play down the probable prognosis by withholding important facts. Although there are differences of opinion as to what constitutes "important" or "probable," certainly all would agree that a 50% chance of the occurrence of an event is important information, and this is even more true if the probability is near 90%. Only remote possibilities, such as one chance in ten, could be envisaged as defensibly withheld, especially since medical decisions are frequently based on the tenth and ninetieth percentiles.

That the parents have the right to know all the facts is becoming daily more clear; in fact, a recent ruling of the New York State Board of Regents makes medical records and reports accessible to patients.[80] To withhold any fact or probability puts the clinician in a judgmental position difficult to defend, since there is little agreement even among colleagues as to which facts can be withheld in a given case. To communicate everything of importance in an informing interview is thus not only to give the family their just due, but also to give the clinician a solid defensive posture. (A description of the form of the informing interview at a MR center may be found helpful.)[76]

Obviously, the precise manner of communicating the information to the family must be tempered by the nature of the individuals concerned. Some parents may require several sessions to assimilate difficult or painful information, and some may promptly reject it outright. It is particularly important to discuss thoroughly issues related to brain damage. The consequences of such action are far-reaching for both child and parents.[86] For example, parents may diminish their efforts to change the child's behavior in the belief that the behavior as well as the brain damage is irreversible. They may needlessly seek medications to effect behavioral change, reasoning that a physical agent which has affected their child's behavior requires a form of control beyond that of ordinary behavior management methods. The child may internalize these views with important consequences for his self-image and adult behavior. To the layman, terms such as damage, disability, organicity convey such a strong implication of permanence and lack of control that their use, even when justified, must be accompanied by a particularly clear explanation of the range of management methods known to be effective in a given case. A probable prognosis should be given whenever possible.

Clinicians should view the duty of informing the parents as much a part of the diagnostic process as is a blood analysis. Time should be devoted to open-ended discussion of the diagnosis and management sufficient to satisfy the parents' needs. There is no reason why a leisurely separate visit for an informing interview is less legitimate than for any other purpose. This is general practice at most institutional facilities.

REFERENCES

1. Adams, J. Adaptive behavior and measured intelligence in the classification of mental retardation. *American Journal of Mental Deficiency*, 1973, 78, 77–81.

2. Adams, J., McIntosh, E. I., & Weade, B. L. Ethnic background, measured intelligence, and adaptive behavior scores in mentally retarded children. *American Journal of Mental Deficiency*, 1973, 78, 1–6.

3. Adler, L. L. (Ed.). Issues in cross-cultural research. *Annals of the New York Academy of Sciences*, 1977, 285.

4. American Association on Mental Deficiency. *A.A.M.D. Adaptive Behavior Scale.* Washington D.C.; Nihira, K., Foster, R., Shellhaas, M., & Leland, H. 1974.

5. American Psychiatric Association. *Diagnostic and Statistical Manual of Mental Disorders* (2nd ed.) Washington, D.C., 1968.

6. Anastasia, A. Four hypotheses with a dearth of data: Response to Lehrke's "A theory of x-linkage of major intellectual traits." *American Journal of Mental Deficiency*, 1972, 76, 620–622.

7. Balla, D. Relationship of institution size to quality of care. *American Journal of Mental Deficiency,* 1976, *81,* 117–124.

8. Balthazar, E. *Balthazar Scales of Adaptive Behavior.* Champaign, Ill.: Research Press, 1971.

9. Bayley, N. *Bayley's Scales of Infant Development.* New York: Psychological Corp., 1969.

10. Benton, A. L. Minimal brain dysfunction from a neuropsychological point of view. In F. de la Cruz, B. H. Fox, & R. H. Roberts (Eds.), *Minimal brain dysfunction. Annals of the New York Academy of Sciences,* 1973, *205,* 29–37.

11. Birch, H. G., & Gussow, J. D. *Disadvantaged children: Health, nutrition and school failure.* New York: Grune & Stratton, 1970.

12. Block, J. D., & Rubin, L. Bilateral rapid forefinger oscillation: Age norms 4–75 years, and aging characteristics. In preparation.

13. Block, J. D., & Silverstein, L. Application of bioengineering and biofeedback methods to the young CP. In preparation.

14. Center for Disease Control. Congenital malformations surveillance report. Washington, D.C.: Public Health Service, U.S. Department of Health, Education and Welfare.

15. Clausen, J. Mental deficiency: Development of a concept. *American Journal of Mental Deficiency,* 1967, *71,* 727–745.

16. Clausen, J. The continuing problem of defining mental deficiency. *Journal of Special Education,* 1972, *6,* 97–106.

17. Clements, S. D. *Minimal brain dysfunction in children* (National Institute of Neurological Diseases and Blindness (NINDS) Monograph No. 3). Washington, D.C.: U.S. Government Printing Office, 1966.

18. Cohen, M. J. The right to treatment. In J. Wortis (Ed.), *Mental retardation and developmental disabilities: An annual review* (Vol. 8). New York: Brunner/Mazel, 1976.

19. Denckla, M. B. Development of speed in repetitive and successive finger-movements in normal children. *Developmental Medicine and Child Neurology,* 1973, *15,* 635–645.

20. Dingman, H. F., & Tarjan, G. Mental retardation and the normal distribution curve. *American Journal of Mental Deficiency,* 1960, *64,* 991–994.

21. Doll, E. A. *Vineland Social Maturity Scale.* Minneapolis: American Guidance Service, 1953.

22. Downs, M. P., & Sterritt, G. M. A guide to newborn and infant screening. *Archives of Otolaryngology,* 1967, *85,* 15–22.

23. Fraiberg, S., & Freedman, D. A. Studies in the ego development of the congenitally blind child. *The Psychoanalytic Study of the Child,* 1964, *19,* 113–168.

24. Frankenburg, W. K., & Dodds, J. *The Denver Developmental Screening Test Manual.* Denver: University of Colorado Press, 1968.

25. Frisk, M., Wegelius, B., Tenhuven, T., Widholm, O., & Hortling, H. *The problem of dyslexia in teenage. Acta Paediatrica Scandinavica,* 1967, *56,* 333–343.

26. Gesell, A. *Gesell Developmental Schedules.* New York: Psychological Corp., 1949.

27. Gittelman, M., & Birch, H. G. Childhood schizophrenia: Intellect, neurologic status, perinatal risk, prognosis and family pathology. *Archives of General Psychiatry,* 1967, *17,* 16–25.

28. Gold, M. W. Research on the vocational habilitation of the retarded: The present, the future. In N. R. Ellis (Ed.), *International Review of Research in Mental Retardation* (Vol. 6). New York: Academic Press, 1973.

29. Goldman, R. D., & Hartig, L. K. The WISC may not be a valid predictor of school performance for primary-grade minority children. *American Journal of Mental Deficiency,* 1976, *80,* 583–587.

30. Granat, K., & Granat, S. Below-average intelligence and mental retardation. *American Journal of Mental Deficiency,* 1973, *78,* 27–32.

31. Grant, W. W., Boelsche, A., & Zin, D. Developmental patterns of two motor functions. *Developmental Medicine and Child Neurology,* 1973, *15,* 171–177.

32. Griffiths, R. *The abilities of young children.* London: Child Development Research Centre, 1970.

33. Grossman, H. J. (Ed.). *Manual on Terminology and Classification in Mental Retardation.* Washington, D.C.: American Association on Mental Deficiency, 1973.

34. Gunzberg, H. C. *Progress Assessment Charts for Children Unsuitable for Education at School.* London: National Association for Mental Health, 1965.

35. Hatcher, R. P. The predictability of infant intelligence scales: A critical review and evaluation. *Mental Retardation,* 1976, *14,* 16–20.

36. Holm, V. A., & Thompson, G. *Selective hearing loss: Clues to early identification.* Seattle: University of Washington Press, 1971.

37. Holmes, L. B., Moser, H. W., Halldorsson, S., Mack, C., Pant, S. S., & Matzilevich, B. *Mental retardation: An atlas of diseases with associated physical abnormalities.* New York: Macmillan, 1972.

38. *International Classification of Diseases* (8th rev. ICDA). Public Health Service. No. 1693, U.S. Dept. of Health, Education and Welfare. Washington: U. S. Government Printing Office, 1968.

39. Jacobs, J. F., & DeGraaf, C. A. Expectancy and race: Their influences on intelligence test scores. *Exceptional Children,* 1973, *40,* 108–109.

40. Jan, J. E., Robinson, G. C., & Scott, E. A multidisciplinary approach to the problems of the multihandicapped child. *Canadian Medical Association Journal,* 1973, *109,* 705.

41. Jedrysek, E. Recent French literature: Psychoeducational aspects. In J. Wortis (Ed.), *Mental Retardation: An Annual Review* (Vol. 3). New York: Brunner/Mazel, 1971, 146–159.

42. Johnson, R. C. Prediction of independent functioning and of problem behavior from measures, of IQ and SQ. *American Journal of Mental Deficiency,* 1970, *74,* 591–593.

43. Kamin, L. J. *The science and politics of IQ.* Potomac, Md.: Erlbaum, 1974.

44. Kanner, L. *A history of the care and study of the mentally retarded.* Springfield, Ill.: Charles C. Thomas, 1964.

45. Kaufman, A. S. A new approach to the interpretation of test scatter on the WISC-R. *Journal of Learning Disabilities,* 1976, *9,* 33–41.

46. Koppitz, E. M. *The Bender Gestalt test for young children.* New York: Grune & Stratton, 1963.

47. Koppitz, E. M. *The Bender Gestalt test for young children* (Vol. 2). New York: Grune & Stratton, 1975.

48. Krishef, C. H. State laws on marriage and sterilization of the mentally retarded. *Mental Retardation,* 1972, *10,* 36–38.

49. Lambert, N., Windmiller, M., Cole, L., & Figverda, R. *AAMD Adaptive Behavior Scale: Public School Version,* American Association of Mental Deficiency, Washington, D.C., 1975.

50. Lehrke, E. A theory of x-linkage of major intellectual traits. *American Journal of Mental Deficiency,* 1972, *76,* 611–619.

51. Loehlin, J. C., Lindzey, G., & Spuhler, J. N. *Race differences in intelligence.* San Francisco: W. H. Freeman, 1975.

52. Lubs, H. A., & Ruddle, F. H. Chromosomal abnormalities in the human population: Estimation of rates based on New Haven newborn study. *Science,* 1970, *169,* 495–497.

53. MacMillan, D. L., Jones, R. L., & Meyers, C. E. Mainstreaming the mildly retarded. *Mental Retardation,* 1976, *14,* 3–10.

54. McCall, R. B., Hogarty, P. S., & Hurlburt, N. Transitions in infant sensorimotor development and the prediction of childhood IQ. *American Psychologist,* 1972, *27,* 728–747.

55. McKusick, V. A. *Mendelian inheritance in man* (4th ed.). Baltimore: Johns Hopkins, 1975.

56. Meier, J. (Ed.). Screening and assessment of young children at developmental risk. Department of Health, Education and Welfare, Pub. No. 73–90. Washington, D.C.: U.S. Government Printing Office, 1973.

57. Mercer, J. R. Labelling the mentally retarded. Berkeley: University of California Press, 1973.

58. Mercer, J. R. The myth of the 3% prevalence. In *Sociobehavioral studies in mental retardation* (Monograph No. 1). Washington, D.C.: American Association on Mental Deficiency, 1973.

59. Nielsen, H. H. *A psychological study of cerebral palsied children.* Copenhagen, Munksgaard, 1966.

60. Nielsen, H. Psychological appraisal of children with cerebral palsy: A survey of 128 reassessed cases. *Developmental Medicine and Child Neurology,* 1971, *13,* 707–270.

61. Office for Handicapped Individuals, *Programs for the handicapped.* U.S. Department of Health, Education and Welfare. Washington, D.C.: U.S. Government Printing Office.

62. President's Committee on Mental Retardation. *Mental Retardation and the Law.* U.S. Department of Health, Education and Welfare. Washington, D.C.: U.S. Government Printing Office.

63. Primrose, D. A. The changing pattern of admissions to a mental deficiency hospital. *Health Bulletin* (Edinburgh), 1974, *32,* 1–3.

64. Richards, B. W. Health and longevity. In J. Wortis (Ed.), *Mental retardation and developmental disabilities: An annual review* (Vol. 8). New York: Brunner/Mazel, 1976.

65. Rockwell, W. Curtis Brewer can do nothing for himself . . . *Today's Health,* December, 1975.

66. Rodriguez, J., & Lombardi, T. P. Legal implications of parental prerogative for special class placement of the MR. *Mental Retardation,* 1973, *11,* 29–31.

67. Rose, G. H., & Tanguay, P. E. Developmental neurophysiology. In J. Wortis (Ed.), *Mental retardation and developmental disabilities: An Annual Review* (Vol. 7). New York: Brunner/Mazel, 1975.

68. Rutter, M. Psychiatric causes of language retardation. In M. Rutter & J. A. M. Martin (Eds.), *The child with delayed speech.* (Clinics in Developmental Medicine, No. 43). Philadelphia: Lippincott, 1972.

69. Rutter, M., Graham, P., & Yule, W. *A neuropsychiatric study in childhood.* (Clinics in Developmental Medicine, Nos. 35/36.) Philadelphia: Lippincott, 1970.

70. Schapiro, B., Vukovich, K. R. Early experience effects upon cortical dendrites: A proposed model for development. *Science,* 1973, *167,* 292–294.

71. Schrag, P., & Divoky, D. *The myth of the hyperactive child.* New York: Pantheon, 1975.

72. Schwartz, R. H., & Flanigan, P. J. Evaluation of examiner bias in intelligence testing. *American Journal of Mental Deficiency,* 1971, *76,* 262–265.

73. Shaffer, D. Psychiatric aspects of brain injury in childhood: A review. *Developmental Medicine and Child Neurology,* 1973, *15,* 211–220.

74. Sheridan, M. D. What is normal distance vision at five to seven years? *Developmental Medicine and Child Neurology,* 1974, *16,* 189–195.

75. Silverstein, A. B. Note on prevalence. *American Journal of Mental Deficiency,* 1973, *77,* 380–382.

76. Stephens, W. Interpreting mental retardation to parents in a multidisciplinary diagnostic clinic. *Mental Retardation,* 1969, *7,* 57–59.

77. Taft, L. T. Mental retardation: An overview. *Pediatric Annals,* 1973, *2,* 10–24.

78. Tarjan, G., Wright, S. W., Eyman, R. K., & Keeran, C. V. Natural history of mental retardation: Some aspects of epidemiology. *American Journal of Mental Deficiency,* 1973, *77,* 369–379.

79. Terman, L. M. *The measurement of intelligence.* New York: Houghton Mifflin, 1916.

80. Text of state rules for professions. *New York Times,* July 29, 1977.

81. Touwen, B. C. L., & Prechtl, H. F. R. *The neurological examination of the child with minor nervous dysfunction.* (Clinics in Developmental Medicine, No. 38.) Philadelphia: Lippincott Co., 1970.

82. Trotter, S. Massive screening set for nation's poorest children. *APA Monitor,* 1975, *6,* 1.

83. VanderVeer, B., & Schweid, E. Infant assessment: Stability of mental functioning in young retarded children. *American Journal of Mental Deficiency,* 1974, *79,* 1–4.

84. Werner, E. E., Bierman, J. M., & French, F. E. *The children of Kauai.* Honolulu: University of Hawaii Press, 1971.

85. Werry, J. S. Studies on the hyperactive child. IV. An analysis of the minimal brain dysfunction syndrome. *Archives of General Psychiatry*, 1963, *19*, 9–16.

86. Whalen, C. K., & Henker, B. Psychostimulants and children: A review and analysis. *Psychological Bulletin*, 1976, *83*, 1113–1130.

87. Wiegerink, R., & Simeonsson, R. J. Public schools. In J. Wortis (Ed.), *Mental retardation and developmental disabilities: An annual review* (Vol. 7). New York: Brunner/Mazel, 1975.

88. Williams, H. Congenital colour blindness and its detection in children. *Developmental Medicine and Child Neurology*, 1974, *17*, 247–251.

89. Williams, R. L. The silent mugging of the black community. *Psychology Today*, December, 1974.

90. Windle, C. What's in a name? In *Sociobehavioral Studies in Mental Retardation* (Monograph No. 1). Washington, D.C.: American Association on Mental Deficiency, 1973.

91. Zimmerman, I. L., & Woo-Sam, J. Research with the Wechsler Intelligence Scale for Children. *Journal of Clinical Psychology*, Monograph Supplement No. 33, 1972, p. 5–44.

COMMON SCHOOL-RELATED
PROBLEMS AND ISSUES

Gaston E. Blom, M.D.

This chapter will focus on school problems of middle childhood that frequently come to the attention of the pediatrician or family physician. Most of these problems concern general adjustment and adaptation to school while others can be more specifically identified. Some of the common specific problems include school phobia, hyperactivity, and learning disabilities.

Parents will frequently initiate contact with the physician about school difficulties because schools have encouraged them to obtain medical assessment and advice from a physician. The pediatrician is frequently one of the first and early contact persons for school problems, and in many instances he may be able to deal with them without psychological or psychiatric referral. In order for these efforts to be more effective, however, collaboration between the physician and the school are important. Unfortunately, this kind of professional collaboration does not sufficiently exist; nor does it exist with regard to other professionals in public or private practice, such as mental health professionals.[1] A number of reasons for this state of affairs within the training and practice of child professionals are here presented.[4]

PSYCHOLOGY OF MIDDLE CHILDHOOD

As a basis for dealing with school issues and problems, it is helpful to have some practical understanding of the psychology of middle childhood. Middle childhood covers the chronological age span of 6 through 11 years of age, representing the elementary school years. However, one should view middle childhood in the whole context of child development, i.e., events that precede and follow the middle childhood years. Because development is variable for individuals and is characterized by regressions and progressions, one sees children in whom delay in earlier issues in development may still be present or in whom accelerations to later issues can occur. Many psychological theories of development provide frames of references to an understanding and response to behaviors; all of them should be viewed in relation to biological growth, maturation, and function. It is highly important that the intactness of body structures and their functions be assessed as possible contributory factors in school problems.

In addition, attention should be given to a child's constitutional temperament. Temperament consists of enduring behavioral response styles and activity patterns that have their origin in early life.[25,6] Innate characteristics of the child interact with the environment of people and things. Psychological adjustment from this viewpoint is seen in terms of goodness of fit between the child and the environment. This judgment applies not only to the infant and his parents but also to the child of school age and his teacher.

Regarding psychological theories, emphasis should be placed on their operational usefulness in understanding and dealing with psychological behaviors. One may use theories in combination, especially in relation to school problems. Psychosocial development[14] and learning theories[26] are particularly relevant to each other, and competence theory should also be stressed.[27] This theory postulates that from the beginning of life a child's world is one of action. The child learns about himself, others, and inanimate objects through actions and their consequences. Successful and pleasurable experiences give rise to a feeling of efficacy, and an accumulation of such experiences results in a sense of competence and self-esteem. This action-based theory calls attention to the importance of training for skill acquisition and maintenance in any effort at remediation.

Many lines of development deal with specific areas of behavioral functioning. Any one of these lines, particularly the major ones (motor, cognitive, language, and emotional), has the potential of functioning as an organizer of development beyond its own area. This may occur spontaneously or may be the basis for remedial intervention.

Consider, for example, language development. Training in language skills (oral language, reading and writing) may influence other areas of development. It has been demonstrated that training in verbal mediation (talking to one's self) may improve behavioral control and cognitive problem-solving.[16,18] Another example which can be considered is motor development. Body motor training may not only improve body skills but lead to an increase in self-esteem, improved peer relations, gratifications in play and game situations, and greater confidence in dealing with problem areas.[10] Improved relationships and conflict resolution achieved through psychotherapeutic efforts may have an extended organizing influence. Moreover, the appropriate use of medication may influence physiological or constitutional elements and facilitate broader behavioral organization. In this psycho-bio-educational approach sensible multiple interventions may focus on one or more developmental lines to foster organizing effects.

Developmental concepts need to take sociocultural influences on behavior into consideration. Behavior is strongly contextually determined—therefore influenced—by environmental settings of people and things. A large number of studies indicate the influence of family structure and methods of socialization on child behavior as well as that from school, neighborhoods, and subcultures.[8]

From a practical viewpoint, one can assess adjustment to real life areas in middle childhood according to descriptive manifest behaviors. These include academic learning, body and motor skills, hobbies and special interests, group participation, social skills with others, friendship with peers, play opportunities, comfortableness as a child with adults, knowledge of and experience with the world, and standards and values in behavior. A training-treatment approach deals with these behavioral areas by providing opportunities for their development through skill training as well as by dealing with those factors which interfere with their acquisition.

Whatever be the initiating factors of problem behaviors, such behaviors have their own consequences. Consequences, moreover, have a powerful influence in maintaining problems and over time it may be difficult to separate primary from secondary factors. Dealing with consequences may have a major role in changing behavior.[3]

In summary, this psychology of middle childhood emphasizes a developmental point of view. In addition, a number of theories and concepts can be successfully integrated to provide understanding an approaches to child behavior. Those which have been briefly discussed include: temperament, psychosocial development, learning theory, competence, developmental lines, sociocultural influences, and assessment of real life areas. Such a collective view of middle childhood considers both training and treatment approaches to problem remediation.

GOING TO SCHOOL: A DEVELOPMENTAL STEP

Development is an evolving differentiation of the personality towards higher levels of adaptation and efficiency in functioning. As this applies to behavior, it involves feeling, thinking, and action. Psychological development proceeds when the maturational and developmental readiness of a child can benefit and respond to appropriately defined and presented tasks, expectations, and experiences.

Going to and attending school presents a series of tasks and experiences where in a number of challenges, opportunities, and changes are presented.[21] There are cognitive tasks, such as attention, memory, thinking with a reality focus, and acquisition of subject-matter knowledge. There is language use for communication and learning to read. There are motoric expectations including body control, motor planning, and involvement in group games. There are emotional tasks of relating to other adults and peers, cooperation, acquisition of realistic achievements and skills, more separation and independence from the family, coping with newness and anxiety, emotional control and acceptance by others in terms of what one can do rather than who one is.

For most children, the transition from a family/home-centered environment to a school/neighborhood-centered environment proceeds without difficulty, or with but transitory emotional difficulties. Characteristically, these children look forward to challenges and newness, cope and master these situations, and eventually respond with security, competence, and pleasure. When maturation and development have proceeded along an average time table and when there have been earlier preparatory life experiences as well as opportunities and support for new experiences, such a happy transition is much more likely to occur.

However, such favorable factors do not exist for many children. Some of them have experienced maturational and developmental lags, or suffered challenges too difficult or inappropriately timed. Others have had family, home, and neighborhood experiences strikingly different from school environment expectations.

At one extreme, a child may have been overprotected, indulged, and the center of attention at home. He lacks the freedom, comfort, and inner resources to engage and respond positively to the new situations and requirements of school. At the other extreme, a child may have not received sufficient protection and guidance at home, having been allowed and expected to negotiate for himself. Such a child may find difficulty in meeting school expectations such as being quiet, sitting still, tolerating frustration, and using language. In both extremes, the children have discordant school-home experiences that present difficulties for them. Furthermore, parents and school professionals will find these children difficult to understand and to help unless the discrepancies are clarified and modified.

Stressful experiences in life, fate events, may also impinge on the child and his family and thus influence the child's reactions to school life. Family moves may upset the predictability and stability of school, neighborhood, friendships, and home. There may be deaths or illness in family members; parent separation and divorce may occur (although many one-parent families function very adequately). A birth of a sibling may present stress to the child and family. One or both parents may be unemployed, adding economic stress to the family. Events that directly affect parents only will yet be reflected in their response to their children.

Some children experience disturbing life events not as discrete and single experiences but as multiple and continuous. Children exposed to such disorganized family-life experiences often lack organization in their own behavior; not surprisingly, they will find school expectations difficult to meet. Some of these children may be helped to find in school more stability, predictability, and consistency than exist at home.

Edith (8 years of age) was a girl of average intelligence who showed fluctuations in academic performance and in aggressive and resistive behaviors in third grade. It was found that there were frequent fights and separations between her parents, and on these occasions Edith displayed disorganized behavior at school. Attempts were made to resolve parental conflict with only minimal success, although the parents were able to see that their behavior caused Edith anxiety and distress. With school counseling Edith was slowly able to share her fears as to what might happen at home. Her teacher became sensitive to her emotional state on coming to school and, after acknowledging her concerns, encouraged her to focus on school work and activities as a way to feel better and be successful. With support and encouragement Edith was able to deal with school realities. Edith's disorganized behavior diminished considerably.

In dealing with school problems, it is helpful if the pediatrician or family physician has some awareness of school expectations, an individual child's maturational and developmental readiness for such expectations, the nature of the transition from home to school, discrepant home-school environments, and stressful life experiences. With such information a physician, together with school personnel, may be able to develop appropriate plans for assistance to the child and his family. Such plans might include a modification in school expectations, socialization to the school culture, short-term counseling to parents and children around a specific issue or event, social service support, parent education and guidance, employment referral, and referral for mental health services.

The Nature of Schools

Schools have considerable variability in the make-up of their culture, their staffs, and the children who attend.[24] Expectations differ and the nature of problem behaviors will also differ in various schools—inner urban elementary schools are not the same as suburban schools. Apart from these clear distinctions, however, there are more subtle variations, which will present quite different environmental problems to individual children. For example, a school wherein a high percentage of the students have above-normal intelligence will put greater stress on a child with average or borderline intelligence than a school wherein there are more peers of his own ability level. Schools with a high turnover of children in a given year (the average turnover in one school district in a western city was 33% for an academic year) do not present conditions of stability and continuity in teaching, so important for many children.

An inhibited, quiet child may find a school that has a great deal of physical contact and fighting particularly upsetting, but in contrast, a more aggressive child may find an orderly, quiet, structured school environment difficult to adapt to and might become the focus of school and peer dissatisfaction and rejection. Of course, it may not be possible—or desirable—to change schools; it nevertheless helps to know their special environmental impingements on children. One can then sometimes help an individual child to deal with them more effectively through direct discussion, guidance, and support at home and at school.

The question also arises regarding the good fit of a particular child with a particular teacher. Certain teachers may have difficulty tolerating and managing certain kinds of behavior, or dealing with the specific behaviors of an individual child. Sometimes, such a situation can be resolved by constructive discussion with school personnel (if the matter is tactfully approached, without blame). Other times, it may be helpful to consider a class change (if one is fairly sure about incompatibility). However, this resolution is not always easily accomplished because of understandable teacher concerns, such as a reflection on his competence, or possible negative evaluation by others.

For many years, schools have been the target of both rational and irrational criticisms by individual parents, parent groups, and many sectors of society. Schools are pulled by multiple forces in a pluralistic society; different philosophies of education exist. In such a climate, it is understandable that positive family-school relations may suffer. Even though such relations are complex, it is possible for physicians to function as a mediator or facilitator in solving problems between an individual child and his family and the individual school.

The physician may intervene directly or through school mediators such as school nurses and social workers. When factors interfering with school adjustment are more objectively understood, school personnel are more often than not empathic, willing to solve problems, and to strengthen the parent-child-teacher alliance.

Family–School Relations

It is important to recognize that parents can bring to the school situation their own problems, anxieties, and conflicts. Frequently, the parents' negative childhood experiences of learning, schools, and teachers become activated through the problems of their own child. If the child has persistent problems, parents can become caught in the web of anxieties, resentment, and guilt. It is not easy for the school to avoid being defensive, to sort out what is rational and irrational about complaints, and to deal with parental reactions in constructive ways.

Home visits and school visits may often bridge the gaps in understanding and may foster an alliance for problem-solving.[13] However, when both home and school feel threatened, mistrustful, defensive, and blamed, visits and contacts will be dominated by negative feelings, and building an alliance will be difficult. In these situations the pediatrician, as an outside person, may be able to mediate between the school and the family by providing an opportunity for both parties to express their concerns and to discuss negative experiences. The pediatrician need not over-identify with family or school in this procedure, but he may be able to reduce the tension so that an alliance can be fostered.

On the one hand, school and other child professionals may view deviant behaviors as a result of family experience and child-rearing. However, this viewpoint fails to recognize that the child is an individual who responds both to his inner world and to outer events in individual ways. Such recognition does not deny the importance of family influence, nor the influences of psychosocial and economic stress in which so many parents and their children live. These stresses are compounded by a child with school problems; this, in turn, results in greater demands on parents. Under such circumstances families may not display strengths, resources, and capacities that schools expect them to have. To attend a school meeting or appointment, to take a child to a physician or clinic, or to schedule a home visit may mean loss of income and unattended children at home. It is not that responsibilities should not be expected of parents, but that they need to be framed in realistic and empathic ways.

On the other hand, parents and nonschool professionals may not recognize the circumstances, problems, and difficulties of schools and teachers. Schools are frequently scapegoated for many problems in society; accountability expectations in academic achievement may not be realistic; communities are reluctant to vote increases in school taxes; teachers and school professionals are often viewed as having easy jobs with long vacations. Teachers are expected to deal effectively in management and instruction with large classes of children whose abilities and behaviors differ widely, for six hours a day. Teachers have little time for instructional planning, often must plan at home, evenings and weekends. Teachers are often not sufficiently prepared in preservice education for the realities of their work, yet inservice education is frequently seen by parents as unnecessary.

Discussion groups with parents of children with learning and behavior problems report issues and problems with schools from the parental point of view.* Some of the more frequent remarks of parents include the statements which follow.

1. We are never informed about good things that happen or progress that is made.
2. School people stand up for each other even when someone is wrong.
3. They don't listen and understand where we are although they don't have to agree.
4. Schools are not geared to work with children who do not fit into their mold.
5. We often end up talking with someone who doesn't know our child.
6. Problem children and their parents are individuals too.
7. Certain families get pegged and their children suffer.
8. Our opinions as parents don't count with school people.
9. Schools throw their responsibilities right back on parents.
10. The important issues, such as learning, are ignored.
11. The school sees child problems as the responsibility of mothers and not fathers.

In discussion groups, elementary teachers report issues and problems with families whose children have school problems.† Teachers frequently make statements such as those which follow.

1. My opinions about their child don't count.
2. Parents don't treat me as a professional person.
3. They don't listen and try to understand what I am saying.
4. They blame me because their child isn't learning.
5. It is difficult to get them off the defensive.
6. They don't seem to realize that I have 29 other children to teach and manage.
7. Parents expect me to be mother and therapist as well as teacher.

---

* Ekanger, C. Unpublished data, 1970.
† Blom, G. Unpublished data, 1972.

8. They don't give me credit for trying.
9. Parents are hard to get to school to talk about problems.
10. I wish they would just teach a class and see what it is like.
11. They don't realize that I'm a person too.

As can be seen from these reports, the issues for parents and teachers concerning children with school problems either parallel or interact with each other. One can understand how family-school relations become adversarial, confronting, uncooperative, and competitive. Some children may complicate the picture by pitting parents and teachers against each other and thus remove themselves from responsibility for their own problems.

The Pediatrician's Role

Since the pediatrician, or family physician, will frequently be contacted about general school adjustment problems of children, one should examine what he can appropriately be expected to do. When the school recommends that a parent seek the help of the pediatrician, the parent may sometimes be able to clarify the reason for referral; at other times, however, the school may not have made its questions explicit. In such cases, with parental consent, the pediatrician should contact a school professional to ascertain the school's concerns or questions. Without school information, the pediatrician may not find any physical abnormalities or deviant functions, thus obtain a limited perspective on the child and the problem, and be less helpful as a result.

What are the kinds of information can a pediatrician obtain that will assist school, family, and child with school adjustment problems? A list would include the following:

1. A current assessment of body structures and functions, and general health status.
2. Special tests, procedures, and consultation indicated from medical history, physical findings, or both.
3. Current behaviors of the child that are considered problems.
4. Health and developmental history, including an estimate of temperament.
5. Impressions of current development in terms of learning, body motor skills, language, individual interests, peer relations, family relations, play activities, group participation, social skills, behavioral standards, and neighborhood adjustment.
6. Important life events and his reactions to them.
7. Home-school congruencies and incongruencies.
8. Strengths and stresses in the family situation.
9. Views of the child and his family regarding the school.
10. Direct observation of the child with and without his parents including attempts to discuss problems directly with him.

From such a comprehensive assessment a pediatrician will be able to contribute information about health status and intactness of body structures and functions, past or present developmental events that may contribute to the problem, findings from special tests and consultation, an estimate of the nature and degree of behavior disturbance (transitory, long standing, or related to situational events), contributions to the problem from home and other environmental sources, disparate (or similar) views of the child at school and at home and possible indication for psychoactive medication.

The expectation of this degree of participation by pediatricians in school adjustment problems may seem too demanding of time and energy. However, most parents not only appreciate this involvement but are willing to pay for the time that it takes. If conferences at school or in the pediatrician's office are not possible, then phone calls or conferences with a school contact person may be a satisfactory alternative. Schools often report that they experience difficulty in obtaining written or oral reports from physicians. The participation of various professionals who know the child and family will facilitate problem identification and clarification, treatment and training strategies, and possible referral needs. The pediatrician can further implement this process by clarifying for both parents and child some of the possible causes for the problem behaviors; such clarification may provide relief and mastery through improved understanding of the problem. In some instances, remediation may be accomplished through short-term counseling of the child and his parents or by encouraging parents to discuss identified problem areas with the child.

There are, of course, problems more severe in nature and complexity; these need to be referred to other resources. First, the determination for such referral needs to be made. Then, if referral is considered necessary, the pediatrician needs to discuss the reasons for referral with the parents. Furthermore, the parents' feelings about referral will need discussion. In addition, someone needs to communicate tactfully with the child about the relevant assessments and recommendations and to deal with his feelings about them. The use of private or public referral sources will depend on family income and preference as well as the availability of professional resources in a community. The pediatrician can be a most useful mediator, interpreter, and facilitator between the family and community resources.

Today, most public schools have special child professionals who can provide important direct services to children and their families. These include counseling, language remediation, body motor-skill training, and special academic assistance within regular or modified school programs. If more intensified and specialized remediation is necessary, schools have special education programs with specific admission criteria.

Specialized services outside of the school may also be necessary. For example, a disorganized, unstable family may need the assistance of social services. Mental health referral of a child and family may be indicated under the following situations:

1. When short term and less intensive measures are not resulting in progress;
2. When emotionally disturbed behaviors are of longer duration than a few months, and are of high intensity and frequency;
3. When conflict has existed between the child and his parents for some time;
4. When the disturbed behaviors are associated with difficulties in other developmental areas of the child's life.

Whenever specialized services are utilized, families appreciate the continued interest of the pediatrician for support, reassessment, and possible changes in program.

SPECIFIC SCHOOL PROBLEMS

School Phobia

A common identifiable behavioral disturbance in children during first grade is school phobia. "Phobia," in a sense, is a misnomer because the psychological issues involved are those of separation from home. The symptom picture includes one or more of the following: forms of somatic distress (lack of appetite, abdominal pain, headache, sore throat, fatigue, vague body complaints, and vomiting), crying and clinging behaviors, direct fears about school, and anxious behaviors. These symptoms are usually manifested in the morning before going to school and relieved by not attending school. Frequently, the mother or parent responds to the child's symptoms with anxiety, uncertainty, impatience, and frustration—all reactions that accentuate the child's symptoms.

With milder symptoms, the child will often attend school but may show evidence of persistent anxiety that may interfere with the ability to learn and adjust to the school environment. In subtle forms, school attendance may be irregular, and so the child will not keep up with his classmates. In more severe school phobia, the child does not attend school. The teacher's response to a child's anxious behaviors, in many cases, may influence their future directions; a combination of tolerance, understanding, and firmness frequently resolves the anxiety. In either persistent mild or severe forms, early intervention is needed to prevent the development of secondary consequences, such as failure to keep pace with academic and social developmental progress in the classroom.

School phobia is one of the few behavioral disorders that is as frequent in girls as in boys, in intact as in unstable families. It appears to be more common in first-born children. Investigation will often reveal that the child has experienced previous separation problems in kindergarten and preschool, in staying at home with a babysitter, and in going to bed by himself. A few children may not have been previously exposed to appropriate separation experiences, and some may have had stressful separation experiences. Going to school—and especially first grade—represents a separation event and a step of independence.

Psychological study of a child's school phobia usually indicates that the relationship between the involved child and parent can be characterized as overly close and mutually dependent.[15] The parent may have had similar fears of school as a child, and a similar attachment to his own mother. In other words, the child-parent relationship of today may frequently repeat the parent-child relationship of yesterday. In addition to closeness, both child and parent may have difficulty in expressing natural feelings of anger towards the other, or if they do express them, anxiety and guilt follow. The silent or open concern for the welfare of each other in separated situations expresses the wish for mutual protection as well as the concern that angry feelings will hurt the partner.

With this background of separation difficulty, overly close parent-child attachment, and problems in expressing and dealing with anger, situational events at home may accentuate concerns about dependency and anger. These might include the birth or presence of a younger sibling, parental discord, or parent illness or separation. In a predisposed child, anxiety may be intensified by the unaccustomed freedom of expression and interactions at school.

School phobia is to be contrasted with truancy. Truancy, i.e., absence from school without permission, is more frequent in boys of any ordinal position in the family. Truancy occurs throughout the middle childhood years in families where stability, organization, and guidance are lacking or inconsistent. The truant child may show early patterns of premature independence. The truant child will not show much distress or conflict except for the anxiety of being caught. The truant child will frequently show poor academic performance, problems in emotional control, and low fustration tolerance. While early intervention in truancy is as important as in cases of school phobia, in order to prevent subsequent development of academic difficulties and antisocial behaviors, the nature of the intervention is very different. In truancy, one provides firm support, structure, and expectations to the family as well as to the child. An adult relationship at school that is warm, friendly, and yet firm can be helpful. It is desirable to create a school experience that is gratifying and successful, which may mean designing special and appealing experiences. The goal is the identification of the child with socialized characteristics of an adult through a pleasurable relationship. This may also be achieved through a long-term therapeutic relationship with a mental health professional. The child needs to be held accountable for unsocialized behavior in a consistent, firm, but concerned manner. When the truancy pattern becomes well established, it may require the constructive use of legal authority to expect school attendance. Such children need consistent, rewarding, but firm relationships to adults at home (if possible) at school, or in therapy.

In school phobia the treatment approach is different, because the child experiences conflict and distress. A medical evaluation to make certain there is no illness and to reassure the parents and the child about health status is advisable. Short-term counseling of the parents in order to verbalize the experience and origins of their feelings and concerns will prepare for the use of behavioral measures, the treatment of choice.[11,3] When given an opportunity, some children may be able to verbalize and to use play to express their concerns within a short period of time. The behavioral measures that are then developed consist of gradual clear steps in going to school for increasing lengths of time with necessary support from parents, peers, and teacher that is gradually withdrawn. In addition, rewards may be added for the successful accomplishment of each step. The purpose, steps, and rewards are openly clarified with the child.

The parent may need the periodic support and guidance of the physician (by phone, perhaps) as the program proceeds. It is important that the parent consistently reward the desired behavior of going to school. Parental attention and reward after school should be stressed rather than parental concern and distress before school, for the latter can reinforce not going to school. It is likewise important not to make staying home highly desirable and rewarding. Sometimes a friendly peer can accompany the child to school, but in some instances the parent may need to go with the child. Whatever sensible procedural steps and measures are developed should be honestly, openly, and consistently contracted for with the child. If there is failure in a step (the first one is the most difficult), then one starts afresh the next day or the step can be altered by providing more temporary support. Contact with the school is important by physician or by parent so that their understanding, cooperation, and participation are involved in program implementation.

In the great majority of instances, a behavioral approach will be successful within 4 to 6 weeks. When no (or insufficient) progress is being made and discussion with the school nurse, social worker, or psychologist does not provide further helpful behavioral steps and procedures, then a mental health referral is indicated. Some followup information about the child's progress in school adjustment is indicated after he returns to school. The goal is not only return to school but also adjustment to and satisfaction from school life. This is illustrated in the case of Tim.

Tim, (10 years of age) an only child, had been reluctant to attend school since first grade. As a result, his mother drove him to and from school almost every day. At home he was somewhat of an isolate who collected stamps and had no friends. The parents had made three family moves during Tim's elementary years, which meant changes in school and neighborhood. Although Tim attended school because of his mother's special efforts, he avoided the playground and ate lunch in his classroom. He was able to perform grade-level academic work but since he was in the bright-normal to superior intelligence range, his average performance was less than his capabilities. Because of his persistent behaviors of reluctance, avoidance, inhibition, and isolation, therapy was recommended with parent participation. His mother revealed that not only was she fearful as a child but also had found the recent family moves disruptive. She, too, felt lonely and isolated without friends, and had experienced the moves as losses in security. Tim's father had been insensitive to the feelings and needs of his wife and son, being caught up in ambitious business activities. It took some time before Tim could express fearful and angry feelings directly. Then the school, in slow steps, encouraged Tim to eat lunch with his classmates, to attend gym, and to stay on the playground. Prior to those steps, his mother gradually stopped driving him to school.

Hyperactivity

Hyperactivity is descriptive of a body motor behavior and constitutes a disturbance when excessive and frequent. It is often associated with short attention span, distractibility, and strong reactivity to stimuli. Hyperactivity is reported to be present in 3–10% of elementary school children to a moderate to severe degree, and is reported three to nine times more frequently in boys than in girls. What constitutes hyperactivity is a judgment based on observation of behavior, a judgment that may not be commonly agreed to by parents, teachers, and other professionals. It is important that professionals recognize that hyperactivity may not exist in a special observational setting (an office), while it does appear in other contexts of classroom and home. A number of behavioral scales have been developed to objectify hyperactivity; [9,19] some have practical usefulness in establishing the presence of hyperactivity and in providing a baseline from which change can be followed. It is also possible to single out a specific hyperactive behavior (e.g., out of seat at school or in and out of room at home), count the frequency of that behavior in a given time interval, and provide a baseline rating on which change can be measured.

In addition to the presence and frequency of hyperactive behavior, certain characteristics may discriminate different types of hyperactivity: purposelessness, driveness, brain damage, constant movement, and periodic activity are among those that should be ascertained. The presence of anxiety and fears should be noted as well as situations which increase or decrease activity.

The tendency to overestablish hyperactivity in children does not mean that it is not important. It often interferes with learning at school, socialization, and the development of other important skills and acquisitions (coordinated body movement, emotional control, and the like). Hyperactivity produces consequence reactions in peers and adults in the child's environment which further exaggerate problems, for a hyperactive child tends to generate excitement and stimulation in his environment. Hyperactivity is often identified at school age when increased requirements and expectations, such as sedentary activity increased attention span, and frustration tolerance are made. Yet the behavior may have existed prior to school age without presenting major difficulties.

Hyperactive children clearly represent a heterogenous group; this is one of the reasons that it is difficult to evaluate the literature on the topic. Attempts are being made to discriminate types of hyperactivity according to different causes and patterns.[23] Listed are some of the different types of hyperactivity which have been cited.

1. Normal activity not tolerated by parents or teachers.
2. Situational causes such as environmental stress, excessive stimulation, classrooms with large numbers of students, psychological and physical abuse or neglect.
3. Inadequate diet or food intake; exposure to lead.
4. Developmental patterns, i.e., temperamental high activity pattern or response style from an early age.
5. Anxiety-based hyperactivity, often periodic in nature with evidence of fearfulness.
6. Hyperactivity as one of a number of behaviors associated with general psychological disturbance, e.g., depression, autism.

7. Minimal brain dysfunction often characterized by purposeless, driven motor behavior.

If possible, steps should be taken to discriminate as to type of hyperactivity. A past and present history should include specific behavior descriptions as well as quantitative and qualitative characteristics of what is considered hyperactive behavior. Descriptions from both home and school are important, and symptom check lists may be used to objectify clinical judgments further. A physical examination provides an opportunity to observe behavior, reaction to stimuli, and performance on various refined sensory and motor tasks. The latter tasks are often referred to as *soft sign neurological evaluation*.[22]

The presence of abnormal findings on soft sign evaluation together with a history of perinatal problems, febrile seizures, and a persistent pattern of overactive and hyperactive responses may suggest minimal brain dysfunction.[10a] An electroencephalogram may show borderline findings in about 30% of such children. A diagnosis of minimal brain dysfunction is made on a configuration of symptoms and signs, test findings, and historical data. Minimal brain dysfunction constitutes about 10% of the hyperactive child population.[7]

Treatment should be related to the type of hyperactivity. In some instances, medication is not indicated, but when it is used, it should be viewed as modifying its behavior, not affecting its cause. It can facilitate the child's benefit from therapeutic, teaching, training, and environmental measures, but it should not be considered as a solitary approach to remediation. The type of medication selected can sometimes, but not always, be based on the assessment of type of hyperactivity. The use of tranquilizing medication may be considered in anxiety– and psychosis–based hyperactivity. Stimulant medication, such as ritalin and dexedrine, is the most frequently used and leads to symptom improvement in one-third to two-thirds of cases reported in the literature. If medication is used, it should consist of a dosage adequate to insure a clear symptom response. Monitoring makes certain that the medication is taken and that the child's behavioral response is adequately assessed. Periodic medication holidays are advisable[12] but not until after several months of medication use.

Special diets for hyperactivity are questionable, although adequate and regular food intake are important. It is very easy for such children to establish a somewhat haphazard life style when they need special guidance, care, stimulus management, structured experiences, rest periods, and shorter time expectations. Verbal mediation training may facilitate emotional control, motor control, and academic problem-solving. Behavioral training and behavior modification may foster desirable and adaptive behaviors. Some children benefit from psychotherapy when anxiety, psychological disturbance, and consequential reactions exist. Parents also benefit from counseling, guidance, and advice.

The few existing followup studies on hyperactivity indicate that hyperactivity decreases by age and especially by puberty. However, academic problems and severe adjustment problems frequently continue or worsen.[20] This is particularly true when medication has not been consistently taken. Hence, if medication is monitored and thoughtfully used, together with teaching and therapeutic methods when indicated, the outcome is much more successful.[17]

Learning Disabilities

The usual plural form of the term *learning disabilities* implies that there are many. There is no consistent or uniform clinical picture in children with learning disabilities; considering them specific, therefore, is not warranted. The concept has been developed, primarily by psychologists and educators, for children who from the start of school show difficulties in learning and who, in particular, demonstrate a discrepancy between capacity and performance in academic tasks. Often, the usual medical and psychological evaluations do not clarify the nature of the problem. Official definitions that have evolved combine academic and cognitive malfunctioning in the presence of adequate academic instruction. Various etiologies may be included: emotional disturbance, social disadvantage, sensory and motor handicaps, and mental retardation. Many other entities are discussed in relation to learning disabilities: perceptual handicap, minimal brain dysfunction, dyslexia, developmental aphasia, and others.

It is, of course, easier to discuss the difficulties of definition than to offer solutions. Learning disabilities comprise a variety of syndromes which have as a common manifestation learning performance(s) below expectation level by age, grade, and intelligence. It may be possible to identify the difficulty in a particular academic performance area such as reading, mathematics, both reading and mathematics, and in specific subject-content areas (history, science, or social studies). Difficulties in specific subject-content areas are more usually associated with psychological disturbance, unless reading difficulty interferes with the learning of subject matter. One should try to distinguish among factors that are causative, consequential, or concomitant (the latter not related to the learning disability but of possible importance). Emotional factors often play an important consequential role in academic failure.

It can be useful to differentiate groups of learning disabilities according to their nature.

1. Retardation. There is a lag or slower development of performance skills, but learning processes are not disordered or deviant.
2. Failure to perform. There is evidence that learning has and is taking place, but for motivational reasons a child will not perform.
3. Interfering behaviors. Short attention span, distractability, anxiety, hyperactivity, depression, inhibition, low frustration tolerance, and behaviors reflecting emotional disturbance interfere with learning.
4. Deviant learning process mechanisms. Auditory, visual, language, or motor processes are different from the normal at any developmental level.

While these four groups appear distinct, mixtures are common and particularly so when the disability has been manifest for some time. Most professionals would consider the deviant learning process group a true learning disability.

There are a number of possible factors which initiate a learning disability. In addition, they frequently set up an ongoing process that, together with subsequent events, presents a complex clinical picture. Both initiating factors and subsequent events are multiple, interacting, and additive. The overt learning disability, once established, tends to have an autonomy which merits special educational measures, for later learning that is based on difficulties in earlier learning only compounds the disability.

A multidisciplinary assessment of both initiating and contributory factors is important. An evaluation should consider not only causes but remediation measures as well. The pediatrician's role here again involves a developmental history and careful physical examination to assess the intactness and functioning of body structures and symptoms. Often clear abnormalities may not be demonstrated in the physical assessment; however, various possible biological contributions should be considered: atypical seizures, hearing and visual impairments, neuromotor and sensorimotor deviations, metabolic disorders, minimal brain dysfunction or damage, genetic family history of learning problems, developmental irregularities, and perinatal abnormalities. Consultation with medical specialists is sometimes warranted. It is important to rule out mental retardation, although this condition usually has been evident to the pediatrician and parent earlier in terms of uniform slowness in motor, language, cognitive, and emotional development. A evaluation can be further established by intelligence testing if it has not already been done.

Even though other professionals can contribute to the understanding of the disability, the pediatrician's ongoing interest in the child and family is indicated. Later reassessment may be necessary as development proceeds, and continued support to the child and family is important. Medications may be useful at times for specific symptoms; counseling or referral may be useful for psychological assistance. Parents may need help in considering the various treatment and training procedures advocated or publicized (some of which are exploitative and lack a rational basis).

There may be times when the pediatrician, school, and other community resources together do not have a sufficiently clear understanding of the learning disability in a particular child. Referral to a developmental evaluation center or service, under educational or medical sponsorship, may be helpful. Such facilities have professionals from various disciplines who can contribute to an understanding of the learning disability as a developmental disorder. These disciplines usually include pediatrics, psychiatry, medical specialties, psychology, physical therapy, occupational therapy, language therapy, and audiology. Such professional collaboration may provide a more refined assessment of biopsychological functions in various developmental areas and may be able to suggest further teaching and treatment measures.

From management and treatment points of view, it is important to recognize areas of strength for the child and to foster them, for academic progress often consists of slow gains over time. Attention should be given to successful and pleasurable nonacademic skills and experiences. Parents need to know what they can do to help their child with his remediation program. Too many well-meaning program elements may overburden the child and family. Siblings in a family may react adversely to the special efforts and attention given to a learning-disabled child. The learning-disabled child is aware of being different from other children and may have a variety of emotional reactions as a result. It can be difficult to maintain motivation to learn, but support and understanding can help.

An example of a boy with a learning disability who made fairly successful progress is Dick.

Dick, 10 years of age, was in a special education program for two years. He demonstrated both inhibited motor behaviors and occasional periodic aggressive outbursts against other children. His father, employed in an outdoor occupation, expected a great deal of assertive behaviors from him at an early age. He wanted Dick to go fishing, hunting, camping, and to play contact sports. Dick had clumsy and awkward motor behaviors. His father was disappointed that his son did not fulfill his own ambitions and expectations. Pediatric evaluation showed a electroencephalogram without a seizure pattern and with a number of soft neurological signs. Dick had average intelligence with lower verbal skills than performance skills; he demonstrated visual perceptual difficulties that interferred with reading in terms of word recognition and reading speed. He was two grades below grade level in reading. Because of both inhibited and uncontrolled motor behaviors and suggestive signs of minimal brain dysfunction, ritalin medication was tried, and resulted in more evenly modulated motor behaviors. Because of motor clumsiness, body motor training focused on graded skills training without the expectation that he needed to meet his father's ambitions. Dick and his parents were seen in regular counseling. In reading, he received more assistance in phonic approaches and worked at levels wherein he could experience success. Slow academic gains were made so that Dick could eventually return to a public classroom, one grade behind his expectation level. He remained on ritalin medication for 18 months. This was withdrawn for a summer and resumed for another school year. A 3-year followup indicated that he was adjusting well without medication, doing average academic work.

In other publications, the writer has stressed the importance of a biopsycho-educational approach to learning disabilities.[2,5] This approach uses assessments and remediations from both training and treatment professions. It can be applied through the use of a problem-oriented scheme in which significant developmental and environmental areas are assessed, problem statements are developed in these areas when indicated, and diagnostic and intervention strategies are instituted for them. The scheme provides a comprehensive picture and approach to remediation with a broad developmental orientation. Areas in this problem-oriented scheme include affective, cognitive, academic, interpersonal, language, sensorimotor, child-rearing, family, and medical.

SUMMARY

This chapter has focused on common school-related problems and issues for children in middle childhood that frequently come to the attention of the pediatrician. Some of the problems fit into a more general category of behavioral adjustment and psychological adaptation to school while others are more clearly identified entities: school phobia, truancy, hyperactivity, and learning disabilities. The role of biological factors and intactness of body structure and function is important to consider in the assessment of the child with general or specific school problems. In order for the pediatrician or family physician to be more effective in dealing with these types of problems some understanding of development and developmental theory is needed. The developmental step of going to school, the nature of schools, and the quality of family-school relations are also important to understand. The extent and limitations of the pediatrician's role in assisting children and their families with school related problems have been described. The pediatrician can be an important mediator and facilitator in fostering constructive family-school relations and in developing a problem-solving approach to school problems.

REFERENCES

1. Berkowitz, H. A preliminary assessment of the extent of interaction between child psychiatry clinics and public schools. *Psychology in the Schools*, 1968, 5, 291–295.
2. Blom, G. E. The psychoeducational approach to learning disabilities. *Seminars in Psychiatry*, 1969, 1, 318–329.
3. Blom, G. E. A psychoanalytic viewpoint of behavior modification. *Journal of the American Academy of Child Psychiatry*, 1972, 3, 165–176.
4. Blom, G. E. Experiences at the interface of child psychiatry and special education: Implications for training and practice. Paper presented at the annual meeting of the American Academy of Child Psychiatry, St. Louis, Missouri, October, 1975.
5. Blom, G. E. *Psychoeducation: Eclectic and integrated approaches to learning disabilities.* *Acta Symbolica*, 1975, 6(3), 95–124.
6. Brazelton, T. B. *Infants and mothers: Differences in development.* New York: Delacorte, 1969.

7. Brazelton, T. B. *Doctor and child.* New York: Delacorte, 1976.

8. Clausen, J. A. Family structure, socialization, and personality. In M. L. Hoffman (Ed.), *Review of child development* (Vol. 2). New York: Russell Sage, 1966.

9. Conners, C. K. A teacher rating scale for use in drug studies with children. *American Journal of Psychiatry,* 1969, *126,* 884–888.

10. Cratty, B. J. *Perceptual motor behavior and the educational process.* Springfield, Ill.: Charles C Thomas, 1969.

10a. de la Cruz, F. F., Fox, B. H., & Roberts, R. H. (Eds.): Minimal brain dysfunction. New York: New York Academy of Sciences, 1973.

11. Edlund, C. V. A reinforcement approach to the elimination of a child's school phobia. *Mental Hygiene,* 1971, *55,* 433–436.

12. Eisenberg, L. Principles of drug therapy in child psychiatry with specific reference to stimulant drugs. *American Journal of Orthopsychiatry,* 1971, *41,* 371–379.

13. Ekanger, C. A., & Westervelt, G. Contributions of observations in naturalistic settings to clinical and educational practice. *Journal of Special Education,* 1967, *1,* 207–213.

14. Erikson, E. H. *Childhood and society* (2nd ed.). New York: Norton, 1968.

15. Gardner, G. E., & Sperry, B. M. School problems: Learning disabilities and school phobia. *American Handbook of Psychiatry* (2nd ed.) (vol. 2). New York: Basic Books, 1969.

16. Jensen, A. R. Verbal mediation and education potential. *Psychology in the schools,* 1966, *3,* 99–109.

17. Laufer, M. W. Long term management and some follow-up findings on the use of drugs with minimal cerebral syndromes. *Journal of Learning Disabilities,* 1971, *4,* 518–522.

18. Meichenbaum, D. H., & Goodman, J. Training impulsive children to talk to themselves. *Journal of Abnormal Psychology,* 1971, *77,* 127–132.

19. Miller, L. C. School behavior checklist: An inventory of deviant behavior for elementary school children. *Journal of Consulting Clinical Psychology,* 1972, *38,* 134–144.

20. Minde, K., Weiss, G., & Mendelson, N. A 5-year follow-up study of 91 hyperactive school children. *Journal of American Academy of Child Psychiatry,* 1972, *11,* 595–610.

21. Moore, T. Difficulties of the ordinary child in adjusting to primary school. *Journal of Child Psychology and Psychiatry,* 1966, *7,* 17–38.

22. Paine, R. Syndromes of minimal cerebral damage. *Pediatric Clinics of North America,* 1968, *15,* 779–784.

23. *Pharmacotherapy in children.* Washington, D.C.: National Institute of Mental Health (Pub. #HSM73–9002), 1973.

24. Sarason, S. B. *The culture of the school and the problem of change.* Boston: Allyn and Bacon, 1971.

25. Thomas, A., Chess, S., & Birch, H. G. *Temperament and behavior disorders in children.* New York: New York University Press, 1968.

26. Werry, W. S., & Wollersheim, J. P. Behavior therapy with children: A broad overview. *Journal of American Academy of Child Psychiatry,* 1967, *6,* 346–370.

27. White, R. W. *Ego and reality in psychoanalytic theory.* (Psychological Issues, vol. 3.) New York: International Universities Press, 1963.

PSYCHOSIS IN INFANTS
AND CHILDREN

Robert T. Miller, M.D.
Eleanor Galenson, M.D.

It is important that practicing pediatricians be familiar with the nature of early childhood psychosis. They are among the professionals who ordinarily first come in contact with these severely disturbed children, especially in the preschool age group. Because prognosis improves dramatically with early diagnosis and intervention, the prompt detection of psychosis, particularly under 3 years of age, should be regarded as a pediatric emergency. Therapeutic techniques are currently available which can bring about substantial improvement in the psychotic child's behavior and psychic functioning, although they are unfortunately not curative as yet.

EARLY ONSET PSYCHOSIS AND LATE ONSET
PSYCHOSIS

One of the dominant themes in current thinking about childhood psychosis has been the attempt to distinguish early onset psychosis (onset prior to 3 years of age) from late onset psychosis (onset after 6 to 7 years of age). For reasons which are not understood, it is rare for a psychosis to begin between the ages of 3 and 6 years. The main question under study has been whether this bimodal clustering of the onset of psychosis in early and later age groups signifies a discontinuous pathological process, that is, whether early onset psychosis and late onset psychosis are in fact different illnesses.[44]

This chapter stems from work done at the Rousso Therapeutic Nursery, Albert Einstein College of Medicine (New York), directed by Dr. Galenson. The authors are indebted to the staff of the Nursery, especially Ms. Cathy Shapiro, chief teacher-therapist, and Dr. Jan Drucker, chief psychologist, without whose dedication and perseverance this work could not have gone forward.

Clinical studies comparing the two groups have looked for the presence or absence of such factors as remissions, perinatal complications, seizures, psychosis in adult family members, mental retardation, and differential sex distribution. Such studies, however, have not yet provided a clear answer.[41]

For the pediatrician, however, the importance of the distinction lies in the fact that a completely different symptomatic picture is found in the two age groups. Symptoms of late onset psychosis indicate that a partially integrated psychic structure has already developed. Behavior is often organized and complex, but at the same time bizarre and seemingly without purpose. Phantasy activity is present but florid and unrestrained, leading to the formation of delusions and hallucinations. Disordered thinking, such as loose associations and blocking, may also occur.[35] In general, then, the symptomatology of late onset psychosis shares many features with that of schizophrenic psychosis found in adults, and it approximates the adult syndrome more and more closely with advancing age.

In contrast, the symptomatology of early onset psychosis is both less organized and less familiar to pediatricians and is therefore more difficult for them to identify. Since early and rapid intervention in early onset psychosis is much more crucial for its ultimate prognosis than it is for late onset psychosis, this chapter will emphasize the diagnosis and treatment of early onset psychosis. However, to illustrate the late onset form, a brief clinical description follows.

T.B. was first seen at 8 years of age because she had started "to behave like a dog." She was the fifth of eight children who ranged in age from 6 years older to 5 years younger than she was. The family was intact, and the father was regularly employed. Pregnancy and delivery were uneventful, and her developmental milestones were within normal limits, according to her mother's account of them. Although she had always been a friendly, outgoing child, she had been bossy and possessive, and these characteristics tended to involve her in fights with her friends. There had not been excessive fear of separation, of strangers, or any other important fears. However, she had rocked herself to sleep each night from early infancy and was still doing so at the time of referral. There was also a history of intense and prolonged mouthing of objects in the early years. Although T.B. was not a disobedient or stubborn child, she had a way of aggravating her parents by involving herself in activities that would require their attention—leaving a faucet running, for example.

At 6 years of age, she had become increasingly restless and rebellious, began to use foul language, and developed "a fantastic love for dogs." During the next two years, she became increasingly involved with dogs, seeming to prefer them to people. She used her lunch money to buy food for stray dogs and would bring them home daily. Gradually, she began to provoke the dogs to attack other children.

At the time of the first clinical evaluation, she had been observed walking on all fours, barking and biting other children. It was evident that her thinking was now totally dominated by fantasies about dogs. She seemed to believe she was a dog, thought she could understand and communicate with dogs, and said she loved dogs because no one but dogs loved her. Her affect was both labile and inappropriate: States of rage could be immediately followed by intense outbursts of hysterical laughter. She was hospitalized for evaluation and was referred to a children's inpatient service where she responded to a therapeutic regime consisting of phenothiazine, individual psychotherapy, and structured activities.

EARLY ONSET PSYCHOSIS

Psychosis in children under 3 years of age was first described by Kanner[32] as a syndrome of behaviors which includes withdrawal of interest from the environment, panic reactions to changes in the environment, ritualistic activities, fascination with inanimate objects, and disturbance in language development. More recently, Mahler and Gosliner[37] have separated out two subgroups of early onset psychosis—the autistic group and the symbiotic group—each characterized by a particular quality in the relationship between infant and mother.

According to Mahler, the two forms of early onset psychosis can be related to normal developmental stages.[36] In normal development, the infant first shows attachment to a specific person, usually the mother, between the ages of 2 to 4 months.[38] In this earliest relationship, the infant becomes aware of the presence of a nurturing person, but makes no distinction between "himself" and "other" or between stimuli that originate within him and those that originate in the environment. Mahler refers to this early relationship as *normal symbiosis*, stressing the infant's omnipotent experience of being joined with the mother as a dual unity. Prior to normal symbiosis the infant has formed no bonds with the mothering person;[38] this earlier stage of development Mahler refers to as *normal autism*.

In Mahler's view, the fundamental disturbance in both forms of early onset psychosis lies in the psychotic child's inability to utilize or to perceive the mothering person as an organizer of and a living buffer for reality and internal milieu.[36] Whatever the etiology of this disturbance may be—constitutional factors or very early psychological trauma—it prevents the establishment of a mutual mother-infant relationship that can sustain the normal emotional and cognitive development of the infant. (For purposes of clarity, the two clinical subtypes of early onset psychosis, the autistic and the symbiotic, will be discussed separately in this chapter. In practice, however, what is usually seen in a given child is a mixture of autistic and symbiotic features, with a predominance of one type of defense or the other.)

In autistic psychosis no viable relationship between infant and mother exists. Behaviors that indicate the development of an emotional bond between infant and mother either do not appear at all (primary autism) or appear for a short period of time and then fade out (secondary autism). Characteristically, there is absence of recognition of the mother's face or voice. No special smile for her develops. There is no anticipation of maternal behavior, and no mutual visual fixation or other reciprocal interchange with the mother. Stranger or separation anxieties fail to appear. It is the absence of these normal evidences of the development of a special relationship between mother and infant rather than the presence of dramatic symptomatology that is often the first indication of serious trouble. Pediatricians should therefore, routinely include questions relating to the presence or absence of attachment behaviors such as those just described in the course of well baby checkups.

In symbiotic psychosis, a first relationship is made by the infant, though in a severely distorted form. Within an intensely ambivalent attachment to the nurturing person, the infant feels threatened by separation and abandonment on the one hand and by engulfment and obliteration on the other. The psychosis is marked by either intense panic states or by a retreat into an autistic shell (secondary autistic psychosis).

Preliminary data indicate that autistic psychosis occurs four times more frequently in boys than girls, while symbiotic psychosis occurs four times more frequently in girls than boys.[24] Whether this is a reflection of sex-linked genetic makeup, or of different vulnerabilities built into early boy-mother and girl-mother relationships is a moot point.

OTHER FORMS OF PSYCHOSIS

These two types of early onset psychosis, together with the schizophreniclike late onset psychosis, account for the great majority of psychoses seen in children. Depressive psychoses and manic psychoses are virtually nonexistent in childhood, even when manic-depressive illness, which tends to be familial, is present in adult family members. In infancy, severe depressive states can be seen in response to prolonged separation from caretakers[8,61] (see discussion of differential diagnosis in this chapter).

In rare instances symptoms of psychotic intensity, such as poor reality testing, can be part of an overall clinical picture that does not resemble that of either early or late onset psychosis. In another rare condition, Heller's dementia infantalis, progressive and severe mental deterioration starts in the third or fourth year of life. The changes begin with restlessness, stereotyped and anxious behavior, loss of language, and eventually lead into complete dementia and often death. The disease is frequently associated with encephalitis or cortical degeneration secondary to lipoidosis or leukodystrophy.

AUTISTIC PSYCHOSIS

Children with autistic psychosis characteristically show no awareness of the "other." Feelings are discharged in a diffuse manner and seem not to be directed at or related to specific persons or events. This typical behavior can be observed in such diverse forms as incessant shrieking, aimless and stereotyped activity, and spontaneous and prolonged temper tantrums. Since they have not found sufficient satisfaction in the relationship to a nurturing person, autistic infants use their own bodies for relief of tension and as their primary source of pleasure. There is much sucking behavior, self-stroking, as well as head-banging, rocking, self-biting and other self-inflicted injuries that do not appear to be experienced as painful by the child.

Just as autistic children show no awareness of the "other," they show no awareness of the "self." Behavioral evidence derived from studies of normal development indicate that infants' growing awareness of themselves and their mothers proceed side by side. For example, while normal infants are exploring the face, mouth, hand, and other bodily aspects of their mothers, they are exploring these features of their own bodies in remarkably parallel fashion. With the onset of crawling at about the age of 6 or 7 months, of walking at the age of 12 to 15 months, normal infants begin actively to control the distance between themselves and others. By the age of 18 months they are aware of the genital difference,[25,51] and by the age of 24 to 26 months, they have attained bladder and anal sphincter control.

In contrast to normal infants, autistic infants show no interest in exploring their mother's body or their own, nor do they show a response to their mirror image.[24] They remain unaware of their own defecation and urination.[23,50] They are in constant and aimless motion.

The perceptual functioning of autistic children is severely disturbed, with hyper-responsive and hyporesponsive states existing side by side. In the visual mode: although their ability to navigate successfully in space indicates intact vision, nevertheless they do not engage in eye-to-eye contact with others, lack visual attentiveness, and demonstrate typical "blindisms." In the auditory sphere: they do not startle in response to a loud noise, do not react to verbal commands or indeed to the human voice itself. This lack of auditory responsiveness often leads to an initial diagnosis of deafness, but these same children may become intensely disturbed by background auditory stimuli or may put their ear down to the floor to hear their own scratching noises of only marginal intrusiveness.

There may be a similar dichotomy of response to tactile and painful stimuli. Objects placed in the hand simply drop away, yet painful experiences, such as injections or accidental burns, produce no apparent reaction. At the same time, there may be much rubbing of surfaces or head-banging.

In summary, the entire perceptual apparatus seems unavailable for the reception of external stimuli, and is instead focused upon self-initiated or internal sources of stimulation.

Autistic children also show disturbances in motility. Aimless, constant wandering is interspersed with periods of bizarre posturing, whirling, rocking, swaying, lunging, darting, and a variety of ritualistic motions, as well as with periods of immobility. In effect, motor discharge has little or no organized quality and seems predominantly to be either a response to inner stimuli[23] or an effort at self-stimulation.

Language development in autistic children is typically quite deviant. Frequently, there is a history of reduced babbling in the early months. Characteristically, such children acquire three or four words between 10 and 14 months of age. These words, which usually include "mama," "dada," and "no," then drop out and further language development is generally absent. If speech develops at all, echolalia and pronoun reversals are common features. The course of early speech production and comprehension is of considerable clinical importance, since the quality of language development is one of the most sensitive indicators of both the degree of emotional disturbance and the ultimate prognosis.[17,58]

A deficient inner language, or nonverbal symbolic system, is indicated by a lack of gestural communication and mime, delay in imitation, a paucity of imaginative play, and a failure to use toys as semisymbolic representations of experience.[1,57] Another precursor of symbolic activity, the transitional object—the common "security blanket"—which normally appears around the age of 9 months is either completely absent, or present in the profoundly distorted form of the psychotic fetish.

Autistic children show a general asynchrony of developmental milestones. Characteristically uneven and out of phase with each other, the developmental lines of these children, such as those for social relationships, motoric activity, language acquisition and physical growth, are marked by peaks, plateaus, delays, precocities, and occasionally by extraordinary but isolated capacities, e.g., phenomenal feats of memory, rather than by the even and steady progressions of normal development.

On the basis of a variety of questionnaires and psychometric techniques, the parents of autistic children are described in the literature as being no different as a group from other parents in regard to their general personality characteristics and socioeconomic status. However, on the basis of information gathered during long-term psychotherapeutic work with these mothers,[22,24] there would seem to be a high incidence of maternal depression occurring some time during the first 12 to 18 months of the infants' life. Moreover, emotional (if not actual) physical withdrawal of the mother from the child has been quite evident in many of the mother-child pairs treated in the Einstein nursery[24] as well as in other nurseries.[22]

S.B.* was the only child of parents in their early 20's. Pregnancy, delivery, and the neonatal period were medically unremarkable. Mrs. B. had wanted a girl, and she burst into tears when informed that her baby was a boy. She had wanted to breast-feed but "did not have enough milk." During the first few months of life, S. was a sluggish eater, and Mrs. B. responded either by crying and ignoring the baby or by shouting profanities at him and occasionally even hitting him.

The mother felt that from birth on, S. was never a cuddly baby. He smiled for the first time at the age of 1 month, but he never developed a smile specifically for his mother or father. The usual stranger anxiety and separation anxiety of the second half of the first year of life did not appear. He began to use two pacifiers at once, one carried in his mouth and the other inserted in a nostril. His mother first began to worry about his lack of eye contact with her and his unresponsiveness to her speech when he was about 1 year old. At the age of 14 months he started to eat crayons and rip papers, and at the age of 18 months he began to rock incessantly when put into his crib at night. Early on in the second year of life, he began to spend most of his waking hours watching television, especially commercials.

S.'s gross motor landmarks were within normal limits, although he did not hold his milk bottle by himself until he was 1 year old. He may have said "mama" several times at the age of 10 months, but otherwise speech did not develop. He showed no capacity for either independent or reciprocal play.

At the time he was first evaluated (at the age of 2 years), he was in constant, purposeless motion interrupted only by frequent agitated outbursts, which were accompanied by animal-like shrieks. He showed no recognition of his parents, had no response to physical pain, and rarely focused visual and manual attention on one object simultaneously. When he wanted something, he directed his mother's hand toward it, as if it were an extension of himself. He had no speech and had never been seen to imitate communicative gestures, such as "bye-bye."

THE SYMBIOTIC PSYCHOSIS

In contrast to the autistic child, in whom little, if any, relationship to humans has been established, the symbiotic child has established a relationship with his mother, but one which is so intensely ambivalent and unstable that development does not proceed beyond this stage.

As already described, Mahler, Pine, and Berman[38] view the age of 2 to 3 months as the critical period when the normal infant first establishes a specific attachment to the caretaker. The infant becomes aware of his caretaker, but only as a part of a dual unity with himself, without boundaries distinguishing them. This is followed, at the age of 5 to 8 months, by a second critical period during which the sense of unity weakens and a dual process of separation (defining boundaries) and individuation (developing autonomous functioning) begins.[38] The dawning awareness of separateness is signaled by the onset of stranger anxiety and the appearance of an attachment to a transitional object. At this time the child also begins to do things for himself (e.g., hold his bottle, finger feed himself), to crawl, to reach for what he wants, and to be an active partner in peek-a-boo games. Separation anxiety becomes increasingly apparent, reaching a peak around 12 months of age.[4] In the same period, babbling becomes specific to sounds found in the family's native language.

---

* The writers are indebted to Ms. Cathy Shapiro, Jan Drucker, Ph.D., and Stavroula Beratis, M.D., for making this information available.

According to Mahler's description,[36] children with the predominately symbiotic psychosis have a relationship that is governed by an intensely ambivalent hostile dependency. Their delusion of omnipotent fusion with the mother must be maintained at all costs, and any push to separation and independent functioning brings intense anxiety. These children cling to their mothers, desperately resisting separation. Yet, in an instant, they may hit or bite the mother quite violently. They suffer from intense temper tantrums, but, unlike the undirected tantrums of autistic children, these are almost always related to some frustration imposed by the mother. These children often appear to be extremely fearful, for any emerging sense of self brings intense anxiety with it. For example, awareness of bowel and bladder functioning often brings panic, since loss of stool or urine is tantamount to loss of body part or of mother herself.

Perception is not interfered with to the degree found in autism, but perceptual disturbances may occur as partial regressions to the autistic state take place.

In contrast to the diffuse motoric discharge found in autism, motility is generally inhibited in predominately symbiotic psychotic children, save when separation is threatened.

Symbolic or language development is also less severely affected than in autistic children. Various levels of communicative speech and gesturing are reached, and some primitive use of toys may occur.

Parents of children with symbiotic psychosis have been found to have a characteristic pattern of unpredictability in their relationship with their infants.[24] This unpredictability ranges from a smothering overconcern at one moment to an isolating abandonment at another. These parents, like those of the autistic children, seem to be reenacting parts of their own childhood experience.

Z.* was 3 years and 3 months of age when referred to the therapeutic nursery because of atypical behavior. She seemed reduced to a state of panic if her mother left her, even with a familiar baby sitter. She had not been able to make friends. Her only language consisted of guttural sounds, and her play was disorganized and without theme.

Z. was an only child, planned for but ambivalently desired by her parents. Pregnancy and delivery were unremarkable. Her mother described Z. as a demanding, temperamental, screaming baby from her earliest days. However, neither parent held or spoke to her very much. Marked separation anxiety began before the end of her first year, but she showed no affectionate responses to anyone before the age of 2 years.

At the time of evaluation, she enjoyed being passively carried by her mother, but did not mold comfortably to her body contour. She had moments of good eye contact and of reciprocal social interactions and was observed to imitate the movements of those around her—all signs of early attachment and differentiation. However, she became agitated whenever her mother left her field of vision. Also, although she seemed to be aware of her own hands, she would push her mother's hands towards objects she wanted rather than reaching for them herself, as if her mother were an extension of herself. She had an aversion to being touched and the peculiar habit of shaking her own hand. She did not discriminate edible from inedible substances.

Her gross motor coordination was good. Visual-motor coordination was inconsistent: While she had trouble opening the lid to a box, she could pick up raisins from the floor with dexterity. Failure at tasks did not seem to evoke frustration.

Play activity was almost completely unfocused and disorganized and semisym-

---

* The writers are indebted to Mrs. Barbara Fields for making this information available.

bolic play was nonexistent. She was uninterested in toys except for their direct need-gratifying value; for example, she masturbated on the rocking horse while in a deep reverie state. No recognizable words were present at the time of evaluation, although by the age of 18 months, according to her parents, she had acquired at least ten words. Apparently a profound regression in her use of language had taken place at about 2 years of age.

Z. had actively resisted her mother's attempts at toilet training and clearly enjoyed being diapered. She would retain her stools for 4 to 5 days at a time, especially when angry or when she was separated from her mother. Although temper tantrums were a daily occurrence, head-banging and rocking were not present.

DIFFERENTIAL DIAGNOSIS

Although the clinical picture of early onset psychosis might seem to be a fairly specific one, differential diagnosis may nevertheless be difficult, particularly in the early phases of the disorder. Early onset psychosis must be differentiated from the following clinical entities.

Developmental Aphasia

The full relationship between early onset psychosis and developmental aphasia is unclear[13] (see the section on pathogenic mechanisms in this chapter). Children with aphasia often show behavioral patterns that may be confused with those seen in early onset psychosis, in addition to their receptive and expressive language dysfunction. Such behaviors include distractibility, hyperactivity, aggressiveness, silliness, seclusiveness, and social immaturity. They also suffer from memory deficits and impairment in their capacity for abstract thinking, and may have variability of performance on psychological testing. Whether these characteristics are secondary to the communication difficulties experienced by aphasic children or are a result of a common central disorder that also leads to impairment of language functioning is not known. Other features which blur the distinction between aphasia and early onset psychosis are their common natural histories (early onset, delayed acquisition of language, continuing language deficit, and social problems) and their propensity to occur in some families simultaneously.

Certain characteristics in the verbal and nonverbal symbolic systems, however, permit a differential diagnosis to be made.[1] In early onset psychosis, words are used with idiosyncratic or personalized meanings ("fifty-five" to signify "grandmother"), in a concrete and literal sense (one child, whenever asked to put something down, would place it on the floor), and with little or no apparent communicative intent. In addition, psychotic children—as opposed to aphasics—tend to reverse pronouns ("I" for "you"); to echo the speech they hear; to respond to unintelligible sounds; to have few difficulties in articulation, although oddities of inflection, tone, pitch, and stress may be present; and to have a normal short-term memory span. In the nonverbal area, psychotic children are distinguished by a greatly reduced capacity for using and understanding gestures in communication—many cannot even point—by a paucity of imaginative play, by a failure to use toys as semisymbolic representations of experience, and by an absence of imitation.

Establishing the differential diagnosis between early onset psychosis and aphasia, while sometimes difficult, is important because markedly different prognoses and therapeutic approaches are implied.

Mental Retardation

Because psychotic children have delayed development and because they often show low IQ scores on psychological testing, the question of mental retardation often enters the differential diagnosis. In general, however, the classical picture of mental retardation as seen, for example, in Down's syndrome, does not resemble that of early onset psychosis. In the mentally retarded group, the children tend to follow the ususal developmental sequence of initial maternal attachment and later separation and individuation from the mother, but at a slowed pace. They do not tend to show the disturbed or deviant behavior patterns found in the psychotic group. In the cognitive area, mentally retarded children have a pattern of global deficit; psychotic children often show more limited, specific deficits. (The evaluation of the cognitive functioning of children with early onset psychosis is taken up more fully in this chapter in the discussion on pathogenic mechanisms.)

Sensory Deficits

Major sensory deficits can lead to secondary emotional responses as well as ego disturbances. Such a combination gives a clinical picture that may be confused with autism or symbiotic psychosis.

DEAFNESS

Deaf infants may show many of the behaviors found in early onset psychosis. These include not only unresponsiveness to sound, delay in language development, and failure to develop semisymbolic play with toys, but also exaggerated separation anxiety, poor impulse control, low frustration tolerance, and hypermotility. In contrast to autistic children, however, deaf children usually show behaviors indicating that a significant attachment to the mother has been achieved. Furthermore, the diagnosis of deafness can be confirmed by audiological examination in children as young as 1 to 2 months of age, if it is carried out by experienced personnel.[52] Nevertheless, in some cases, differential diagnosis may be extremely difficult. Deafness and early onset psychosis can, of course, coexist. The incidence of early onset psychosis in the deaf population is the same as it is in the hearing population.

BLINDNESS

The blindisms that occur in children with complete or partial blindness can be confused with the hand-gazing seen in autism but it tends to be less stereotyped. Furthermore, blind children typically show evidence of having established a better maternal attachment, and they interact with their social environment. Blindness can coexist with early onset psychosis. In fact, the incidence of early onset psychosis is significantly greater in the blind population than it is in the sighted population.

Organic Brain Syndromes

Specific organic brain syndromes in association with which autism has been known to occur include the following: perinatal cerebral anoxia; neonatal central nervous system infections such as rubella, toxoplasmosis, and syphilis; metabolic disorders such as PKU, cerebral lipoidoses, and Addison's disease; hypsarrythmia; syndromes characterized by evidence of central nervous system dysfunction, including abnormal EEG findings and "soft" or "hard" neurological signs; and retrolental fibroplasia.

Seizure Disorders

Alterations in consciousness and behaviors caused by seizure activity must be distinguished from psychosis. This is easily managed in general, because of the episodic nature of the seizure activity. However, continuous seizure activity or seizures that have permanently altered brain function may cause problems in differential diagnosis. Autism and seizures may coexist, and seizures become increasingly frequent in autistic children as they approach adolescence. About 25% of all children suffering from autism have been reported to develop seizures, even though most of the children in this seizure-prone group had been found to have normal neurological examinations and EEG's during their earlier years.[57] Both grand mal and psychomotor seizures have been reported to occur in psychotic children.

Maternal Deprivation

Actual absence of a mothering person usually does not lead to either autistic or symbiotic psychosis. If the deprivation is chronic, as is the case with institutionalized children, an across-the-board delay in the acquisition of motor and social skills, of speech, and of the adaptive use of toys is seen, rather than the uneven motor, social, and speech development seen in psychotic children.[47] However, self-stimulatory activity, such as rocking and posturing, can occur in institutionalized children; in addition, they attach themselves indiscriminately to any person in the environment. Such behaviors can cause diagnostic uncertainty because they are also present in early onset psychosis. A differentiating point is that when good maternal care is made available to institutionalized children, these behaviors as well as the general development delay respond significantly. Improvement is often dramatic in scope and rapidity, although there is usually some residual impairment in the capacity for forming emotional relationships, in aspects of impulse control, in the capacity for elaboration of play and fantasy, and in language skills. Rapid improvement of this type is not characteristically seen in the young psychotic child.

Acute maternal deprivation occurring after the 6th month of life, whether it be due to the death, psychological withdrawal, or temporary absence of the mother can result in a distinct syndrome, anaclitic depression, which differs from psychosis.[61] Infants first become weepy, demanding, and clinging; these behaviors are followed by psychomotor retardation, weight loss, and persistent crying. Finally, after 2 or 3 more months of such deprivation, there is quiet whimpering and facial rigidity, lethargy and apathy as despair appears to set in. Death may ultimately ensue.

ETIOLOGY

The various theories of causation of early onset psychosis may be grouped as follows: theories of environmental causation; theories of an intrinsically atypical organism; theories that involve either of these possibilities acting independently; and theories which involve these possibilities acting together.

Environmental Causation

Recent studies have made it clear that the quality of maternal response during the first days of life[9,27,34,60] and the first weeks of life[2,40] can determine fundamental patterns of infant behavior (e.g., the organization of motor activity into a homeostatic, tension-reduction feedback system with the mother) as well as basic physiological properties of the infant (e.g., muscle tone and circadian rhythm.) The rather stable behavioral and psychophysiological patterns which emerge from the early mother-infant interactions may be established so soon that they appear to be genetic or neurophysiological in origin rather than the result of experience. The clinical entity of deprivation dwarfism, for example, demonstrates the critical role that experience may play in determining the balance of complex neuroendocrinological mechanisms.[46] To date, however, no particular form of maternal (or family) behavior has been demonstrated to be the specific cause of childhood psychosis.

Atypical Organism

Theories of an intrinsically atypical organism draw on a wide array of data. A genetic influence is suggested by the 2% incidence of autism in the siblings of autistic children, an incidence which is 50 times greater than that in the general population.[56] Twin studies consistently show a much higher concordance rate for autism in monozygotic twins than in dizygotic twins.[21] The difference between the concordance rates is even greater if concordance for cognitive impairment and language delay is included with concordance for autism. This finding suggests that autism reflects one form of a continuously distributed abnormal characteristic, and that the part that is inherited is a cognitive abnormality which includes but is not restricted to autism.

On the other hand, comparison of the discordant pairs of twins, both monozygotic and dizygotic, shows that most often the autistic member, but not the normal member, has had a history of birth trauma. This finding clearly demonstrates the important role of nongenetic factors in the etiology of autism and is broadened by reports of monozygotic twins, delivered without apparent birth trauma, who have been reared in psychologically disparate postpartum environments and who turn out to be discordant for autism.* Overall, the data suggest that in some instances a genetic factor may be etiologically predominant, in other instances an environmental factor is predominant, and that in still other instances the two must act together for autism to arise.

Hauser, DeLong, and Rosman[28] using air contrast studies, have demonstrated unilateral enlargement of the left temporal horn in 14 out of 16 autistic children. Boullin, Coleman, O'Brien, and Rimland[7] have found an increased efflux of serotonin

---

* Kerman, S. Personal communication.

from platelets of autistics and were able to corroborate in blind fashion the diagnosis of 6 of 7 patients with infantile autism.

Psychological testing of older children with early onset psychosis has consistently shown lowered IQ scores.[16,58] About 40% of cases have an IQ under 50, 30% between 50 and 70, and 25% within normal limits. The etiological significance of this association, however, remains unclear. In the first place, there is the group of autistic children who have normal IQ's. Secondly, there are some reports that IQ improves with successful treatment. Thirdly, the motivation of autistic children in taking the tests has been called into question.[42] Lastly, because of difficulties in administration, IQ tests have not been done on subjects under the age of 4 to 5 years.

Autistic children show a pattern of rapid-eye-movement (REM) sleep similar to that of young infants, and they tend to suppress vestibular nystagmus during visual fixation.[56] The significance of these findings is not clear.

The association of early onset psychosis with perinatal complications, neurological abnormalities, and abnormal EEG results has not been reliably documented, despite a multiplicity of studies.

Theories of Dual Origin

Goldfarb proposes an etiological dualism between constitutional and environmental factors.[26] In some families of psychotic children (not limited to early onset psychosis), he found what he referred to as *parental perplexity*, a paralysis of parental functioning characterized by extreme uncertainty, passivity, lack of spontaneity and empathy, and absence of clear, assertive direction. He feels that these parental qualities lead to unfamiliarity and unpredictability in the child's experiences, which in turn bring on terror and avoidance. In these families, the disturbed children showed few stigmata of neurological impairment. In families not showing a pattern of parental perplexity, however, the disturbed children preponderantly showed signs of neurological impairment.

Theories of Interaction

An interaction between constitutional and environmental factors is proposed by many workers. Ruttenberg[53] found in his studies of early onset psychosis that 50–90% of the children had birth histories suggestive of congenital anomalies or birth trauma, while 50–75% showed "soft signs of maternal rejection."

Mahler[36] proposes a "complementary series" of etiologies that would range from constitutionally predisposed infants for whom "good enough" mothering does not suffice to counteract the inborn deficit in the ability to utilize mothering for homeostasis, to constitutionally intact infants subjected to severe psychological trauma during the normal autistic or symbiotic stages of development. The unique aspect of Mahler's theory, however, is that it stresses the interaction of both constitutional and acquired factors with the circular processes between mother and infant that normally lead to the child's differentiation and individuation.

Etiology of Late Onset Psychosis

Inasmuch as late onset psychosis clinically resembles adult schizophrenia, it seems plausible that some of the recent dramatic findings relating to the etiology of the latter might apply to the former as well. In a now classic study, Kety, Rosenthal, Wender, et al.[33] demonstrated that the biological parents of children who had been adopted as infants and who became schizophrenic adults showed a concentration of "schizophrenic spectrum" disorders significantly greater than that found in the adoptive parents of either the schizophrenic or nonschizophrenic offspring. This study presents the strongest evidence to date of a genetic component in the etiology of adult schizophrenia.

Biochemical studies have revealed evidence that antischizophrenic drugs block central nervous system (CNS) dopamine receptors, and that amphetamine, which can produce a psychosis resembling schizophrenia, acts by potentiating dopamine at synaptic endings in the brain. These findings have led to the dopamine hypothesis, which proposes that an overactivity of CNS dopamine synapses leads to the behavioral changes seen in schizophrenia. The transmethylation hypothesis is based on the fact that many hallucinogenic substances, such as mescaline, are methylated metabolites of naturally occurring brain compounds, such as dopamine and serotonin; and that many of the enzyme systems necessary to carry out this transmethylation process are present in the brain. However, no direct evidence exists yet for this theory.

Other etiological factors that have been proposed for late onset psychosis are the following: failure in ego development (for either constitutional or environmental reasons), specific deficits in perception and cognition, excessive physiological reaction to mild stress, deviant systems of family interaction, and socioeconomic variables.

PATHOGENIC MECHANISMS

A variety of pathogenic mechanisms have been proposed for the early onset psychoses, including disorders of interpersonal relationships, disorders of rate and sequence of CNS maturation, disorders of sensorimotor integration and disorders of production and comprehension of language.

Disorders of Interpersonal Relationship

Microanalysis of home movies taken of children with early onset psychosis before they have developed overt symptoms shows mothers actively avoiding eye-to-eye contact with their infant as early as 4 to 5 months of age,[24,39] in contrast to the congruence in gaze behavior between mother and infant that occurs in normal development.[31] This suggests that disruptions in maternal attachment behaviors may contribute to the production of early onset psychosis. Ethological support for this conclusion comes from the work of Harlow who has shown that early and prolonged interference with mother-infant attachment behavior in primates can lead to autistic-like behavior (withdrawal, self-directed behavior, aggressive outbursts).[27]

Several recent reports have correlated the presence of overt or covert maternal depression during the autistic or symbiotic phase of infant development with the occurrence of early onset psychosis.[22,24,48,62] The pathogenic significance of the single factor of postpartum depression remains in question, however, since mothers of infants with impairments such as congenital malformations experience reactive depressions which are not associated with psychosis in the children, and since many infants whose mothers are depressed do not develop psychosis.

Various types of maternal or parental psychological profiles have been proposed as being specific for early onset psychosis: tension and anxiety in the face of infant demands,[6] hostile rejection of the infant,[5] parental perplexity,[26] intolerance of the feeling of intimacy stimulated by a symbiotic union.[24] None of these parental patterns, however, have been found to result exclusively or invariably in early onset psychosis.

Dysmaturation of the Central Nervous System

Dysmaturation of the CNS reflecting a form of encephalopathy has been proposed by Bender as the pathogenic mechanism of all the psychoses, including early onset types. She postulates an embryonic plasticity "reflected in every phase of child development, vegetative, motor, perceptual, intellectual, emotional and social, affecting every level of adaptive function, integration and behavior."[3] The behavioral phenomena demonstrated by psychotic individuals at various stages in their life are viewed by Bender as attempts to defend against this primary disturbance. Thus, symptomatology may vary depending on the nature of the stress, developmental level, and compensating or decompensating defenses. Fish, Wile, Shapiro, et al.,[20] applying Bender's ideas, claim to have successfully predicted the occurrence of psychosis in childhood on the basis of their neurological examination during the newborn period.

Disorders of Sensorimotor Integration

Theories emphasizing deficiencies in sensorimotor integration posit that the behavioral manifestations of early onset psychosis are a consequence of the difficulty of making meaningful patterns out of chaotic perceptual stimuli. Some of the integrative deficits proposed have included excessive or inadequate sensory stimulation due either to variations in constitutional sensitivity or unusual maternal behavior;[64] inability to transpose perceptual information from one modality to another;[14] an imbalance between the excitatory and inhibitory influences in the CNS, resulting in faulty modulation of sensory input and motor output;[43] an inability to relate new stimuli to past experiences;[49] hyperactivity of the reticular activating system leading to a reactive effort to reduce sensory input;[30] and, a primary interference in the development of the normal hierarchy of intersensory integration, specifically the shift from proximal receptors (smell, touch) to distance receptors (vision, hearing).

Central Language Disorder (Developmental Aphasia)

Autistic children perform poorly on tasks requiring language skills and related temporal processing skills.[55] They are impaired in their use of concepts and abstraction, are generally limited in their powers of coding and categorizing, do poorly in sequential logic, and make little use of meaning in their memory processes. In view of these deficits and the typical clinical picture of delayed and deviant language development, it has been proposed that autism arises on the basis of a language disorder and is part of the spectrum of developmental receptive aphasias.[12] A related view proposes that autism arises on the basis of disorders of a variety of specific cognitive functions which are components of the language function itself but extend beyond it.[55] Thus, the absence of gesture, of imitation and mime, and of imaginative play all indicate that deficits in coding and sequencing extend beyond the verbal sphere to the nonverbal symbolic sphere.[45] Moreover, it has been demonstrated that autistic children have great difficulty in recognizing sequences in nonverbal modalities such as tone or color.[29] Overall, they have greatest difficulty in processing temporal sequences and less difficulty with visual-spatial[56] sequences, manipulation, and kinesthetic cues.

It remains uncertain to what extent these cognitive deficits bring about the social and behavioral abnormalities seen in autism. Rutter, however, has made a case for the view that the disturbances in affect are simply secondary phenomena.[54] He offers the following observations.

1. Autistic children, although they do poorly on verbal tasks, can perform well on nonverbal ones, indicating the presence of motivation to perform tasks within their capacity.
2. Social deprivation, per se, leads to impairment of verbal production, but does not usually affect language comprehension to as great a degree.
3. The degree of the initial severity of disturbance of affect is only weakly associated with outcome, while the degree of initial language impairment is strongly associated with outcome.
4. Language disturbances almost always precede the onset of other symptoms.

DeMeyer has suggested that different forms of early childhood psychosis may depend on if and to what degree central language dysfunction is coupled with an inability to carry out crossmodal perceptual transfer.[15]

PROGNOSIS

Without treatment, the prognosis of early onset psychosis is grave.[58] Roughly, 60% of autistic children have a poor outcome (little independent functioning, severely disturbed behavior), 25% have a fair outcome (some independent functioning associated with behavioral difficulties and a need for supervision), and 15% have a good outcome (full independent functioning).

The best predictor of good outcome is the development of language comprehension during the preschool years and of speech by the age of 5 years; the most accurate predictor of poor outcome is the presence of a low IQ (less than 60–75). Normal IQ tends to be associated with the presence of language, and about half of these children with normal IQ go on to have a good outcome. The more speech—of any kind, however deviant—present at the time of initial diagnosis, the better the prognosis.[16] The occurrence of seizures, which ultimately appear in about 25% of all autistic children and almost always in children with IQ's less than 65, worsens the prognosis, as does evidence of specific brain dysfunction. Prognosis worsens also with symptoms that are globally more severe and more numerous.

The clinical course is generally stable from middle childhood, with a continuation of whatever level of improvement or deterioration has been evident by then. Exacerbations may occur during adolescence, and the onset of seizures is usually followed by deterioration. Hallucinations, delusions, and thought disorder ordinarily do not appear as these children reach adolescence and adulthood, although a few cases of early onset psychosis have been reported to develop into typical adult schizophrenia.[48,64]

The few autistic children who reach a level of independent functioning as adults remain introverted and aloof, and lack empathy and social judgment. They continue to have varying degrees of difficulty with abstract concepts and the sequencing of ideas. Their speech is flat in tone, and is formal, somewhat pedantic, in style.[56] They are said to have usual adult sexual feelings but lack the social involvement for sexual relationships. Marriage is virtually nonexistent.

TREATMENT

Successful treatment of early onset psychosis depends on early diagnosis and intervention. This point cannot be stressed enough and is the major reason for alerting pediatricians to the early symptom picture of this illness. Many different therapeutic approaches have been attempted: family therapy, psychotherapy for parents, psychotherapy for children, behavior therapy, speech therapy, special education, day treatment, residential treatment, medication (including psychotropic drugs, hormones, megavitamins and even LSD), and electroconvulsive therapy. None of these techniques has brought consistent results. In the opinion of many workers, the response to treatment is determined more by the degree of impairment than by the type of treatment. Nevertheless, a growing body of clinical evidence suggests that the psychodynamically-oriented therapeutic approach which employs a three-way relationship among parent, child, and therapist (as described originally by Mahler[36] and elaborated by Galenson, Drucker, Miller, et al.[24]) offers a realistic hope for improvement—especially if started before the eighteenth month of life.[10,18,24,63]

Tripartite Psychotherapy

The conceptual framework for this model is that early onset psychosis, whatever its specific etiology and pathogenic mechanism, is characterized by a disturbance in interpersonal relationships in which the child cannot use his mother as a need-satisfying object. The major therapeutic technique consists of slowly enabling the child to use the therapist as a new symbiotic partner who allows and helps the child to reexperience and live through in corrective fashion with her the early phases of psychic life that are so crucial for separation/individuation and for establishing autonomous function. A "corrective symbiotic experience" of this nature aims at and fosters the establishment of body-image integrity, improvement in the relationships to the mother and to others, and the development of absent or distorted ego functions.[36] In addition the therapist encourages a reexperiencing of important past and forgotten feelings in the mother, whose difficulties in relating to her infant almost always can be traced back to her own childhood experience.

The first stage of treatment involves encouraging the child to enter a symbiotic relationship with a substitute mother. In so doing the therapist must avoid approaching the child too intrusively, and thereby throwing him into a panic. The therapist must slowly make himself part of the child's experience as a need-satisfying and comforting agent. At this stage the therapist represents a "mothering principle."[36] He does not yet represent a distinct and separate human person for the child, but rather a benign environment dimly perceived by the infant as being consistently responsive to his needs.

The therapist uses whatever interactions present themselves to establish this mothering principle unintrusively. For example, brief but repeated physical contact through tactile, rhythmic, vocal, and kinesthetic modalities as well as reflection of the child's behavior to him by way of imitation has been used successfully.[24,53] Naturally occurring events, such as feeding, holding, washing, and diapering, offer the opportunity to establish the presence of a benign, caring environment. Other therapeutic interventions in the early stages of treatment which serve to build this initial symbiotic relationship involve the therapist's function as an auxiliary ego, that is, providing the child with those particular ego functions necessary for the separation/individuation process. These include the capacity to evaluate reality (reality testing), the capacity to modulate feelings and impulses (inhibition of discharge of impulses), the capacity to ward off threatening stimuli (stimulus barrier), and the capacity to maintain attention and concentration (cognitive functioning).

In the later part of this first stage of treatment, when the child has accepted the therapist as mothering principle, the therapist leads the mother into the same kind of relationship with her child. Establishing this transfer is almost as delicate a process as making the first contact with the child, because parents regularly develop intense guilt, resentment, and anxiety in regard to assuming the restitutive symbiotic role. This reaction seems to be part of the pathological equilibrium between a mother and her psychotic child,[36] and in general seems to have its roots in conflicts going back to the mother's early childhood.[22,24]

In the second stage of treatment, by maintaining his role as a need-satisfying object, the therapist fosters an awareness of himself and the mother as distinct, specific, whole people. As this attachment to a specific other solidifies, the child develops a corresponding awareness of and investment in a distinct self with an increasing sense of separateness. He begins to show evidence of building an integrated mental image of his body. Thus, for the first time, the child is able to localize the origins of sensations to certain parts of his body, e.g., to the mouth[53] or to the rectum,[23] to the outer environment or to the internal milieu.[36]

The reciprocal development of an emotional attachment to specific people and a sense of his own body becomes the basis for further growth in cognitive, motor, and perceptual skills that can then be called upon to help control and channel various impulses. Such advances include the acquisition of communicative speech, the capacity to defer immediate gratification or to substitute one form of gratification for another,[36] and the attainment of certain cognitive skills. It is not unusual for dramatic developmental spurts to occur once a symbiotic attachment occurs. On the other hand, a child may do little without the auxiliary ego support of the mother figure for a prolonged period, often 3 or more years.[24,53] During this period, he is reliving and coming to understand the traumatic experiences that have disturbed his development. The child is helped to master the intense anxiety and hostility thus evoked by means of body contact and play, as well as through verbal communication with the therapist. Eventually, the child takes over control by means of adaptive-defensive mechanisms rather than by means of his former autistic withdrawal.

S.B.,* the autistic child described earlier, was treated in the Albert Einstein College of Medicine Therapeutic Nursery for a period of 2½ years beginning at the age of 2 years. During the first year of treatment S. emerged from his autistic shell and formed a solid symbiotic relationship with his therapist. The relationship was established primarily through the use of extensive and repetitive physical contact of every variety. For example, he would smear lotion on his therapist's skin as well as on his own, and she would do likewise. A beginning differentiation of self from other was indicated by the appearance of separation anxiety, and he developed fairly consistent mutual visual contact with his therapist. His restlessness lessened, and for the first time he became aware of his mouth, hands and legs.

---

* The writers are indebted to Ms. Cathy Shapiro, Dr. Jan Drucker, and Dr. Stavroula Beratis for making this information available.

During the ensuing 1½ years of treatment, as S. established firmer body boundaries and a better sense of self, he gradually gave up certain aspects of his delusional omnipotent union with therapist and mother; more autonomous functioning developed in its place. Although separation anxiety intensified with his increasing differentiation from his mother, S. began to develop ways of coping with it. For example, he repeatedly initiated games of separation and reunion such as peek-a-boo. An increasing awareness of internal state was demonstrated as he showed sadness and cried with tears for the first time. He became able to defer gratification or accept substitute gratifications, and showed a capacity to plan. Anal and urinary awareness then emerged, several years later than in the normal child. Although physiologically it was clearly within his capacity to exert sphincter control, he stubbornly refused, reinforcing his sense of independence in this way. Finally, he was able to shift his interest away from himself and his therapist (and mother) and to begin to explore the environment at large. By the end of the year, these forays into the world dominated the clinical picture and were accompanied by a zest and a joy that suggested a "love affair" with the world, a euphoric curiosity usually seen early in the second year of life in normal development.

On the other hand, S. still showed major deficits. Although he shifted from his original perpetual shrieking to normal babbling and jargon, he developed no words or communicative speech. A deficit in symbolic functioning in general was indicated by the absence of communicative gestures, thematic play, and deferred imitation. Relationships with his peers remained rudimentary and charged with disruptive anxiety.

Thus, while S. made considerable progress in treatment, he still remained severely impaired in functioning and continued to require his therapist as his symbiotic partner and auxiliary ego. His mother was virtually unable to act in this capacity in the early part of treatment. Instead, she exposed S. to overwhelming stimulation, e.g., genital stimulation. At other times, she failed to respond to his needs because she was so absorbed in her own fantasies; she could not, for instance, protect him from dangerous encounters. The situation became critical midway in treatment when S. began to show appropriate independent behavior derived from his attachment to his therapist, but at a point when his mother could not yet tolerate her role as a symbiotic partner. Several accidents—all fortunately without sequelae—indicated how potentially vulnerable S. was at this time. Further therapeutic work with the mother, in large part revolving around her relationship with her own mother, enabled her to free herself enough from her rage at S. to look after his physical safety at least.

Involving the mother in the therapeutic process, making it a tripartite one, is always a significant element of the treatment situation.

Other Therapeutic Modalities

Behavior modification as a treatment modality has become increasingly popular because it is nonverbal and requires little conceptualization on the part of the child. This approach tends to be pragmatic, more directed toward simple improvements in behavioral repertoire and social skills than in giant strides toward cure. The underlying assumption behind the behavior modification approach is that the autistic child has not withdrawn from social contact because of anxiety, but has failed to develop social skills because of a range of cognitive, perceptual, and language disorders. In contrast to dynamically oriented therapies, behavioral modification calls for the therapist to actively intrude upon the child in order to engage in deliberate interaction.[59]

Many examples of the successful alteration of various maladaptive behaviors have been described in the literature. The long-term social benefit of these changes, however, remains unknown. There is some evidence that a home-based approach,[56] counseling of parents,[56] and the facilitation of attachment behaviors[59] improves the effectiveness of the behavior modification approach; such evidence suggests a convergence with the dynamically oriented therapies.

Recent reports have suggested that sign language can be taught to children with early onset psychosis, with significant improvement in disturbed behavior.

A variety of drugs has been used experimentally in the treatment of early onset psychosis, but none has brought about consistent improvement in clinical state.[11]

Treatment of Late Onset Psychosis

Psychotherapy, in either a residential or outpatient setting, in conjunction with a variety of ancillary supporting services such as structured activity groups and special educational curricula, continues to be the major therapeutic approach to late onset psychosis. A few programs employ the educational experience itself as the definitive intervention.[19] Neuroleptic drugs give inconsistent results in late onset psychosis, in contrast to their predictable effect in adult schizophrenics; when they are effective, it is usually by bringing about a reduction in psychomotor excitement. Electroconvulsant therapy and psychosurgery are rarely employed.

CONCLUSION

The early onset psychoses of autism and symbiosis are distinct clinical entities with symptomatology easily recognized if looked for, and quite different from that seen in the schizophrenic-like late onset psychosis. Depressive or manic psychosis rarely, if ever, occurs in childhood.

For early onset psychosis, a treatment approach has been described that can—at least sometimes—bring significant improvement, although it is arduous, costly, and must be of long duration. Since prognosis can improve dramatically with earlier diagnosis and intervention, early onset psychosis should be viewed as a pediatric emergency. Pediatricians, as well as other child care professionals, are well advised to be familiar with the syndrome.

REFERENCES

1. Bartak, L., Rutter, M., & Cox, A. A comparative study of infantile autism and specific developmental receptive language disorder. *British Journal of Psychiatry*, 1975, *126*, 127–159.

2. Beebe, B., & Stern, D. Engagement-disengagement and early object experiences. In N. Freedman & S. Grand (Eds.), *Communicative structures and psychic structures*. New York: Plenum, in press.

3. Bender, L. Childhood schizophrenia: A clinical study of 100 schizophrenic children. *American Journal of Orthopsychiatry*, 1947, *17*, 40–56.

4. Benjamin, J. Further comments on some developmental aspects of anxiety. In H. Gaskill (Ed.), *Counterpoint: Libidinal object and subject.* New York: International Universities Press, 1963.

5. Bettelheim, B. *The empty fortress.* New York: Free Press, 1967.

6. Boatman, M., & Szurek, S. A clinical study of childhood schizophrenia. In D. Jackson (Ed.), *Etiology of schizophrenia.* New York: Basic Books, 1960.

7. Boullin, D., Coleman, M., O'Brien, R., & Rimland, B. Laboratory predictions of infantile autism based on 5-HT efflux from blood platelets. *Journal of Autism and Childhood Schizophrenia,* 1971, *1*(1), 63–71.

8. Bowlby, J. *Attachment.* New York: Basic Books, 1969.

9. Brazelton, T. B., Tronick, E., & Adamson, L. Early mother-infant reciprocity. In *Parent-infant interaction.* Ciba Foundation Symposium #33 (new series). North Holland: Elsevier, 1975.

10. Call, J. Prevention of autism in a young infant. *Journal of American Academy of Child Psychiatry,* 1963, *2,* 451–459.

11. Campbell, M. Pharmacotherapy in early infant autism. *Biological Psychiatry,* 1975, *10,* 399–423.

12. Churchill, D. Relation of early infantile autism and early childhood schizophrenia to developmental language disorders of childhood. *Journal of Autism and Childhood Schizophrenia,* 2, 182–193.

13. Cohen, D., Caparulo, B., & Shaywitz, B. Primary childhood aphasia and childhood autism: Clinical, biochemical, and conceptual observations. *Journal of Child Psychiatry,* 1976, *15,* 604–645.

14. DeMeyer, M., Alpern, G., Barton, S., et al. Imitation in autistic, early schizophrenic and nonpsychotic subnormal children. *Journal of Autism and Childhood Schizophrenia,* 1972, *2,* 264–287.

15. DeMeyer, M., Barton, S., & Norton, J. Comparison of adaptive, verbal, and motor profiles of psychotic and nonpsychotic subnormal children. *Journal of Autism and Childhood Schizophrenia,* 1972, *2,* 359–377.

16. DeMeyer, M., Norton, J., Allen, J., et al. Prognosis in autism. *Journal of Autism and Childhood Schizophrenia.* 1973, *3,* 199–246.

17. Eisenberg, L. Autistic child in adolescence. *American Journal of Psychiatry,* 1956, *112,* 607–612.

18. Etemad, J., & Szurek, S. A modified follow-up study of a group of psychotic children. In S. Szurek & I. Berlin (Eds.), *Clinical Studies in Childhood Psychosis.* New York: Brunner/Mazel, 1973.

19. Fenichel, C., Freedman, A., & Klapper, Z. A day school for schizophrenic children. *American Journal of Orthopsychiatry,* 1960, *30,* 130–143.

20. Fish, B., Wile, R., Shapiro, T., et al. Prediction of schizophrenia in infancy. In P. Hoch & J. Zubin (Eds.), *Psychopathology of schizophrenia.* New York: Grune & Stratton, 1966.

21. Folstein, S., & Rutter, B. Infantile autism: A genetic study of 21 twin pairs. *Nature,* 1977, *265,* 726–728.

22. Fraknoi, J., & Ruttenberg, B. Formulation of the dynamic economic factors underlying infantile autism. *Journal of American Academy of Child Psychiatry,* 1971, *10,* 713–738.

23. Fuhrer, E. The development of a preschool symbiotic psychotic boy. *The Psychoanalytic Study of the Child,* 1964, *19,* 448–469.

24. Galenson, E., Drucker, J., Miller, R., et al. Detection and treatment of early childhood psychosis. Unpublished manuscript.

25. Galenson, E., & Roiphe, H. The emergence of genital awareness during the second year of life. In R. Friedman, R. Richart & R. VandeWiele (Eds.), *Sex differences in behavior.* New York: Wiley, 1974.

26. Goldfarb, W. *Childhood schizophrenia.* Cambridge, Mass.: Harvard, 1961.

27. Harlow, H., & McKinney, W. Non-human primates and psychosis. *Journal of Autism and Childhood Schizophrenia,* 1971, *1,* 368–375.

28. Hauser, S., Delong, G., & Rosman, N. Pneumoencephalographic findings in the infantile autism syndrome. *Brain*, 1975, *98*, 667–688.

29. Hermelin, B. Rules and language. In M. Rutter (Ed.), *Infantile autism: Concept, characteristics and treatment.* Edinburgh: Churchill and Livingstone, 1971.

30. Hutt, S., & Hutt, C. *Behavior studies in psychiatry.* Oxford: Pergamon, 1970.

31. Jaffe, J., Stern, D., & Perry, J. Conversational coupling of gaze behavior in prelinguistic human development. *Journal of Psycholinguistic Research*, 1973, *2*, 321–329.

32. Kanner, L. Autistic disturbances of affective contact. *Nervous Child*, 1943, *2*, 217–250.

33. Kety, S., Rosenthal, D., Wender, P., et al. Types and prevalence of mental illness in the biological and adoptive families of adopted schizophrenics. In D. Rosenthal & S. Kety (Eds.), *The transmission of schizophrenia.* Oxford: Pergamon, 1963.

34. Klaus, M., Trause, M., & Kennell, J. Human maternal behavior after delivery. In *Parent-infant interaction.* Ciba Foundation Symposium #33 (new series). North Holland: Elsevier, 1975.

35. Kolvin, I., Ounsted, C., Humphrey, M., et al. Studies in the childhood psychoses. *British Journal of Psychiatry*, 1971, *118*, 381–419.

36. Mahler, M. *On human symbiosis and the vicissitudes of individuation.* New York: International Universities Press, 1968.

37. Mahler, M., & Gosliner, B. On symbiotic child psychosis: Genetic, dynamic, and restitutive aspects. *The Psychoanalytical Study of the Child*, 1955, *10*, 195–212.

38. Mahler, M., Pine, F., & Berman, A. *The psychological birth of the human infant.* New York: Basic Books, 1975.

39. Massie, H. The early natural history of childhood psychosis. *Journal of Childhood Psychiatry*, 1975, *14*, 683–707.

40. Massie, H. Patterns of mother-infant behavior and subsequent childhood psychosis. *Child Psychiatry and Human Development*, 1977, *7*, 211–230.

41. Miller, R. Childhood schizophrenia, a review of selected literature. *International Journal of Mental Health*, 1974, *3*, 3–46.

42. Morrison, D., Miller, D., & Mejia, B. Comprehension and negation of verbal communication in autistic children. In S. Szurek & I. Berlin (Eds.), *Clinical studies in childhood psychosis.* New York: Brunner/Mazel, 1973.

43. Ornitz, E. Childhood autism: A disorder of sensorimotor integration. In M. Rutter (Ed.), *Infantile autism: Concepts, characteristics and treatment.* Edinburgh: Churchill and Livingstone, 1971.

44. Ornitz, E., & Ritvo, E. Perceptual inconstancy in early infantile autism. *Archives of General Psychiatry*, 1968, *18*, 76–98.

45. Piaget, J. *Play, dreams and imitation in childhood.* New York: Norton, 1962.

46. Powell, G., Brasel, J., & Blizzard, R. Emotional deprivation and growth retardation simulating idiopathic hypopituitarism. *New England Journal of Medicine*, 1967, *276*, 1271–1278.

47. Province, S., & Lipton, R. *Infants in institutions.* New York: International Universities Press, 1962.

48. Reiser, D. Psychosis of infancy and early childhood, as manifested by children with atypical development. *New England Journal of Medicine*, 1963, *269*, 790–797; 844–849.

49. Rimland, B. *Infantile autism.* New York: Appleton-Century-Crofts, 1964.

50. Roiphe, H. Some thoughts on childhood psychosis, self, and object. *The Psychoanalytical Study of the Child*, 1973, *28*, 131–145.

51. Roiphe, H., & Galenson, E. Early genital activity and the castration complex. *Psychoanalytical Quarterly*, 1972, *41*, 334–347.

52. Rubin, M. Hearing aids for infants and children. In M. Rubin (Ed.), *Hearing aids: Current development and concepts.* Baltimore: University Park Press, 1976.

53. Ruttenberg, B. A psychoanalytic understanding of infantile autism and its treatment. In D. Churchill, D. Alpern & M. DeMeyer (Eds.), *Infantile autism: Proceedings of the Indiana University Colloquium.* Springfield, Ill.: Charles C. Thomas, 1970.

54. Rutter, M. Concepts of autism: A review of the research. *Journal of Child Psychology and Psychiatry,* 1968, *9,* 1–25.

55. Rutter, M. Development of infantile autism. *Psychological Medicine,* 1974, *4,* 147–163.

56. Rutter, M. Infantile autism and other childhood psychoses. In M. Rutter & L. Hersov (Eds.), *Child psychiatry, modern approaches.* Oxford: Blackwell Scientific, 1977.

57. Rutter, M., Bartak, L., & Newman, S. Autism: A central disorder of cognition and language. In M. Rutter (Ed.), *Infantile autism: Concepts, characteristics, and treatment.* Edinburgh: Churchill and Livingstone, 1971.

58. Rutter, M., Greenfield, D., & Lockyer, L. A five-to-fifteen-year follow-up study of infantile psychosis. *British Journal of Psychiatry,* 1967, *113,* 1169–1199 (Part I); 1969, *115,* 865–882 (Part 2). *British Journal of Social Clinical Psychology,* 1970, *9,* 152–163 (Part 3).

59. Rutter, M., & Sussenwein, F. Developmental and behavioral approach to the treatment of preschool autistic children. *Journal of Autism and Childhood Schizophrenia,* 1971, *1,* 376–397.

60. Sander, L., Stechler, G., Burns, P., et al. Early mother-infant interaction and 24-hour patterns of activity and sleep. *Journal of American Academy of Child Psychiatry,* 1970, *9,* 103–123.

61. Spitz, R. Anaclitic depression: An inquiry into the genesis of psychiatric conditions in early childhood: II. *The Psychoanalytic Study of the Child,* 1946, *2,* 313–342.

62. Tustin, F. *Autism and childhood psychosis.* London: Hogarth Press, 1972.

63. Wenar, C., Ruttenberg, B., & Dratman, M. Changing autistic behavior. *Archives of General Psychiatry,* 1967, *17,* 26–35.

64. Zaslow, R. Psychogenic theory of etiology of autism. Paper presented at the meeting of the California State Psychological Association, San Diego, January, 1967.

CHILD ABUSE:
A SOCIAL-PSYCHOLOGICAL-MEDICAL
=====DISORDER=====

Edward Goldson, M.D.

INTRODUCTION AND HISTORY

In the United States, approximately one quarter-million cases of child abuse are reported each year.* However, according to most authorities, this number represents only a fraction of the real number of abused children. Indeed, there may be well over one million cases per year.[51] Child abuse is the second most common cause of childhood morbidity and mortality under 5 years of age in the United States.[70] Although most cases can be prevented, child abuse is a sociomedical disorder that remains a significant public health problem in the United States.

The abuse of children is not a new phenomenon. In primitive societies where the struggle for existence of the group was all-encompassing, the individual—particularly the nonproductive child—was often sacrificed for the good of the group. Such sacrifices were determined in part by the purely economic needs of the group, while other abuses were the result of superstition and ignorance. For instance, children born on unlucky days or as twins or with teeth or with congenital abnormalities could be put to death. This may well have been one way of coping with an uncompromising, unknown, and threatening environment. It is of interest to note that in those societies where food was plentiful and the struggle for survival was not so difficult, the degree of abuse and infanticide was lower.[1]

During each phase of societal evolution, particularly in the West, child abuse has taken many forms, including infanticide, mutilation, and exploitation of children by burgeoning industry. However, as time has progressed, its occurrence has declined.[19] At the same time, each civilization has had its advocates for children,[5] including Plato in

---

* Lebsack, J. R., American Humane Association. Personal communication.

400 B.C., Sir Thomas More in the 16th century, and Charles Dickens in the 19th century.[67]

Although child advocacy has existed throughout history, it was not until 1871 that the Society for the Prevention of Cruelty to Children was founded in New York City. This society, which was an outgrowth of the Society for the Prevention of Cruelty to Animals, was the first organization in the United States to become a proponent of children's rights. Finally, Kempe, Silverman, Steele, et al.[44] brought the broad implications of child abuse before the public in 1962. Since this significant publication, in which the term *battered child syndrome* was coined, there has been an outpouring of writing from many disciplines concerned with the care of abused children.

In the forthcoming pages, an attempt will be made to view child abuse in a broad context. The term *abuse* will be used to encompass the phenomena of nonaccidental trauma (NAT) and neglect-failure-to-thrive (FTT) as well as sexual molestation and emotional abuse. However, the focus of this chapter will be on NAT and neglect-FTT. Sexual molestation presents a pattern of psychopathology that is quite different from NAT and neglect-FTT and, therefore, requires a separate discussion. Emotional abuse is the most difficult form of abuse to define or to document.[49] However, it must be considered when dealing with an unloving, hypercritical, unaccepting, and negative home. It is ironic that such desolate environments often meet the physical needs of the child, often exist among the more economically privileged of our society, and yet— perhaps even because of the appearance of care—the abuse often goes unnoticed or ignored.[17] Indeed, this form of abuse can be quite subtle and insidious and can be most destructive, ultimately, to the overall development of the child. Also included in this chapter will be a discussion of the incidence and reporting of child abuse and consideration of the etiology of the disorder. The problems of identification, dynamics, and personality of the parents as well as the personality and development of the children will be considered. Finally, some thoughts on prevention and treatment of child abuse will be presented.

INCIDENCE AND REPORTING

The problem of identification, reporting, and the recognition of the true incidence of abuse is a very critical issue. The Child Abuse Prevention and Treatment Act of 1974 has mandated all segments of society, but particularly those concerned with the care of children, to report suspected abuse. This task frequently falls in the domain of the physician, who may be the one most remiss, however, in fulfilling his legal obligations. Such failure may be the result of a low index of suspicion, a lack of knowledge of proper reporting procedures, or reluctance and discomfort in reporting or relating to abusing individuals.[69,73,54] To date, the majority of reports come from public institutions that serve the indigent and where a high index of suspicion for abuse exists. Children of the affluent may not be so readily identified, since professionals providing child care services to the more well-to-do may not look for or choose to ignore abuse if it occurs. It is this writer's opinion that abuse among children of the more socially and economically privileged is underreported in the United States. Because of poor reporting, our understanding of the incidence and magnitude of the problem is incomplete. Therefore, the 229,360 official reports of child abuse in the United States in 1974 probably reflect gross underreporting. Only 88,000 of these reports were validated and subsequently proven as involving some form of child abuse.* This may be caused in

---

* Lebsack, J. R., American Humane Association. Personal communication.

part by variations in local and state statutes and their judicial interpretation. Twelve states report only physical abuse, not neglect or failure to thrive. This inability to realistically define the magnitude of child abuse remains a roadblock in dealing with this significant sociomedical disorder. Despite these problems, it is recognized that abuse occurs among all racial and ethnic groups, in rural and urban settings, among all socioeconomic groups in the country, and, more commonly, under the age of 5 years.

ETIOLOGY

One way of beginning to analyze such a complex phenomenon as child abuse is to view it from a broad etiological framework. Although every family is unique, there are certain underlying characteristics common to abusive families. Both Gil and Gelles[30,31,32] have looked at sociopsychological models which may be instructive and are worth considering.

Gil identifies three levels of manifestation of abuse. The first level of manifestation is at the societal level where basic social philosophy and attitudes toward human beings are articulated. He suggests that only in an egalitarian society can an unhampered development of children take place. Furthermore, he maintains that the way in which a society views and values its children will determine the degree and level to which it will allow them to develop and achieve their potential. Finally, the degree to which a society condones the use of force to achieve its ends very much determines how it will relate to its children and what rights will be accorded to them. Gil maintains that our society is nonegalitarian, views its children as subservient, and condones the use of force. It is no wonder, then, that abuse does and will occur given such societal attitudes toward children and toward violence.

Gil identifies the second level of manifestation at the institutional level. Institutions are the bearers of societal norms. Abuse at this level may occur in the form of corporal punishment, but it may also take place in a setting in which the child is demeaned and threatened or where spontaneous and creative behavior is inhibited. This is an environment wherein the individual's optimal development is either thwarted, inhibited, or insufficiently promoted by the basic structure of the institution.

Finally, he identifies the third level of manifestation, the interpersonal level of abuse, which is the one that confronts clinicians. This level involves the physical or emotional injuring of a child by the individual charged with his care, either by omission or commission. One might consider this the "final common pathway" of societal as well as institutional abuse. All of these levels of manifestation come to rest in the individual abusive act, which is what comes to the clinician's attention.

NONACCIDENTAL TRAUMA (NAT)

Identification and Characteristics of NAT

In considering the recognition of child abuse, let us first turn to the diagnosis of NAT. NAT is defined as any nonaccidental injury sustained by the child as a result of acts of omission or commission on the part of his caretaker. The obvious physical signs of NAT have been well described by many workers and include fractures, bruises, subdural hematomas, and burns.[4,25,35,40,41,48,74] Less common signs of NAT include sub-galeal hematomas secondary to hair pulling, handprints on the face and other parts of the body following smacking, the semicircular appearance of a human bite, genital injuries secondary to biting or tying of the penis, and tears on the floor of the mouth following forced feeding.[42] Occasionally the child sustaining NAT can present with diffuse, nonspecific neurological signs which disappear during hospitalization.[2] Children have been identified with pseudocyst of the pancreas, rupture of abdominal viscera, or other injuries to abdominal organs secondary to blunt trauma.[59,80] Purtscher retinopathy,[79] hypertonic dehydration,[11] and chloral hydrate ingestion have been associated with NAT.[48] Finally, there is the "whiplash shaken infant syndrome" identified by Caffey[11] in which there are no external signs of injury; on examination of the dead child's brain at autopsy, however, subarachnoid hemorrhages and retinal detachments are present. On radiographic examination it is possible to see metaphyseal avulsions and subperiosteal hemorrhages secondary to traction-stretching stresses on the periosteum induced by grabbing the children by the extremities or thorax and shaking them.[11]

Usually, the child presenting with any of the manifestations of NAT will have an injury inconsistent with the history, or with his developmental level. The kinds of injuries noted above do not occur accidentally! With these considerations in mind, the clinician should begin to suspect abuse. X-rays of the long bones, distribution and nature of the bruises and burns, as well as the history often lead to a correct diagnosis of NAT.[70] Finally, a complete assessment of family functioning can be of great help in recognizing NAT: For example, the parent who frequently seeks medical advice at odd hours for seemingly trivial problems should raise the physician's suspicions with respect to family dysfunction.

Dynamics of NAT

Let us now turn to the dynamics of NAT. One might consider that there are two distinct categories of individuals and conditions which result in NAT (see Fig. 1). The first condition involves psychotic or (at least) severely emotionally disturbed individuals who have bizarre attachments to the child. These attachments may be indeed so bizarre as to actively include the child in the individual's disturbed ideation. The abuse that such individuals perpetrate is an overt, planned physical injury which fulfills a particular need, or which is the result of a distorted perception of the child and his needs. "It is a cold calculation of destruction which in itself requires neither provocation nor rationale."[83] The child may represent some hated individual in the abuser's past or he may be an everpresent threat to the abuser and so must be injured or destroyed. The number of abusers falling into this category is very small compared with those who abuse through faulty parenting, that is, who fail to nurture and protect the child.[55]

The abusers falling into the faulty parenting category can be divided into two groups, the active abuser and the passive abuser.[38,41] Passive abuse results from a lack of understanding of children and their need for protection within the environment. Many of these injuries may appear to be accidental, but on closer examination, they emerge as the result of negligence on the part of the child's caretaker. Active abuse occurs when the abuser lashes out at the child in anger, either having lost control of his or her emotions or wishing to discipline the child. Notwithstanding this theoretical division, I would venture to suggest that a combination of circumstances must exist in order for the abuse to occur.[36]

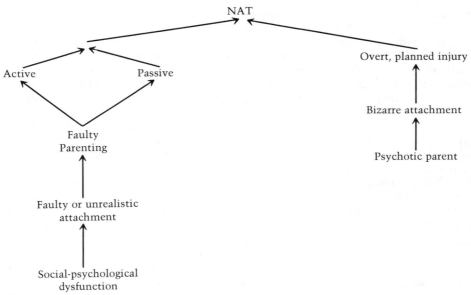

Figure 1.   Dynamic of Non-Accidental Trauma (NAT)

Helfer[39] has presented a model that is helpful in viewing the problem. He suggests that three components must exist for abuse to occur. The first component is the individual's potential for abuse, which is a function of how the parents themselves were treated, the ability of the family to utilize support systems, the relationship between the parents, and how they view the child.

The second component is the child himself and how he functions; for example, the child may be viewed as different because of a birth defect or because his physical or intellectual capabilities are perceived as being inadequate.[70] There is an increased incidence of battering among children born prematurely,[35,45] possibly because of aberrant or inadequate attachment associated with prolonged separation between parent and infant.[44] The child may not have been wanted in the first place, or he may fail to meet the parents' expectations. All of these elements can contribute to how the parents view and treat the child.

The third component is the presence of a crisis: the loss of a job, an argument, an automobile breakdown, or the child's spilling a glass of milk. It is the combination of these three factors that precipitates the loss of control and the striking out at the child. Of course, there are psychological as well as social and environmental determinants that contribute to the outburst. Each determinant plays a variable role in individual situations, each may have its roots in societal or institutional models, yet each is present in every situation of abuse.

Personality of the Parents Involved in NAT

In attempting to understand NAT it is obviously important to consider the personality of the parents involved. From a review of the literature, and (perhaps even more importantly) from clinical experience, one is able to differentiate parents involved in NAT from those involved in Neglect-FTT. Although there are no absolute divisions, some differences are worth considering, particularly when one takes into account the dynamics of NAT and the kind of therapy that should be employed. The individual involved in NAT has been described as being impulsive, immature,[42a] narcissistic, sadomasochistic, aggressive,[77] demanding, and with a low frustration threshold.[15] Furthermore, a significant number of these parents were themselves physically and emotionally abused as children.[70,77] In addition, they are often depressed, uncommunicative, socially isolated, rejected, and rejecting.[81] Finally, they perceive the child as demanding in such a way that neither their own narcissistic needs nor their expectations of the child are fulfilled.

Frequently, there is a reversal of roles, with the child being expected to "mother" the parent, and the adult becoming the child and demanding to remain so.[28] One can easily see how a child could be injured if he did not fulfill the distorted needs of the parent or if he placed the caretaking burden back, rightfully, on the shoulders of the adult. The physically abusive parent's models for parenting were distorted, thus the resultant faulty attachment to their own children. If one places this distortion in attachment, and subsequently a parenting distortion, into a social context in which violence is an accepted means of dealing with stress and frustration, then NAT is no longer a mystery. Instead, one wonders why more parents do not batter their children—which, in fact, may be the case.

Finally, there is the stress in these individuals' lives, the final component of the triad leading to abuse. It has been frequently reported that a significant number of abusing parents live under poor socioeconomic conditions and have unstable homes and many emotional problems.[20,24,32,75] However, it should be emphasized that NAT can and does occur in the more affluent segments of American society, for many of the same socioeconomic stresses and psychological antecedents are present, albeit to a different degree and at a different level.

Characteristics of the Child with NAT

As with the abusive parent, there appear to be differences between neglected children who go on to FTT and those children who sustain NAT. Children who sustain NAT have been described as being stubborn, negativistic, apathetic[37] and in many ways unappealing. This may not be the way they started in life, but it is often the way they present to the professional. On admission to the hospital they may cry very little; if they do, there is a hopeless quality to their distress, no expectation of being helped. They are initially wary of physical contact and often present with a characteristic behavior which Ounsted has named "frozen watchfulness."[56] This behavior is characterized by little chatter or smiling in the presence of adults. Instead, these children gaze-fixate and are often silent even when subjected to painful stimuli. Ounsted sees this behavior as an adaptation to the unpredictable behavior of a loved and loving parent who, without provocation, becomes an aggressor.[56] However (and this has been borne out by our clinical experience), many of these children soon become manipulative and controlling while searching out and assessing their environment; they tend to seek things from individuals they perceive as being in control. Moreover, these children relate to such caregiving and supportive persons only on a very superficial level. As adults, they often have distorted interpersonal relationships and often abuse their own children.

From a cognitive point of view, many of these children grow up with intellectual deficits. Some of these deficits are the result of the physical injury sustained and the lack of effective therapy; others are related to the kind of environment to which they have been subjected.[39] The children who sustain central nervous system (CNS) injuries are certainly at high risk for having permanent neurological damage, intellectual handicaps, or both.[7,71] Even those children who escape CNS damage, however, have been found to have cognitive deficits suggesting that there are powerful environmental forces which affect the child's development.[21,53] The development of language appears to be most affected.[53,71] It is interesting to note that the abused children who do not sustain severe NAT do not go on to have growth failure or other significant physical problems. There is also a suggestion that when these children are compared to children sustaining neglect-FTT they do better cognitively,[21] particularly if there have been appropriate intervention and support.

NEGLECT-FAILURE TO THRIVE (FTT)

Identification and Characteristics of Neglect-FTT

While the diagnosis of NAT can be relatively simple, the recognition of neglect-failure-to-thrive presents a much more difficult task. FTT can be defined as a child's failure to maintain his or her expected growth pattern when there is no known underlying disease process causing such failure. Neglect is more difficult to define since it is impossible to quantify it. Rather, neglect is a complex of behaviors. One sees children who are unkempt, dirty, appear undernourished, and yearn for human warmth. The parents do not interact with their children in any meaningful manner; for example, the mother may not touch or cuddle her infant or speak to it with any warmth or change in vocal inflection. These children can be identified as being neglected.

In recognizing some of the pitfalls of a neglect-FTT diagnosis, it is worth noting that there are several physical signs associated with maternal deprivation, one of the antecedents of neglect-FTT. Hypotonia[9] and an infantile posture of tonic immobility[46] characterized by flexed elbows, abducted humerus, and pronated hands positioned at the side of the head all have been associated with neglect and deprivation. Neglected children may present with disturbances of sleep and elimination, e.g., enuresis, as well as significant autoerotic and self-mutilating behaviors.[61] These are some of the outward signs of maternal deprivation and neglect; they may be present long before failure to thrive occurs. Although FTT is not always the inevitable outcome of neglect, it is this writer's opinion that FTT is the end of a continuum which includes maternal deprivation and neglect.

Dynamics of Neglect-FTT

Neglect-FTT presents a different set of conditions from that of NAT (see Fig. 2). Based on experience in working with parents whose children sustain neglect-FTT, it appears that, under some circumstances, the basic mother-child attachment and bonding is absent, resulting in maternal deprivation, lack of positive or negative stimulation, and a lack of the delivery of basic care for the child.

Another route to the same outcome involves the situation in which attachment and bonding are present, albeit tenuous, but can be easily broken as a result of social or economic stress. In the former instance, the mother is profoundly emotionally disturbed. In the latter instance the potential for the development of normal attachment exists but deleterious socioeconomic conditions, maternal depression, or isolation destroy what tenuous attachment exists. The final common pathway in both of these

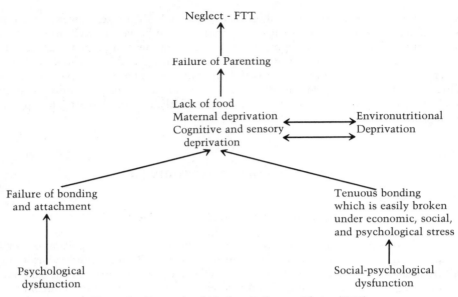

Figure 2.   Dynamic of Neglect-Failure to Thrive (FTT)

circumstances is the chronic failure of parenting that ultimately leads to neglect and, in severe circumstances, to failure-to-thrive, even death.

Personality of the Parents Involved in Neglect-FTT

The personalities of neglecting parents are somewhat different from those of parents who physically injure their children. In the first place, neglecting parents, because of their own inadequate childhoods, either fail to bond with their children or have very weak attachments which fail under stress. This is in contrast to the aberrant attachments that exist among parents who physically injure their children. Many of the neglecting parents have been described as being inadequate, anxious, passive individuals who have had very poor object relationships and poor parenting themselves.[24,50] However, these neglecting parents have very little overt psychopathology and do not tend to lose control and thus act out aggressively against the child.[62] Instead, they seem to have an inability to adapt to change, or to understand and respond to the needs of the child.[24] A most striking behavior is their lack of verbal and emotional interaction with their children.[62] If one assumes that parents and children reciprocally influence each other's behavior,[8,50] the synchrony that normally develops between parent and child is disturbed among parents who do not relate meaningfully to their children and who finally neglect them.

There seems to be a subtle, yet striking, difference between the basic parent-child relationship of the parent of the child with neglect-FTT and of the parent of the child who sustains NAT. The neglecting parent has no meaningful relationship with the child, while the physically abusive parent has a relationship (albeit a distorted one). In many ways physically abusive parents may be more amenable to therapy than parents who neglect in that the former are reachable and very often have great concern for their children. The parent who is not attached, or at most tenuously bonded, may be far more difficult to reach and help.

Characteristics of the Child with Neglect-FTT

Children with neglect-FTT demonstrate different behavioral and developmental characteristics from children who sustain NAT. The most striking aspect of the adult-child relationship in this abusive situation is the lack of relationship. The effect of this lack of interaction was recognized almost thirty years ago by Spitz[76] when he described anaclitic depression in institutionalized children who, essentially, had been emotionally neglected. His work has been reaffirmed by Bowlby[6] who went a step further in recognizing that the outcome for these neglected children was precarious, and that many of them grew up to be socially deviant and emotionally crippled. Coleman and Provence[16] described several children who behaved like institutionalized children, but who were living at home in very poor emotional environments. Finally, Provence[65] studied the developmental outcomes of institutionalized children and found them to be intellectually and physically delayed when compared with children raised in average homes.

Children with neglect-FTT are in many ways similar to the institutionalized children described above. These children have poor physical growth and may even present with abnormal posturing and other neurological signs such as hypotonia. They tend to be apathetic, quiet, cry very little, have poor appetites and histories of feeding problems, do not relate to their physical or emotional environments, and are quite passive.[10,34] One often finds them lying in bed, staring off into space with very depressed and anxious expressions on their faces. Two authors have identified disturbances in sleep and eating patterns, enuresis, and disturbed interpersonal relationships.[61] However, a number of these children, particularly those who have not become totally depressed and withdrawn from their environments, may be voracious eaters who gain weight rapidly during hospitalization or while in a wholesome home. When this occurs, the children soon begin to interact with their environments and relate to individuals appropriately.

One might consider a number of explanations as to why these neglected children fail to thrive. There are circumstances, of course, in which the child is simply not fed enough, as may be the case in many deprived families or in those families who have particularly bizarre relationships with their children and starve them. When these children were first identified, however, it was believed that they did have adequate nutrition and that their FTT was psychologically based or was the result of maternal deprivation.[58,76] In an intriguing series of studies, Powell and his coworkers examined a group of children with FTT who had clinical findings of idiopathic hypopituitarism.[63] These children had deficiencies in ACTH and growth hormone which returned to normal when the children were removed from their adverse environments.[64]

Another group of workers identified definite growth hormone deficiency, together with growth retardation, in a group of children who, although they did not respond to replacement therapy, did begin to grow when their environment was changed.[27] Gardner postulated an inhibition of growth hormone secretion in response to emotional stress and resulting sleep disturbances as one cause of FTT associated with neglect and deprivation.[29] Engel and his coworkers found a decrease in gastric secretion in a depressed and withdrawn child who was failing to thrive, and they have suggested a relationship between gastric secretion and emotional state.[22] Patton and Gardner also identified changes in intestinal absorption associated with emotional disturbances.[57] Conceivably, these changes in gastrointestinal function could alter the absorption of foodstuffs and result in decreased utilization of seemingly adequate nutrients. Looking at the arguments for an endocrine effect versus a gastrointestinal effect on growth, the common denominator appears to be a lack of adequate food.[68,82]

The observations noted in the preceding discussion suggest that a child's emotional state affects his physiological function. If this is accepted, it follows that there could be changes in growth hormone secretion, gastric secretion, and the secretion of other growth-promoting hormones such as thyroid hormone. In turn, these changes could influence the utilization of nutrients even in the presence of adequate food intake. On the other hand, the child's depression, as well as the conflict with or withdrawal from his environment could explain a decreased appetite, leading to decreased food intake which results in growth failure. In summary then, it is highly plausible that all of the above observations and explanations for neglect-FTT can play different roles in different children with the final common pathway being inadequate nutrition either because of poor physiological utilization of nutrients or simply because there is not enough food to eat.[13,18,66,78]

After all is said and done, however, the critical issue concerning children who sustain neglect-FTT remains the effect that these experiences have on their development. Without intervention, we find distorted and disturbed individuals who often do not function well in society, either socially or intellectually. These individuals may be the victims of what Chase has called "environutritional deprivation."[12] From a physical point of view, these children often demonstrate cerebellar dysfunction and growth retardation. Sadly enough, unless appropriate intervention occurs early in life these deficits may not be reversible.[66,71] This irreversibility may be related to critical periods of brain growth that occur in the first year of life and can be hampered by environutritional deprivation.[12] Intellectual impairment often accompanies physical growth failure among these children. The child's overall development is delayed, with deficits most evident in tasks requiring verbal and neurointegrative skills and abstract thinking.

Finally, children with neglect-FTT are emotionally damaged. They often become individuals who do not develop bonds with adults or children, who are superficial and indiscriminate in their relationships, and are often depressed and isolated. Ultimately, these individuals may well repeat the cycle of physical, sensory, cognitive, and emotional deprivation with their own children.

NAT AND NEGLECT-FTT: DUAL CONSIDERATIONS

In the preceding pages, I have attempted to present NAT and neglect-FTT as two distinct phenomena. However, the reader must bear in mind that there are children who sustain both NAT and neglect-FTT. These children are, of course, at greatest risk for all of the problems previously noted. Furthermore, one might suggest that all the dynamics of NAT and neglect-FTT are also applicable to this situation and probably exist in various combinations. If one accepts this proposition, then one can see that the final component of abuse is what Martin calls the "abusive environment."[52] This is defined as an environment with excessive punishment, obvious rejection, and hostility toward the child, an environment that is understimulating and apathetic to the needs of the growing child.

As part of this environmental complex, one must consider the physical and social conditions under which such families live. Although many abusive families may be economically and socially well-off by United States standards, more of these families are poor. They are frequently in the lower socioeconomic groups, have inadequate housing, poor medical care, considerable marital discord, high unemployment, and little education. Furthermore, they seem to be unable to reach out to existing services and to deal with the bureaucracy they must encounter to get help.[14,33,71] Such considerations further highlight the need to examine both the environment in which abuse occurs and the specific psychological dynamics that are invariably a part of the abusive pattern. An understanding of the psychological as well as social and economic conditions is critical if one is to understand abuse.

THERAPY AND PREVENTION

In recognizing the issues just discussed, one naturally looks to the modes of prevention and therapy that are possible for both the child and the family. First, the abuse must be identified and the appropriate personnel involved. The key to identification is an interdisciplinary approach wherein physicians, social workers, nurses, law enforcement personnel, lawyers, and other health care professionals are aware of the complexity of the problem and are able to relate to each other and to the family in a positive, supportive, and constructive manner.[26,42a] The conditions and needs of the family must be identified and appropriate steps must be taken to protect the child from further abuse as well as to protect the family from abusing the child. Second, a relevant program of intervention tailored to the needs of the particular family must be instituted and maintained. This program may entail the removal of the child from the home, individual or group therapy for the parents, maintenance of the child in the home with supports to the parents, or intervention into the socioeconomic situation of the family in order to relieve the stress. Most important: There must be continued involvement, assessment, and followup once intervention has begun. One of the major causes of failure of the work with abusing families is the temporary—often critical and punitive—involvement of professionals, followed by withdrawal and lack of followup and support. Such counterproductive and destructive behavior on the part of agencies is invariably destined to result in recurrent abuse. It is imperative that a program be developed for the individual family, and that the program be continued until it is decided that it is no longer needed or is not effective. Constant evaluation and assessment, together with continuity, are essential for success.

It is all well and good to recognize abuse and institute therapy—the real goal is to prevent abuse. Up to the present time, society and its representatives have only been patching up wounds. It is now incumbent upon us to look at ways and means of preventing abuse. In this regard, Gil's[31] concept of an egalitarian versus a nonegalitarian society is again instructive. He maintains that in a nonegalitarian society we can only ameliorate the problem, not prevent abuse from occurring (a stance quite possibly correct, although pessimistic indeed).

Nevertheless, it is our role and mandate as health care professionals at least to attempt to prevent abuse. Several ideas may be worth brief consideration. First, by looking at the process of parenting and by identifying those parents who are having difficulty with their parental roles in the prenatal as well as the perinatal period, one may be able to intervene before abuse occurs. Second, it must be recognized that infants, particularly premature infants, are at higher risk for abuse. Such a situation is most likely the result of poor parent-child attachment related to the separation,[23] the uncertainty as to whether the child will survive, the parents' sense of guilt and of loss of a normal child, and the fact that these small infants are more difficult to care for. It is also often related to the youth of the parents and the association of youthful parentage with prematurity.

Recognizing the above, steps must be taken to ameliorate the devastating effects of separation, to prevent estrangement, and to foster positive attachment by making the infant, despite his prematurity, more available to the parent. This may mean changing medical practice regarding visiting in hospitals (particularly in intensive care units) and then providing situations where, once the child is no longer critically ill, he can be cared for by his parents in a nonintensive, relaxed, supportive environment.

Parents are not simply created; on the contrary, parenting is the result of a learning and maturational process. Perhaps we should reconsider the models we provide for parenting and begin to develop parenting programs geared not only to the teenager, but to the younger school child. The establishment of respite centers for parents under severe stress is another means of supporting parents before they abuse their children.

Finally, we should reconsider how society views its young and how it deals with conflict. Despite our protestations to the contrary, we are not a child-oriented society. Consequently, the needs of parents and children are not a high societal priority. Until this changes, we may well continue only to respond to the crisis of abuse rather than to deal with the underlying causes.

ACKNOWLEDGEMENTS

Appreciation is extended to Drs. Harold Martin and Susan Goldberg for their critical review of this manuscript and their helpful comments and to Ms. Maewyn Ballard for preparation of the manuscript.

REFERENCES

1. Abt-Garrison, A. F. *History of pediatrics.* Philadelphia: W. B. Saunders, 1965.
2. Baron, M. A., Bejar, R. L., & Sheaff, P. J. Neurologic manifestations of the battered child syndrome. *Pediatrics,* 1970, *45,* 1003–1007.
3. Bennie, E. H., & Sclare, A. B. The battered child syndrome. *American Journal of Psychiatry,* 1969, *125,* 141–151.
4. Birrell, R. G., & Birrell, J. H. W. The maltreatment syndrome in children. *Medical Journal of Australia,* 1966, 2, 1134–1138.
5. Bloch, M. Dilemma of "battered child" and "battered children." *New York State Journal of Medicine,* 1973, 73, 799–802.
6. Bowlby, J. Maternal care and mental health. *Bulletin of the World Health Organization,* 1951, *3,* 355–534.
7. Brandwein, H. The battered child: A definite and significant factor in mental retardation. *Mental Retardation,* 1973, *11,* 50–51.
8. Brazelton, T. B. Infants and mothers: Differences in development. New York: Delacorte/ Seymour Lawrence, 1969.
9. Buda, F. B., Rothney, W. B., & Rabe, E. F. Hypotonia and the maternal-child relationship. *American Journal of Diseases of Children,* 1972, *124,* 906–907.
10. Bullard, D. N., Glasser, H. H., Heagarty, M. C., & Pivchik, E. C. Failure to thrive in the neglected child. *American Journal of Orthopsychiatry,* 1967, *37,* 680–690.
11. Caffey, J. The whiplash shaken infant syndrome: Manual shaking by the extremities with whiplash-induced intracranial and intraocular bleedings, linked with residual permanent brain damage and mental retardation. *Pediatrics,* 1974, *54,* 396–403.
12. Chase, H. P. Undernutrition and growth and development of the human brain. In J. D. Lloyd-Still (Ed.), *Malnutrition and intellectual development.* Lancaster, England: MTP Press, 1976.

13. Chase, H. P., & Martin, H. P. Undernutrition and child development. *New England Journal of Medicine*, 1970, *282*, 933–939.

14. Cherry, B. J., & Kuby, A. M. Obstacles to the delivery of medical care to children of neglecting parents. *American Journal of Public Health*, 1971, *61*, 568–573.

15. Cohen, M. I., Raphling, D. L., & Green, P. E. Psychologic aspects of the maltreatment syndrome of childhood. *Journal of Pediatrics*, 1966, *69*, 279–284.

16. Coleman, R., & Provence, S. Developmental retardation (hospitalism) in infants living in families. *Pediatrics*, 1957, *19*, 285–292.

17. Cottle, T. J. Rich kids have problems, too. *New York Times*, July 7, 1975.

18. Cravioto, J., DeLicardie, E. R., & Birch, H. G. Nutrition, growth and neurointegrative development: An experimental and ecologic study. *Pediatrics*, 1966, *38* (Suppl. 2), 321–333.

19. DeMause, L. Our forebearers made childhood a nightmare. *Psychology Today*, 1975, *8*, 85–88.

20. Ebbin, A. J., & Gollub, M. H. Battered child syndrome at Los Angeles County General Hospital. *American Journal of Diseases of Children*, 1966, *111*, 600–612.

21. Elmer, E., & Gregg, G. S. Developmental characteristics of abused children. *Pediatrics*, 1967, *40*, 596–602.

22. Engel, G. L., Reichman, F., & Segal, H. A study of an infant with gastric fistula. I. Behavior and the ratio of total HCl secretion. *Psychosomatic Medicine*, 1956, *18*, 374–398.

23. Farnaroff, A. A., Kennell, J. H., & Klaus, M. H. Follow-up of low birth weight infants: The predictive value of maternal visiting patterns. *Pediatrics*, 1972, *49*, 287–290.

24. Fischhoff, J., Whitten, C. F., & Petit, M. G. A psychiatric study of mothers of infants with growth failure secondary to maternal deprivation. *Journal of Pediatrics*, 1971, *79*, 209–215.

25. Fontana, V. J., Donovan, D., & Wong, R. J. The "maltreatment syndrome" in children. *New England Journal of Medicine*, 1963, *269*, 1389–1394.

26. Fontana, V. J., & Robison, E. A multidisciplinary approach to the treatment of child abuse. *Pediatrics*, 1976, *57*, 760–764.

27. Frasier, S. D., & Rallison, M. L. Growth retardation and emotional deprivation: Relative resistance to treatment with human growth hormone. *Journal of Pediatrics*, 1972, *80*, 603–609.

28. Galdson, R. Observations on children who have physically abused their parents. Paper presented at the 121st annual meeting of the American Psychiatric Association, New York, May, 1965.

29. Gardner, L. I. Deprivation dwarfism. *Scientific American*, 1972, *227*, 76–82.

30. Gelles, R. J. The social construction of child abuse. *American Journal of Orthopsychiatry*, 1975, *45*, 363–371.

31. Gil, D. *Violence against children: Physical child abuse in the United States*. Cambridge, Mass.: Harvard, 1970.

32. Gil, D. Unraveling child abuse. *American Journal of Orthopsychiatry*, 1975, *45*, 346–356.

33. Giovannoni, J. J., & Billingsley, A. Child neglect among the poor: A study of parental adequacy in families of three ethnic groups. *Child Welfare*, 1970, *49*, 196–204.

34. Glasser, H. H., Heagarty, M. C., & Bullard, D. M. Physical and psychological development of children with early failure to thrive. *Journal of Pediatrics*, 1968, *73*, 690–698.

35. Goldson, E., Cadol, R. V., Fitch, M. J., et al. Nonaccidental trauma and failure to thrive: A sociomedical profile in Denver. *American Journal of Diseases of Children*, 1976, *130*, 490–492.

36. Green, A. H., Gaines, R. W., & Sandgrund, A. Child abuse: Pathological syndrome of family interactions. *American Journal of Psychiatry*, 1974, *131*, 882–886.

37. Green, A. H., Gaines, R. W., & Sandgrund, A. Psychological sequelae of child abuse and neglect. Paper presented at the 127th annual meeting of the American Psychiatric Association, Detroit, May, 1974.

38. Gregg, G. S., & Elmer, E. Infant injuries: Accident or abuse. *Pediatrics*, 1969, *44*, 434–439.

39. Helfer, R. E. The etiology of child abuse. *Pediatrics*, 1973, *51*, 777–779.

40. Helfer, R. E., & Kempe, C. H. *The battered child.* Chicago: University of Chicago, 1968.

41. Holter, J. C., & Friedman, S. B. Child abuse: Early case finding in the emergency department. *Pediatrics*, 1968, *42*, 128–138.

42. Kempe, C. H. Uncommon manifestations of the battered child syndrome. *American Journal of Diseases of Children*, 1974, *129*, 1265.

42a. Kempe, C. H., & Helfer, R. E. (Eds.). Helping the battered child and his family. Philadelphia: J. B. Lippincott Co., 1972.

43. Kempe, C. H., Silverman, F. N., Steele, B. F., et al. The battered child syndrome. *Journal of American Medical Association*, 1962, *181*, 17–24.

44. Klaus, M. H., Jerauld, R., Kreger, N. C., McAlpine, W., Steffa, M., & Kennell, J. H. Maternal attachment: Importance of the first post-partum days. *New England Journal of Medicine*, 1972, *286*, 460–463.

45. Klein, M., & Stern, L. Low birthweight and the battered child syndrome. *American Journal of Diseases of Children*, 1971, *122*, 15–18.

46. Krieger, I., & Sargent, D. A. A postural sign in the sensory deprivation syndrome. *Journal of Pediatrics*, 1967, *70*, 332–339.

47. Lansky, L. L. An unusual case of childhood chloral hydrate poisoning. *American Journal of Diseases of Children*, 1975, *127*, 275–276.

48. Lauer, B., tenBroeck, E., & Grossman, M. Battered child syndrome: Review with 130 patients with controls. *Pediatrics*, 1974, *54*, 67–70.

49. Laury, G. V., & Meerlo, J. A. M. Mental cruelty and child abuse. *Psychiatric Quarterly* (Suppl.) 1967, *41*(2), 203–254.

50. Leonard, M. F., Rhymes, J. P., & Solnit, A. Failure to thrive in infants: A family problem. *American Journal of Disabled children*, 1966, *111*, 600–612.

51. Light, R. J. Abused and neglected children in America: A study of alternate policies. *Harvard Educational Review*, 1973, *43*, 556–598.

52. Martin, H. The child and his development. In C. H. Kempe & R. E. Helfer (Eds.), *Helping the battered child and his family*. Philadelphia: Lippincott, 1972.

53. Martin, H. P., Beezley, P., & Kempe, C. H. The development of abused children. *Advances in Pediatrics*, 1974, *21*, 25–73.

54. Mindlin, R. L. Child abuse and neglect: The role of the pediatrician and the Academy. *Pediatrics*, 1974, *54*, 393–395.

55. Newberger, E. H. The myth of the battered child syndrome. *Current Medical Dialog*, 1973, *40*, 327–334.

56. Ounsted, C., Oppenheimer, R., & Lindsay, J. Aspects of bonding failure: The psychopathology and psychotherapeutic treatment of families of battered children. *Developmental Medicine and Child Neurology*, 1974, *16*, 447–456.

57. Patton, R. G., & Gardner, L. I. *Growth failure in maternal deprivation*. Springfield, Ill.: Charles C. Thomas, 1963.

58. Patton, R. G., & Gardner, L. I. Short stature with maternal deprivation syndrome: Disordered family environment as cause of so-called idiopathic hypopituitarism. In L. I. Gardner (Ed.), *Endocrine and genetic disorders of childhood*. Philadelphia: W. B. Saunders, 1969.

59. Pena, S. D. J., & Medovy, H. Child abuse and traumatic pseudocyst of the pancreas. *Journal of Pediatrics*, 1973, *83*, 1026–1028.

60. Pickel, S., Anerson, C., & Holliday, M. A. Thirsting and hypernatremic dehydration: A form of child abuse. *Pediatrics*, 1970, *45*, 54–59.

61. Pollitt, E., & Eichler, A. Behavioral disturbances among failure-to-thrive children. *American Journal of Diseases of Children*, 1976, *130*, 24–29.

62. Pollitt, E., Eichler, A. W., & Chan, C. K. Psychological development and behavior of mothers of failure-to-thrive children. *American Journal of Orthopsychiatry*, 1975, *45*, 525–537.

63. Powell, G. F., Brasel, J. A., & Blizzard, R. M. Emotional deprivation and growth retardation

simulating idiopathic hypopituitarism. I. Clinical evaluation of the syndrome. *New England Journal of Medicine*, 1967, *276*, 1272–1278.

64. Powell, G. F., Brasel, J. A., Raiti, D., & Blizzard, R. M. Emotional deprivation and growth retardation simulating idiopathic hypopituitarism: II. Endocrinologic evaluation of the syndrome. *New England Journal of Medicine*, 1967, *276*, 1279–1283.

65. Provence, S. *Infants in institutions: A comparison of their development with family-reared infants during the first year of life.* New York: International Universities Press, 1962.

66. Prugh, D. G., & Harlow, R. G. "Masked deprivation" in infants and young children. In *Deprivation of Maternal Care*. Public Health Papers, World Health Organization. New York: Schocken, 1966.

67. Radbill, S. X. A history of child abuse and infanticide. In R. E. Helfer & C. H. Kempe (Eds.), *The battered child*. Chicago: University of Chicago, 1968.

68. Rutter, M. *Maternal deprivation reassessed.* London: Penguin, 1972.

69. Sanders, R., & Wyman, M. D. Resistance to dealing with parents of battered children. *Pediatrics*, 1972, *50*, 853–857.

70. Schmitt, B. D., & Kempe. C. H. The pediatrician's role in child abuse and neglect. *Current Problems in Pediatrics*, 1975, *5*, 5.

71. Selig, A. L. The myth of the multi-problem family. *American Journal of Orthopsychiatry*, 1976, *46*, 526–532.

72. Silver, H. K., & Finkelstein, M. Deprivational dwarfism. *Journal of Pediatrics*, 1967, *70*, 317–324.

73. Silver, L. B., Dublin, C. C., & Lourie, R. S. Child abuse syndrome: The "gray areas" in establishing a diagnosis. *Pediatrics*, 1969, *44*, 594–600.

74. Smith, S. M., & Hanson, R. 134 battered children: A medical and psychological study. *British Medical Journal*, 1974, *3*, 666–670.

75. Smith, S. M., Hanson, R., & Noble, S. Parents of battered babies: A controlled study. *British Medical Journal*, 1973, *4*, 388–391.

76. Spitz, R. A. Hospitalism. *The Psychoanalytic Study of the Child*, 1946, *2*, 113–116.

77. Steele, B., & Pollock, C. B. A psychiatric study of parents who abuse infants and small children. In R. E. Helfer & C. H. Kempe (Eds.), *The battered child*. Chicago: University of Chicago, 1968.

78. Stoch, M. B., & Smythe, R. M. Does undernutrition during infancy inhibit brain growth and subsequent development? *Archives of Disease in Childhood*, 1963, *38*, 546–552.

79. Tomasi, L. G., & Rosman, P. Purtscher retinopathy in the battered child syndrome. *American Journal of Diseases of Children*, 1975, *129*, 1335–1337.

80. Touloukian, R. J. Abdominal visceral injuries in battered children. *Pediatrics*, 1968, *42*, 642–646.

81. Wasserman, S. The abused parent of the abused child. *Children*, 1968, *14*, 175–179.

82. Whitten, C. G., Pettit, M. G., & Fischhoff, J. Evidence that growth failure from maternal deprivation is secondary to undereating. *Journal of the American Medical Association*, 1969, *209*, 1675–1682.

83. Young, L. *Wednesday's children: A study of child neglect and abuse.* New York: McGraw-Hill, 1964.

INDEX

a
b
c
d
e
8 f
9 g
0 h
1 i
8 2 j